Frontal Lobe Function and Dysfunction

Frontal Lobe Function and Dysfunction

Edited by

HARVEY S. LEVIN
HOWARD M. EISENBERG
ARTHUR L. BENTON

New York   Oxford
OXFORD UNIVERSITY PRESS
1991

Oxford University Press

Oxford   New York   Toronto
Delhi   Bombay   Calcutta   Madras   Karachi
Petaling Jaya   Singapore   Hong Kong   Tokyo
Nairobi   Dar es Salaam   Cape Town
Melbourne   Auckland

and associated companies in
Berlin   Ibadan

Library of Congress Cataloging-in-Publication Data

Frontal lobe function and dysfunction /
edited by Harvey S. Levin, Howard M. Eisenberg, Arthur L. Benton.
p. cm.
Based on a conference held at the University of
Texas Medical Branch at Galveston on Nov. 17–18, 1989.
Includes bibliographical references.
ISBN 0-19-506284-1
1. Cognition disorders—Congresses. 2. Frontal lobes—Congresses.
3. Brain damage—Congresses.
I. Levin, Harvey S. II. Eisenberg, Howard M. III. Benton, Arthur Lester, 1909–
[DNLM: 1. Cognition Disorders—congresses.
2. Frontal Lobe–injuries—congresses.
3. Frontal Lobe—physiology—congresses.
4. Frontal Lobe—physiopathology—congresses.
5. Mental Disorders—congresses.
WL 307 F9343 1989] RC394.C64F76 1991 616.8′4—dc20
DNLM/DLC for Library of Congress   91-2632

9 8 7 6 5 4 3

Printed in the United States of America
on acid-free paper

To Walle J. H. Nauta

Preface

Our purpose in editing this volume has been to present a critical summary of advances in experimental and clinical research on the neuroanatomic organization and functioning of the frontal lobes. It is intended to provide the reader with a synthesis of recent research on the neural circuitry of the prefrontal region, neuropsychologic and metabolic studies elucidating the participation of the frontal lobes in experimental cognitive tasks, and frontal lobe involvement in various neurologic diseases and injuries that impair cognition and alter behavior.

The distinctive roles of the prefrontal region in cognition, memory, and affective functioning have been brought to light by investigators employing neuroimaging techniques and studies of animals and humans following focal cortical excisions. This research has uncovered alterations in delayed response performance, planning, susceptibility to interference effects, and memory organization that are not disclosed by conventional psychological tests. The contributors to this book have also elucidated the behavioral and affective consequences of frontal lobe injury and their impact on rehabilitation.

The scope of the volume encompasses chapters by basic neuroscientists, chapters by neuropsychologists who use experimental cognitive tasks in studying patients with focal lesions of the frontal lobes, and chapters on the involvement of the frontal lobes in various neuropsychiatric disorders including dementia and schizophrenia. It also includes a chapter by Hanna Damasio that provides templates for studying frontal lobe anatomy in humans. In addition, the volume addresses developmental aspects of frontal lobe functioning and theoretical approaches to integrating data collected from neurological patients with knowledge gained from animal research.

We have attempted to provide investigators and clinicians with both a timely review and a useful reference that we hope will stimulate research and new insight into clinical interventions for patients with frontal lobe injury.

We are grateful to Jeffrey House and Stanley George of Oxford University Press for their editorial advice and encouragement, to Donna Dickson, Melanie Meiselbach, and Liz Zindler for assistance in manuscript preparation, and to

Lynn Burke of the Moody Medical Library for providing much valuable reference material.

We are deeply indebted to the Moody Foundation for support of the frontal lobe conference held in Galveston, Texas on November 17–18, 1989 at which the contributions to this volume were first presented.

Galveston   H. S. L.
Galveston   H. M. E.
Iowa City   A. L. B.
June, 1991

Acknowledgments

This volume is based on a conference concerning frontal lobe functioning and recovery from injury which was held at The University of Texas Medical Branch at Galveston on November 17–18, 1989. Support for the conference and preparation of this volume was generously provided by The Moody Foundation of Galveston. Research by the editors that is described in this volume was supported in part by the National Institutes of Health grant NS-21889, Javits Neuroscience Investigator Award. The editors are indebted to Liz Zindler, Melanie Meiselbach, and Anita Padilla for their assistance in coordinating the conference and preparing the manuscripts, to Lynn Burke of the Moody Medical Library for assistance in searching the literature.

Contents

Contributors

HELEN BARBAS
Department of Applied Health
  Sciences
Boston University School of Medicine
Boston, Massachusetts

ARTHUR L. BENTON
Department of Neurology
University of Iowa College of
  Medicine
Iowa City, Iowa

KAREN FAITH BERMAN
Clinical Brain Disorders Branch
Intramural Research Program
National Institute of Mental Health
Neuroscience Center at St. Elizabeth's
Washington, D.C.

PAUL BURGESS
National Hospital
London, England

ANTONIO R. DAMASIO
Department of Neurology
University of Iowa College of
  Medicine
Iowa City, Iowa

HANNA C. DAMASIO
Department of Neurology
University of Iowa College of
  Medicine
Iowa City, Iowa

DAVID G. DANIEL
Neuropsychiatric Research Hospital
Intramural Research Program
National Institute of Mental Health
Neuroscience Center at Saint
  Elizabeth's
Washington, D.C.

ADELE DIAMOND
Department of Psychology
University of Pennsylvania
Philadelphia, Pennsylvania

HOWARD M. EISENBERG
Division of Neurosurgery E-17
University of Texas Medical Branch
Galveston, Texas

MORRIS FREEDMAN
Baycrest Center for Geriatric Care
  and University of Toronto and
  Mount Sinai Hospital Research
  Institute
Toronto, Ontario
Canada

HARRIET R. FRIEDMAN
Section on Neuroanatomy
Yale University School of Medicine
New Haven, Connecticut

JOAQUIN M. FUSTER
Department of Psychiatry
University of California at Los
  Angeles Medical Center
Los Angeles, California

PATRICIA S. GOLDMAN-RAKIC
Section of Neuroanatomy
Yale University School of Medicine
New Haven, Connecticut

FELICIA C. GOLDSTEIN
Emory Neurobehavioral Program
Wesley Wood Hospital
Atlanta, Georgia

KENNETH M. HEILMAN
Department of Neurology
University of Florida College of
    Medicine
Gainesville, Florida

JERI S. JANOWSKY
Department of Psychology
University of Oregon
Eugene, Oregon

ROBERT T. KNIGHT
Department of Neurology
University of California, Davis
Veterans Administration Medical
    Center
Martinez, California

HARVEY S. LEVIN
Division of Neurosurgery D-73
University of Texas Medical Branch
Galveston, Texas

PATRICK McNAMARA
Neurology Service
DVAMC Boston and Boston
    University School of Medicine
Department of Veterans Affairs
Boston, Massachusetts

DAVID NEARY
Department of Neurology
Manchester Royal Infirmary
Manchester, England

MARLENE OSCAR-BERMAN
Aphasia Resource Center
Psychology Service, VAMC, Boston
Boston, Massachusetts

DEEPAK N. PANDYA
Bedford VA Hospital
Department of Anatomy
Boston University School of Medicine
Bedford, Massachusetts

MICHAEL PETRIDES
Department of Psychology
McGill University
Montreal, Quebec
Canada

GEORGE P. PRIGATANO
Neuropsychology
Barrow Neurological Institute
St. Joseph's Hospital & Medical
    Center
Phoenix, Arizona

ROBERT G. ROBINSON
Department of Psychiatry
University of Iowa College of
    Medicine
Iowa City, Iowa

TIM SHALLICE
Psychology Department
University College London
London, England

ARTHUR P. SHIMAMURA
Department of Psychology
University of California
Berkeley, California

JULIE S. SNOWDEN
Department of Neurology
Manchester Royal Infirmary
Manchester, England

LARRY R. SQUIRE
Department of Psychiatry
University of California San Diego
Medical School
La Jolla, California

SERGIO E. STARKSTEIN
Institute of Neurologic Investigation
Buenos Aires, Argentina
Department of Psychiatry
Johns Hopkins University School of
  Medicine
Baltimore, Maryland

DONALD T. STUSS
Rotman Research Institute of
  Baycrest Center
North York, Ontario
Canada

DANIEL TRANEL
Division of Behavioral Neurology &
  Cognitive Neuroscience
Department of Neurology
University of Iowa College of
  Medicine
Iowa City, Iowa

ROBERT T. WATSON
Department of Neurology
University of Florida
College of Medicine
Gainesville, Florida

DANIEL R. WEINBERGER
Intramural Research Program
NIMH—St. Elizabeth's Hospital
Washington, D.C.

DAVID H. WILLIAMS
Division of Neurosurgery
The University of Texas Medical
  Branch
Galveston, Texas

Introduction and Historical Perspective

1
The Prefrontal Region: Its Early History

ARTHUR L. BENTON

This historical sketch deals with the early development of knowledge and concepts about the structure and functions of the prefrontal region, i.e., the region anterior and mesial to those areas of frontal cortex having to do with motor functions (motor cortex and frontal eye fields) and speech (Broca's area). The greater part of the prefrontal region has a characteristic cellular structure, frontal granular cortex, and within the region a number of areas are differentiated from each other on architectonic grounds. However, it is not yet clear that, apart from different afferent and efferent connections with other parts of the brain, this partition into sectors on an architectonic basis in itself possesses basic functional implications. The prefrontal region is simply a topographic concept and, indeed, one whose boundaries vary slightly in the descriptions of different anatomists. It differs from other regions of the cerebral cortex in that its destruction is not associated with loss of basic sensory or motor capacities or with obvious impairment of speech.

What gave the prefrontal region a special significance was the conviction that it provides the neural substrate of complex mental processes such as abstract reasoning, foresight, planning capacity, self-awareness, empathy, and the elaboration and modulation of emotional reactions. Different authors singled out one or another of these defects as the core disability generating the other defects. At the same time the ensemble of defects came to be known as the "frontal lobe syndrome."

This chapter describes, in a necessarily sketchy and fragmentary way, the evolution of ideas about these functions of the prefrontal region from the sixteenth century, when the frontal lobes were first clearly identified, to 1947, the date of a landmark conference in which knowledge and conceptions of frontal lobe function were discussed, particularly as they related to prefrontal leukotomy. More detailed accounts of specific aspects of the broad topic can be found in the monographs of Soury (1899), Kleist (1934), Rylander (1939), Ajuriaguerra and Hécaen (1949), Sanides (1962), Clarke and O'Malley (1968), Meyer (1971), Fuster (1980/1989), and Spillane (1981).

EARLIEST CONCEPTIONS

Gross Morphology

The frontal lobes make their first appearance in the scientific literature as one of three "prominences" (anterior, medial-inferior, posterior) into which Varolio (1573,1591) divided the cerebral hemispheres. Willis (1664) was the first to apply the term "lobes" to these prominences, and Chaussier (1807) proposed the names "frontal," "temporal," and "occipital" to take the place of anterior, medial-inferior, and posterior, respectively. Arnold (1838) introduced the term "parietal lobe," thus forming the modern fourfold classification.

The division of the frontal lobe into component gyri and sulci had to wait until opinion about the significance of the cerebral convolutions underwent a change. Before 1820 anatomists held the pleats and creases of the cerebral cortex in very low esteem indeed (see Schiller, 1965). Called "enteroid processes" by Malacarne and Rolando, they were regarded either as reflecting the manner in which the pia mater succeeded in penetrating into the depth of the brain or as containing minute glands that discharged phlegm or animal spirits into the ventricles. In either case, there seemed to be as little reason to assign names to these bulges and creases as there would be to specify every fold in the intestines. No great care was exercised to depict them accurately, and early illustrations of the convexity of the hemispheres led Rolando to write that they reflected artistic skill more than scientific observation. Later these illustrations provoked Ecker's derisive comment that they reminded him of a bowl of macaroni (Fig. 1–1). No doubt a number of factors—the very limited opportunity to study fresh brains before decomposition, faulty communication between the anatomist and his artist (perhaps combined with the latter's creative imagination), and interindividual differences in the external morphology of the hemispheres—all contributed to this failure to depict any constancy in pattern.

Nevertheless, some major structures attracted sufficient attention to lead to specific identification. Bartholin, Sylvius, and Vicq d'Azyr described the Sylvian fissure (see Baker, 1909), and Reil provided a detailed description of the oval mass at the base of the Sylvian fissure that came to be known as the insula or the island of Reil. By the third decade of the nineteenth century the cortical gyri appeared to some anatomists to be sufficiently constant, in that they formed a recognizable pattern and therefore, to warrant identification. There is no doubt that Gall's placement of his "faculties" in the cortical gyri provided a strong impetus to closer examination. Rolando (1831) himself wrote a paper, "On the Structure of the Cerebral Hemispheres," in which he emphasized the importance of describing the cerebral convolutions and in which he identified the precentral and postcentral gyri surrounding the fissure that now bears his name.

The description of the external surface of the hemispheres in terms of four major lobes and the subdivision of each lobe into its constituent gyri and sulci were then carried forward by anatomists in France, Germany, and Britain, among them Leuret, Foville, Gratiolet, Broca, and Ecker. The work was essentially completed by the middle decades of the nineteenth century. Figure 1–2 reproduces Ecker's illustration of the lateral and superior aspects of the left hemi-

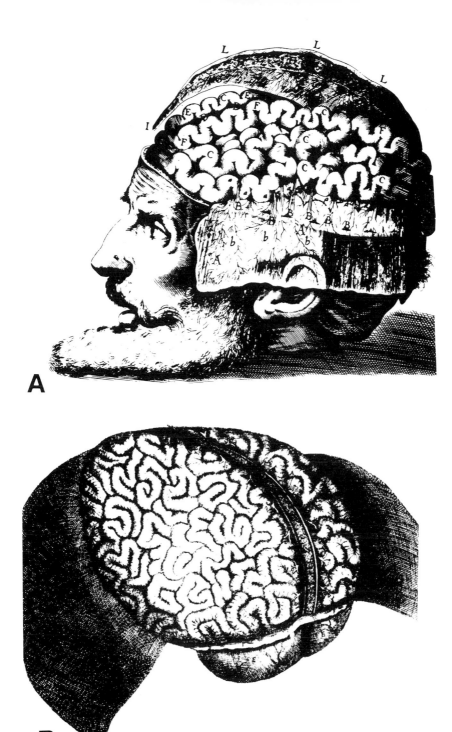

Figure 1–1 **A.** An enteroid process? Illustration by Giulio Casserio in Adriaan Van de Spiegel's *De Humanis Corporis Fabrica* (Venice, 1627). **B.** A bowl of macaroni? Illustration in Vieussens's *Nevrographia Universalis* (Leiden, 1685). (From the Martin Rare Book Room, Hardin Library for the Health Sciences, University of Iowa.)

SULCUS CENTRALIS.

FIG. 1.

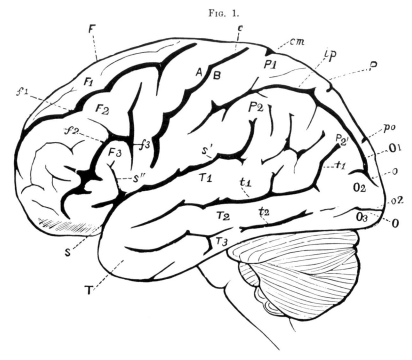

VIEW OF THE BRAIN FROM THE SIDE.

F Frontal lobe ; *P* parietal lobe ; *O* occipital lobe ; *T* temporal lobe.
S Fissura Sylvii ; *S'* horizontal, *S"* ascending branch.
c Sulcus centralis ; *A* anterior, *B* posterior central convolution.
F_1 Upper, F_2 middle, F_3 lower (or third) frontal convolution.
f_1 Upper, f_2 lower, f_3 vertical frontal fissure (sulcus præcentralis).
P_1 Upper, P_2 lower parietal lobule ; P_2 gyrus supramarginalis, P_2' gyrus
    angularis.
ip Sulcus interparietalis.
cm End of the sulcus calloso-marginalis.
O_1 First, O_2 second, O_3 third, occipital convolution.
po Fissura parieto-occipitalis.
o Sulcus occipitalis transversus.
o_2 Sulcus occipitalis longitudinalis inferior.
T_1 First, T_2 second, T_3 third temporal convolution.
t_1 First, t_2 second temporal fissure.

Figure 1–2   Lateral view of left cerebral hemisphere (Ecker, 1869/1873).

sphere in his *Die Hirnwindungen des Menschen* (1869/1873). As will be seen, the three gyri of the convexity of the frontal lobe and their corresponding sulci are clearly shown and labeled. Similarly, the major convolutions of the parietal, temporal, and occipital lobes as well as transitional ridges such as the supramarginal and angular gyri are accurately depicted.

The landmarks on the inferior and medial surfaces of the frontal lobes also were described during the middle decades of the nineteenth century. The gyrus rectus was identified and named by Valentin in 1841. The other orbital and mesial gyri were described by Foville, Leuret, and Gratiolet as well as by Valentin.

Although later workers described many important details (see Meyer, 1971), by 1870 the gross morphology of the cerebral hemispheres was essentially as well known as it is today; Ecker's 1869 sketch could well find a place in a modern textbook of anatomy. Thereafter, interest in the external configuration of the hemispheres waned somewhat as it appeared that the gyri and sulci were merely convenient landmarks that bore no necessary correspondence either to underlying structure as disclosed by neurohistology or to functional properties inferred from animal experimentation and clinical observation.

Functional Aspects

From the earliest periods and extending to the nineteenth century there were two opposing points of view about the functional significance of the cerebral hemispheres. Aristotle was a "cardiocentrist," maintaining that the brain merely served the function of cooling the body heat generated by the heart, which was itself the seat of mentation. However, many "cerebrocentric" theorists regarded the brain as a secretory organ also, their basic concept being that perceptual and cognitive processes took place in the ventricles.

Localization of mental functions in the substance of the brain largely displaced ventricular localization in the seventeenth and eighteenth centuries when the corpus callosum and the corpus striatum were identified as the seat of intellect. The choice of these organs was probably dictated in part on theoretic grounds because of their central location. However, empirical observations, such as those of the eighteenth-century French surgeon La Peyronie, that various parts of the cerebral hemispheres could be damaged without apparent impairment of intellectual function must also have played a role in the localization.

However, in due course, the cerebral hemispheres were accorded some degree of functional significance. Although Willis (1664/1681/1965) localized perception in the corpus callosum, he did regard the cortex as a repository of memory images and not as a mere secretory organ. Basing his conclusions on a detailed analysis of the work of others rather than on his own observations, Swedenborg placed the higher mental faculties in the cerebral cortex and suggested that different cortical regions served different modalities of sensory experience (see Akert and Hammond, 1962; Spillane, 1981). Rolando (1828) believed that consciousness and voluntary action are dependent on the integrity of the cerebral cortex. By the 1830s the concept that the cerebral cortex was the seat of intellect was almost universally accepted. Thus the French clinician–pathologists of that era, in their studies of patients with "general paralysis of the insane," reasoned that lesions of the white matter produced the characteristic motor disabilities, while cortical lesions were responsible for the mental deterioration (see Soury, 1899). Similarly, in his famous *Lehrbuch der Nervenkrankheiten* (1840–

1846, 1853), Romberg implicated cortical disease as the basis of mental impairment.

A related question of equally long standing was whether or not the size and complexity of the cerebral hemispheres could be related to "intelligence." Beginning with Herophilus (ca. 400 B.C.), the majority of observers answered the question positively. Others, such as Thomas Bartholin (1616–1680), voiced an emphatic negative opinion, pointing out that the cerebral convolutions were exceedingly complex in some animals that were not noted for their intellectual capacity. However, when nineteenth century comparative anatomy established the systematic development of the brain along the evolutionary scale, a relationship of the size, complexity, and differentiation of the cerebral hemispheres to "intelligence" was universally accepted. The finding that the most impressive differences between the human brain and that of infrahuman primates consisted in a tremendous development of the prefrontal and posterior parietal regions emphasized the importance of these regions in the mediation of human behavior. With specific reference to the frontal lobes, workers such as Broca and Rüdinger pointed out that the third frontal gyrus, the "organ of speech," reached its full development only in the human brain (see Meyer, 1971).

Intrahemispheric Localization

The early nineteenth century controversy over localization of function within the hemispheres has been recounted many times (e.g., Benton, 1976, 1981; Clarke and Jacyna, 1987; Clarke and O'Malley, 1968; Gibson, 1962; Krech, 1964; Riese and Hoff, 1950; Swazey, 1970; Walker, 1957). A few representative examples illustrating the major trends in thought will be mentioned.

By his placement of "faculties" in discrete parts of the cerebral cortex and his insistence that the brain was an assemblage of organs, each of which subserved a specific intellectual capacity or trait of character, Franz Joseph Gall (Gall and Spurzheim, 1809) made localization of function a central issue in neurophysiology and neuropsychology. Predictably, his radical thesis engendered a mixed reception and a rancorous controversy. It was rejected by many physiologists and clinicians for a variety of reasons, among them the conviction that Flourens was essentially correct in his view that the hemispheres acted as a unit as well as a rejection of Gall's far-reaching claims, materialistic position, and absurd phrenology. In addition, numerous clinical reports of patients with documented hemispheric lesions but with no observable impairment of function fitted in well with Flourens's "mass action" hypothesis, which stipulated that the amount of loss of brain tissue had to reach a critical level before any noticeable symptoms appeared. Most of these reports concerned patients with frontal lobe injuries.

However, clinical observation did impel many clinicians to embrace the basic concept of localization of cerebral function, whatever their attitudes toward Gall's claims might be. Pointing to the discrete deficits, such as monoplegia of an arm or leg, sensory defect without paralysis, and hemiplegia with or without sensory defect, that were produced by stroke, traumatic injury, or tumor, they concluded that specific cerebral centers governing these functions must exist. Postmortem findings disclosing limited areas of loss of tissue supported the conclusion. Nevertheless, no agreement about the precise locus of the crucial lesions could be reached. The state of affairs was well summarized by Andral (1823–1827) as follows: "We cannot yet assign in the brain a distinct seat to the motions of the upper and lower limbs. No doubt such distinct seat exists, since each of these limbs may be paralysed separately, but we do not know it yet" (cited by Spillane, 1981).

The most spirited disagreement over hemispheric localization revolved around Gall's placement of two centers, one for speech articulation and the other for the "memory of words" in the orbital area of the frontal lobes. Bouillaud (1825) expanded the crucial locus to encompass the whole of the "anterior" lobes and for 40 years argued strenuously that a frontal lobe lesion would be found in every patient who had exhibited an "alalia" or an "amnesia for words" during life. The contradictory evidence (i.e., aphasic disorder produced by lesions in the temporal or parietal lobe), which was brought forth by Andral and others, failed to shake Bouillaud, who continually fueled a controversy that was resolved only in the 1860s and 1870s (Benton, 1964).

Thus, by the close of the first half of the nineteenth century there was still uncertainty about whether or not there was differentiation of function within the cerebral hemispheres of the human brain as opposed to the holistic concept that the hemispheres operated as a unit as envisioned by Flourens. The observation that brain-diseased patients showed discrete deficits of different types persuaded clinicians that almost certainly such differentiation was the case, but consistent correlations between these defects and the locus of the presumably causative lesions could not be established. The evidence was particularly ambiguous with respect to the frontal lobes. Case reports describing asymptomatic patients with fairly extensive frontal lesions were not difficult to find, and this led to the concept that from a clinical standpoint the prefrontal region was a "silent area" of no recognizable functional significance. But countering this nihilistic conclusion was not only the conviction that the massive development of the frontal lobes in the human animal must possess some significance but also the indisputable evidence that disease of the region could cause disturbances in the characteristically human capacity of speech.

In 1850 Bigelow published his account of the famous "crowbar case," originally described by Harlow (1848). The young man had sustained the passage of an iron bar (1.25 inches in diameter at the larger end, 3.5 feet in length and 13.5 pounds in weight), which had entered the left frontal lobe and emerged from the right frontal bone near the sagittal suture, leaving a circular opening of about 3.5 inches in diameter and destroying the left frontal lobe and anterior temporal pole, as well in all probability some right frontal tissue. Interest at the time of publication of Bigelow's paper was focused on the patient's survival from such a massive brain injury. Bigelow himself characterized it as "perhaps unprecedented in the history of surgery," and one distinguished surgeon suspected that it was a "Yankee invention" (see Steegman, 1962).

The implications of the "crowbar case" for frontal lobe function were appreciated only in later years after the publication of Harlow's (1868) follow-up report describing the patient's status until his death 13 years after the accident. Phineas Gage did not appear to have suffered intellectual impairment in the narrow sense of the term. His memory and temporal orientation were intact and he was sufficiently competent to secure employment. Four years after his injury he went to South America where he worked for 8 years before returning to the United States a year before his death. Apparently he was self-supporting during all of this period. However, beginning about one month after his injury, he exhibited a remarkable change in personality. Before the injury he was considered to be an honest, reliable, deliberate person and a good businessman. He was now "childish, capricious and obstinate," showed poor judgment, used profane language, and was inconsiderate of others (Macmillan, 1986; Steegman, 1962). In short, he showed a distinctive type of personality change that later authors such as Welt (1888) associated with prefrontal lobe disease.

THE LATE NINETEENTH CENTURY

The closing decades of the nineteenth century, i.e., the 1870s, 1880s, and 1890s, witnessed an extraordinary growth in knowledge of the central nervous system. The discoveries of Broca and of Fritsch and Hitzig, the introduction of antisepsis, and the advances in the development of neurohistologic techniques led to a surge of activity on the part of experimentalists and clinicians on all fronts— anatomic, physiologic, and behavioral—the fruits of which were a deeper and more detailed understanding of the structure and functions of the brain and spinal cord. Among the topics that were pursued most vigorously was the issue of localization of function in the brain. The aspects of this development dealing with the structure and functions of the frontal lobes will be considered.

Anatomy and Physiology

The structure of the upper brain stem and the limbic regions was reasonably well delineated by the early decades of the nineteenth century (see Lewy, 1942; Meyer, 1971). For example, the basal ganglia had been described in detail by Willis (1664), Vieussens (1684), Vicq d'Azyr (1786), and Burdach (1826), the thalamus by Burdach (1826), and the hippocampus by Treviranus (1820). The interests of these early anatomists were not always confined to gross structure but also, at least on occasion, included consideration of the functional significance of the organs, although their pronouncements were necessarily rather vague. Thus Willis wrote that "the corpus striatum represents an exchange between brainstem and cortex" (cited by Lewy, 1942). And Treviranus (1820), having noted the connections between the hippocampus and the olfactory nerve, corpus striatum, and the fornix and having commented that no other convolution is so closely connected with other regions of the brain, drew the following remarkably prescient conclusion: "Therefore, the hippocampus is probably involved with a higher mental function, perhaps that of memory, which is so greatly aroused by olfactory sensations" (cited by Meyer, 1971).

An event of capital importance in fostering the evolution of thought about cerebral structure and function was the discovery by Gratiolet (1854) of the optic radiations arising from the lateral geniculate nuclei and fanning out to the parietal and occipital lobes. His demonstration that there was in fact a cortical terminus for vision above the thalamic level reinforced the nascent idea that the cerebral cortex was indeed the end-station for sensory information. A year later Panizza (1855) established a rough correspondence between lesions in the occipitoparietal region and impairment of vision in both human cases and in dogs subjected to experimental ablations. But his observations, published in a provincial journal with a limited circulation, remained unknown until resurrected some 25 years later and hence they had no influence on contemporary thought (Benton, 1978).

During the latter decades of the nineteenth century many gifted neuroanatomists, among them Betz, Broca, Cunningham, the Dejerines, Edinger, Flechsig, Golgi, Meynert, Nissl, Ramon y Cajal, and Retzius, utilized both gross dissection and newly developed histologic techniques to investigate the central nervous system. Their studies established the basis for modern concepts of the structure and functions of the human brain. In this regard, the work of the Viennese neuroanatomist, Theodor Meynert (1867, 1869, 1877, 1884/1885), was perhaps most influential in shaping the ideas of neurologists and psychiatrists about brain–behavior relationships. Meynert presented a thorough account of brain structures and their possible functional significance with detailed descriptions of the thalamus and its cortical connections, the hypothalamus, the hippocampus, the lateral geniculate nucleus, and the cerebral cortex. He demonstrated the significance of the corpus striatum as a relay station between brain stem and cortex, thus empirically validating the early speculation of Willis. He was the first to describe the nucleus basalis (nbM), which has figured so prominently in current discussions of the neuropathology of Alzheimer's disease and other dementing illnesses. He identified commissural, projection, and corticocortical pathways (later called association tracts) and contributed to knowledge of regional differences in the cellular architecture of the cortex. Overall, his researches proved to be a powerful stimulus to the formulation of concepts about the nature of the neural mechanisms underlying cognitive behavior such as those advanced by Wernicke (1874) and Liepmann (1900).

The Experimental Physiologists

The major feature of the "golden age of cerebral localization" (1870–1890) consisted of the attempts of physiologists to assign specific sensory, motor, perceptual, and cognitive capacities to specific regions of the cerebral cortex through ablation and stimulation experiments. Their findings, conclusions, and disagreements about the functional properties of the frontal lobes will be reviewed by sketching the positions of some of the leading investigators of the period.

Friedrich Goltz (1834–1902), still remembered for his remarkable demonstrations of the behavioral characteristics of dogs deprived of both cerebral hemispheres, is generally regarded as having been a thoroughgoing holist, carrying forth and defending the tradition of Flourens against the accumulating evidence in favor of specialization of function in the cerebral hemispheres. Indeed, he did argue that the size rather than the locus of lesions was the prime determinant of the sensory, motor, and cognitive deficits observed in brain-injured animals and humans. Moreover, using a water-jet technique that destroyed tissue with minimal bleeding but with poor control of extent of lesion, he reported finding that ablation of loci alleged to be the exclusive cortical centers for one or another function did not have the specific effects ascribed to them by the "localizationists" (Goltz, 1888).

In fact, Goltz was far from being a Flourensian antilocalizationist. He expressed himself as being in principle not at all opposed to the concept of localization of function within the cerebral hemispheres, but he did insist that adequate techniques of experimentation and careful observation are required to clarify the issue (Goltz, 1892). For example, he found that a complete unilateral hemispherectomy did lead to disturbances in a dog's motor behavior but not to the hemiplegia predicted by many investigators. His able assistant, Jacques Loeb (1885, 1886), reported that unilateral destruction of Munk's visual cortical area did not produce a contralateral hemianopia but rather a "hemiamblyopia," i.e., a lateralized weakness in visual attention that could be elicited by double simultaneous stimulation, a method that Loeb himself had devised. Moreover, more anterior unilateral lesions could also produce a comparable hemiamblyopia.

With respect to the question of the locus of intelligence, Goltz insisted that it was a property of the whole cerebral cortex and could not be localized in a particular region. Only extensive bilateral lesions produced a reduction in intelligence. The dog with a complete unilateral hemispherectomy was essentially as intelligent as he had been before the operation, although he might suffer from specific motor or perceptual defects. The degree of intellectual impairment was proportional to the amount of bilateral tissue loss. Extensive bilateral lesions, anterior or posterior, produced significant impairment in intelligence with the qualitative characteristics of the impairment differing according to whether the bilateral ablation was anterior or posterior. Smaller lesions had little or no effect.

Goltz reported that bilateral removal of the frontal lobes produced awkwardness in movement, hyperactivity, hyperreflexia, and some diminution in tactile sensitivity. In addition, he noted that the operated dogs very often showed an alteration in character. They were irritable, restless, and aggressive, they had less to do with other dogs, and their intelligence was somewhat impaired. But ablations of smaller size restricted to the prefrontal region did not produce these effects, and this led Goltz and Loeb (1902) to deny that neural mechanisms underlying intelligence or personality traits were situated there.

The Berlin physiologist Hermann Munk (1839–1912), an indefatigable worker, was a dominant figure in the golden age of localization. Through ablation studies on the dog he identified the visual center in the occipital lobes and maintained that incomplete destruction of that region produced a condition that he designated as "mindblindness" and that was later given the name of visual agnosia (Munk, 1878, 1879). His discoveries, initially disputed by some of his fellow physiologists, had a direct influence on the thinking of clinicians who soon published case reports describing cortical blindness and mindblindness that confirmed his conclusions (Benton, 1978). Munk went on to localize cortical centers for somesthesis and audition in the parietofrontal and temporal regions, respectively. He also confirmed the existence of motor (or sensorimotor) centers in the frontal lobes. As for the prefrontal region, he had relatively little to say. He denied that the area was either exclusively or preferentially associated with the exercise of intelligence or any specific mental capacity such as attention, remarking that intelligence was a functional property of the whole cerebral cortex (Munk, 1890). In this respect at least he was in agreement with Goltz.

David Ferrier (1843–1928) was a pioneer localizationist of great prominence whose stimulation and ablation experiments, primarily on monkeys but also on dogs and cats, generated a comprehensive map of the major sensory and motor centers of the cerebral cortex (Ferrier, 1876; 1878/1886). Although some of his own observations would have suggested caution, he placed the cortical visual center in the angular gyrus in opposition to the occipital localization of Munk and others. How Ferrier came to make this unusual inference is not exactly clear; it is possible that either he inadvertently cut the underlying optic radiations in the course of his operations (Starr, 1884; Schäfer, 1888) or he misinterpreted visuomotor disability as absolute blindness (Glickstein, 1985). In any case, in due course he did acknowledge the participation of the occipital lobes in vision and concluded that the visual center occupied the territory of both the angular gyrus and the occipital lobe. His localization of somesthesis in the cerebral cortex was an unusual one. Finding no impairment of tactile sensitivity after extensive lesions of the convex surface of the hemispheres, he reported that experimentally produced lesions in the hippocampal region produced significant loss of response to pressure and pain. The auditory center was localized in the superior temporal cortex and the motor center in the rolandic region. He was one of the few investigators of the period to call attention to species differences, pointing out that the consequences of destruction of the motor area were far less severe in the dog and cat than in the monkey. He found that stimulation of the frontal cortex anterior to the motor area produced no overt responses.

Ferrier made careful observations on monkeys subjected to ablations of the prefrontal region and concluded that the consequences were a "decided alteration in the animals' character and behavior" but one that was "difficult to describe precisely." An observer who had not known the animals before operation might well judge them to be normal, since no sensory, perceptual, or motor defects were evident. But the animals were apathetic, not interested in their surroundings, and they responded only to momentary stimulation. Thus, "while not absolutely demented, they had lost, to all appearances, the faculty of attention and intelligent observation." Ferrier added that these behavioral changes did not appear in every monkey subjected to bilateral prefrontal ablation; in some animals the operation appeared to have no effect, perhaps because of incomplete removal of tissue.

The functional significance of the frontal lobes was the primary concern of the Italian neuropsychiatrist and physiologist Leonardo Bianchi (1848–1927). Beginning in the 1880s he undertook experimental studies extending over three decades on monkeys and dogs subjected to prefrontal ablations (Bianchi, 1895, 1920/1922). Having noted that unilateral ablations were without effect, he described the changes he had observed after bilateral removals. The animals showed no sensory or motor defects but there were profound changes in character. They no longer showed affection for people whom they used to caress, and when approached they were likely to be fearful. They were no longer sociable with other monkeys nor did they engage in play. At the same time they did groom themselves. They were impulsive and when frustrated they became violent. Bianchi offered a broad interpretation of these changes. Bilateral prefrontal ablation "does not so much interfere with the perceptions taken singly as it does disaggregate the personality." The animal is no longer capable of "serializing and synthesizing groups of representations." Their displays of fear and their agitation are direct consequences of this inability to integrate experiences and of their "defective sense of personality." Thus Bianchi saw frontal lobe changes as reflecting disintegration of the total personality rather than a loss of "general intelligence" or of a specific ability.

Comment

Experimental ablations of prefrontal cortex had generated positive results but nevertheless were somewhat ambiguous in that the predicted effects were not always obtained. The possibility of species differences in outcome was largely ignored, a circumstance that itself favored variation in findings. What had been reasonably well established was that whatever behavioral changes were observed came from bilateral destruction, with unilateral ablations usually being without effect. The prefrontal region was still only a unitary topographic landmark to these investigators. Its connections with other regions of the brain were scarcely known nor were there any indications that the region might consist of functional subdivisions. Unlike motor cortex, it was a silent area that was not responsive to electric stimulation.

In spite of their own observations that at least some of their frontally injured animals were hyperactive, irritable, aggressive, and asocial, Goltz and Loeb finally concluded that the region was a silent area. Perhaps, in their view, it was a question of the size of the lesion. In contrast, Ferrier had made some perceptive observations leading him to believe that prefrontally injured monkeys were partially demented and showed personality changes that he found difficult to describe. His observations were significantly extended by Bianchi, who gave a detailed account of these changes and interpreted them as reflecting a profound alteration of personality.

The Clinicians

By 1880 the associations between disease involving the territory of the precentral gyrus and motor disability and between aphasia and lesions of the foot of the left third frontal gyrus and its surround were universally recognized. The existence of the frontal eye fields and the supplementary motor area was to be brought to light only decades later. Three influential contributions in the late 1880s followed Harlow's 1868 paper describing the features of what came to be known as the "frontal lobe syndrome."

The first paper by Moritz Jastrowitz (1888) dealt with the clinical aspects of cerebral localization. In discussing frontal lobe symptomatology, he stated that he had seen a specific form of dementia, characterized by an oddly cheerful agitation, in patients with tumors of the frontal lobe, which he referred to as "so-called moria." He remarked that he had seen several such cases but had not called attention to them because of the difficulty in describing the peculiar condition and because of its inconstant presentation. But he emphasized that moria is found only in some frontal lobe patients and not necessarily only in tumors. "This peculiar disease picture is seen in many general paretics at the beginning of their illness, in senile dementia, in many alcoholics where certainly frontal lobe atrophy also occurs."

Later that year Leonore Welt (1888) wrote a lengthy paper in which she reported a personally observed case and presented a detailed review of earlier literature. Her patient, a 37-year-old man, had sustained a severe penetrating frontal fracture after a fall from a fourth story window. Presumably he had been trying to close the window but being drunk he lost his balance and fell. Physical recovery was swift and uneventful after an operation for removal of bone from the brain. However, beginning about 5 days after the traumatic event the patient showed a remarkable change in personality. He had always been an honest, industrious, cheerful man, skilled in his occupation as a furrier but somewhat given to boasting and a heavy drinker. There was now a complete change in his character. He was aggressive and malicious and given to making bad jokes. He teased other patients unmercifully and played mean tricks on the hospital personnel. He showed no respect for the physicians and threatened to "expose" them in the daily press. His behavior, which became increasingly intolerable, was the subject of almost daily complaints by the hospital personnel.

He exhibited this objectionable behavior for about a month at which time his behavior gradually improved. He was quieter, cleaner, no longer quarreled with everyone, and in a few days he was his old self. He was quite aware of how he had behaved and was genuinely remorseful. He could not explain what had happened to him. After discharge from the hospital he returned to work as a furrier but continued his heavy drinking. Some months later he died from a pleuritic infection. Autopsy disclosed destruction of the gyrus rectus in both hemispheres as well as the mesial sector of the right inferior frontal gyrus.

Having observed that the findings in her patient were consistent with the observations of Goltz and Ferrier as well as with Harlow's case, Welt pointed out that the number of such cases is very small and that far more often prefrontal injury does not produce these peculiar alterations in character. She discussed and tabulated the numerous negative cases of tumor, abscess, trauma, and atrophy of the frontal lobes in the literature that showed no personality changes although a diminution of intelligence was often apparent. Analyzing the eight autopsied cases showing personality change, she found that invariably there was involvement of the orbital gyri. Orbital pathology was also highly probable in two additional cases that had not come to autopsy. At the same time there were cases in the literature in which demonstrated orbital injury had not produced these personality changes. Welt concluded that the presentation of these character changes warrants the inference of orbital pathology. However, the converse was not true; the absence of such changes did not mean that the orbital area was intact.

In 1890 Hermann Oppenheim wrote a comprehensive paper on the clinical manifestations of brain tumors. In the section dealing with frontal lobe neoplasms he called attention to "a psychic anomaly which is perhaps of focal diagnostic value." Referring to Jastrowitz's concept of moria, he remarked that Bernhardt, Wernicke, and Westphal had made similar observations of childishness and inappropriate joking in patients with brain tumors but were unwilling to assign a lesional localization to this peculiar behavior. Hence, he was initially surprised at Jastrowitz's frontal lobe localization but his review of his own cases in fact confirmed it. However, he would not designate the condition as moria or silliness but rather a peculiar addiction to trivial joking of a predominantly sarcastic nature that was in sharp contrast to the patient's prevailing mood. Four patients who exhibited *Witzelsucht* proved to have tumors of the right frontal lobe, three of which had invaded the mesial and basal area. Nevertheless, this type of behavior can be observed in other conditions, as in a patient with chronic uremia whom Oppenheim had seen. This psychic anomaly appears predominantly in frontal lobe tumors. Future observation should be directed to the specific question of how frequently and under what circumstances it may be useful for focal diagnostic inference.

Comment

The studies of Jastrowitz, Welt, and Oppenheim established that distinctive changes in personality and behavior could be related to disease of the prefrontal region, and Welt specifically implicated involvement of the orbital and mesial sectors of that region. The terms moria (stupidity) and Witzelsucht (addiction to joking) are linguistic residues of their observations. Each of these clinicians called attention to a somewhat different combination of behaviors. Welt described a pattern of aggression, bad temper, and viciousness that she compared to Harlow's crowbar case and to the behavior of Goltz's dogs. Jastrowitz emphasized the inappropriate cheerfulness and lack of concern of his patients. Oppenheim was dubious about the reality of the patients' alleged cheerfulness and pointed to the sarcastic, latently hostile nature of the patients' compulsive joking. The frontal (really prefrontal) lobe syndrome is the legacy of these authors' descriptions.

Although this assemblage of behaviors was observed for the most part in patients with tumor of the frontal lobes, all three clinicians maintained that they could occur in other conditions involving frontal lobe pathology such as general paresis and trauma. Bilateral disease seemed to be the rule but this point was not emphasized. Instead the observation was made that involvement of the mesial-orbital area of the right frontal lobe might be of particular importance in the production of the symptoms.

THE TWENTIETH CENTURY: THE FIRST FIFTY YEARS

Anatomy and Physiology

A major development in the early decades of the twentieth century was the rise of cytoarchitectonics, i.e., the systematic study of the cellular structure of the cerebral cortex. Some nineteenth century anatomists had described the internal structure of specific cortical areas and identified four to six layers in them. Cyto-architectonics represented an extension of their observations and the mapping of all the areas. The major investigators in this ambitious and arduous enterprise (which was carried out on the brains of monkeys for the most part) were Campbell (1905), Brodmann (1909), Cécile and Oskar Vogt (1919), and Von Economo (1925) whose maps showed a basic similarity but nevertheless differed considerably in important details such as the number of areas that were identified. No doubt differences in investigative techniques were one determinant of these discrepant findings (Fleischhauer, 1978), and the unreliability of the more elaborate maps was the target of a harsh critique by Lashley and Clark (1946) who pointed out that significant individual differences were ignored and the boundaries between adjacent areas often could not be ascertained with any confidence. In the event, Brodmann's scheme, designating six layers and some 50 areas, was the one generally adopted by anatomists and neurologists. Although there was disagreement about the number and boundaries of these areas, the frontal pole was generally considered to occupy Brodmann areas 9–10, the mesial surface to occupy areas 24 and 32, the orbital surface to occupy areas 11–14 and 47, and the lateral convex surface to occupy areas 45–46. With some exceptions (e.g., area 24), these areas proved to be of the granular type with a clearly identifiable granular layer IV, in contrast to agranular motor cortex in which layer IV is obscured by layers III and V with their dense concentration of pyramidal cells. In any case, these studies demonstrated that the prefrontal region was far from being a homogeneous structure with the implication that its different parts might well have different functional properties.

Opinions differed with respect to the general question of the functional significance of these variations in internal structure of the cerebral cortex. It seemed reasonable to some students that the associations of pyramidal cell layers with efferent or motor functions and of granular layer IV with afferent or receptive functions must have functional implications. But there were so many exceptions to these rules that no strong generalizations could be made. Consequently, Brodmann's areas came to serve simply as topographic landmarks, primarily for the purpose of lesional localization, in the same way as did the cortical gyri and sulci. Only later was evidence adduced that the boundaries of the architectonic areas bore a relationship to the undersurface of the cortical sulci (Sanides, 1962).

At the same time the establishment of the neuron doctrine with its emphasis on directed (as opposed to diffuse) conduction, coupled with continued improvement in techniques of neurohistologic study, spurred investigation of the specific connections between the cerebral cortex (including prefrontal cortex) and other parts of the brain, most notably the thalamus. Many later nineteenth century anatomists, among them Gudden (1870), Monakow (1882, 1895), and the Dejerines (1895–1901), had already shown that experimentally produced lesions in the cortex led to degeneration in diverse subcortical structures. However, the reported findings were conflicting, the mechanisms and pathways involved were not clear, and the possibility that the observed effects had been produced by extraneous factors such as interference to the vascular supply of the subcortical structures had not been excluded. Experimental investigation during the early decades of the century, mainly on the monkey, identified these connections more precisely. Although the bulk of the work was concerned with motor cortex and the temporal, parietal, and occipital lobes, observations on the afferent and efferent connections of the prefrontal regions were also made. Some studies illustrative of the trend of results are reviewed below.

An early study by Beevor and Horsley (1902) found a striking degeneration of frontothalamic fibers in monkeys subjected to limited lesions in the prefrontal region. The only other area to which fibers could be traced from the inexcitable frontal cortex was the upper part of the substantia nigra. Minkowski (1922), describing his own results on monkeys in combination with some observations of his mentor, Monakow, inferred that there were projections from the dorsomedial nuclei of the thalamus to most of the prefrontal region extending to the frontal pole as well as to the prefrontal mesial surface. (In 1934 Pfeiffer reported the complementary observation that the dorsomedial nuclei formed the main termination of fibers from the anterior limb of the capsule.) In addition, Minkowski found that some projections from the anterior part of the globus pallidus reached the prefrontal region. Efferent connections included projections from the frontal pole to the internal capsule and the red nucleus and from the superior frontal gyrus to the rolandic area.

Levin (1936) made almost complete lesions of the prefrontal region of the right frontal lobe in two monkeys and traced the course of degeneration 2 weeks after the intervention. An extensive projection system, most of the fibers of which entered the rostral thalamus, was identified. The origin of these fibers appeared to be area 9 on the convexity of the frontal lobe. In addition, a bundle of fine fibers, apparently arising from the anterior part of the third frontal gyrus, descended to the midbrain (substantia nigra) and pons (dorsomedial pontine nuclei). Walker (1935, 1938) demonstrated that in monkeys the dorsomedial nucleus of the thalamus provides a spatially organized afferent projection system to the prefrontal region, the lateral part going to the upper frontal pole (area 9) and the mesial part going to the orbital area. He pointed out that this nuclear mass and cortical area attain their greatest development in the human brain. Correspondingly, motor cortex is connected in a definite spatial arrangement with lateral thalamic nuclei. Walker also described degenerative changes in the dorsomedial nucleus following ablation of prefrontal cortex, thus confirming Levin's finding of efferent connections between this region and the thalamus.

The introduction of prefrontal leukotomy and allied procedures in the late 1930s provided the opportunity to study the retrograde degeneration and glial proliferation in the brains of patients who had died after operation either as a result of the intervention or from intercurrent disease. The series of reports by Meyer, Beck, and McLardy (1947; Beck, McLardy, and Meyer, 1950; McLardy, 1950) can serve to illustrate the tenor of results on this material. Degeneration of prefrontal-thalamic connections was found in every case, specifically retrograde degeneration in the dorsomedial nucleus. The findings of Walker (1938) of a spatially organized projection from the dorsomedial nucleus to prefrontal cortex in the monkey, e.g., the pars magnocellularis to orbital cortex and the pars parvicellularis to the dorsal convexity, were largely confirmed. And the point was made that a direct hypothalamic-prefrontal connection is probable in view of the established projection of hypothalamic nuclei to the pars magnocellularis, thus providing an anatomic basis for physiologic observations implicating the participation of the mesial orbital prefrontal cortex in emotional and autonomic changes. Lesions of the cingulate gyrus resulted in degeneration of anterior thalamic nuclei and degeneration of prefrontal-pontine pathways was demonstrable although it was not possible to identify the precise origin of these pathways.

Thus the outcome of these and other studies of the period in monkeys and human subjects was to establish definitively that the prefrontal region had rich afferent, efferent, and intracortical ("association") connections. The most prominent of these were the spatially organized links with the dorsal nuclei of the thalamus pointing to differentiation of function within the region. Connections to the basal ganglia, midbrain, and pons were also clearly demonstrable.

Studies of Animal Behavior

The rise of objective animal psychology, exemplified in the behavioral observations of C. Lloyd Morgan (1900), the puzzle box experiments of E. L. Thorndike (1898), and Jacques Loeb's (1902) studies of associative learning, provided a model for subsequent controlled assessment of the behavioral capacities and characteristics of animals with experimentally produced prefrontal lesions. Two series of studies, one by Shepherd Ivory Franz (1902, 1907, 1912) and the other by Carlyle Jacobsen and his coworkers (Crawford et al., 1948; Fulton and Jacobsen, 1935; Jacobsen and Nissen, 1937; 1931, 1935; Jacobsen, Wolfe, and Jackson, 1935), had a major influence on the evolution of thought about the role of the frontal lobes in the mediation of primate behavior.

Franz gave learning tasks, including the Thorndike puzzle box, to monkeys (and also cats) who had been subjected to unilateral and bilateral prefrontal ablations. Having learned the tasks preoperatively, the animals were tested for retention of the habits. Unilateral ablation had no significant effect, the operated animals retaining the habits almost as well as controls. Bilateral ablation produced loss of the habits in most of the animals; a few showed normal retention. However, those animals who had suffered loss of the recently acquired habits relearned them fairly readily. Franz's studies had the effect of inducing an attitude of skepticism on the part of students of animal behavior toward assigning any "higher-level" functions to the prefrontal region. It remained a "silent area" without identifiable behavioral significance.

Jacobsen's ingenious experiments with chimpanzees and monkeys, undertaken some 25 years later, effectively counteracted this rather nihilistic position. In essence he found that prefrontally injured animals exhibited a characteristic pattern of performances on a set of diverse learning tasks. They were not impaired on tasks, such as visual discrimination learning, in which all elements of the stimulus configuration are continuously in full view and that make no demands on short-term memory. In contrast, delayed response tasks, in which the animal is required to keep in mind an environmental event for 10 to 30 seconds in order to respond appropriately, were consistently failed by the animal who had been subjected to a bilateral prefrontal ablation. Jacobsen's findings in primates were readily confirmed and later work (e.g., Finan, 1939; Harlow and

Settlage, 1948; Malmo, 1942) was devoted to the task of identifying basic factors, such as hyperactivity and distractibility, perseverative tendencies, and right-left confusion, that might underlie the failure in performance.

This defect in maintaining a set (in behavioristic terms) or carrying a representation of an environment event in mind over time (in mentalistic terms) was found in varying degrees in other prefrontally injured animals, such as dogs and cats, and rather less consistently in human subjects (see Hebb, 1945; Hebb and Penfield, 1940). Despite the negative findings reported for some patients, the demonstration of a specific type of cognitive defect associated with injury to the region weakened the cogency of "mass action" theories of cerebral functioning and offered promising clues to the understanding of the behavioral changes associated with frontal lobe disease.

The classic description by Jacobsen and his coworkers of a remarkable change in personality and behavior in one animal after a bilateral prefrontal ablation had a more direct and immediate impact on clinical thinking and practice. This female chimpanzee was a sociable, highly emotional animal who was eager to be tested in experimental tasks that brought her food rewards. Preoperatively she became greatly upset when she made errors on a very difficult task and often would fly into a temper tantrum. After a few errors in the course of training she refused to participate further and eventually had to be dragged from her cage to the experimental set-up, a condition that Jacobsen compared to a Pavlovian "experimental neurosis." She was gradually brought back to active participation in the experiments through feeding and play around the apparatus and was given an easy learning task with minimal possibility of failure. After left prefrontal lobectomy she was once again given the difficult task and once again developed an "experimental neurosis." However, after right frontal lobectomy her behavior changed profoundly. She showed a remarkable equanimity in the face of repeated failures on both the difficult and easy tasks. Jacobsen and his coworkers were sufficiently impressed by this postoperative change in the chimpanzee to make it a main point in their summary. "The basic disturbance is also manifest in the affective reactions. An 'experimental neurosis' was established by continued training on a problem situation too difficult for the animal to master. After bilateral extirpation of the frontal areas, the animal no longer had 'temper tantrums' when it made mistakes, and continued training on difficult problems did not evoke an 'experimental neurosis.' On the other hand, behavior suggestive of Witzelsucht which characterizes human cases with similar lesions, was noted" (Jacobsen, Wolfe, and Jackson, 1935, p. 14).

This series of experimental studies was reported by Fulton and Jacobsen in a major symposium on the frontal lobes at the 1935 International Congress of Neurology in London. The report included a description by Jacobsen of the disappearance of his chimpanzee's "experimental neurosis" following bilateral prefrontal lobotomy. After the presentation the Lisbon neurologist Egas Moniz, who was attending the symposium, raised the question of whether it ought not to be possible to alleviate anxiety states in human patients by a comparable surgical procedure (Valenstein, 1986). Since Moniz embarked on the operation of prefrontal leukotomy immediately after his return from London it has been generally assumed that the Fulton–Jacobsen report provided the impetus for his pioneering effort.

Clinical Studies

Clinical investigation during the first two decades of the century generated findings that were not always consistent but that did serve to document the diverse behavioral disorders observed in association with prefrontal injury. Early reports included that of Zacher (1901) who described a 54-year-old man with an illness of undetermined origin (however, he was diabetic with optic neuritis) that was characterized by lengthy periods of poor attention, fatigability, and apathy interspersed with periods during which he exhibited nearly normal behavior. At no time were there indications of speech disorder. However, gross visual impairment referable to the optic neuritis was evident. An outstanding feature of his condition was his lack of concern about his visual disability and hospitalization. Some years later Campbell (1909) also placed special emphasis on the lack of concern shown by his patient with a frontal lobe tumor. A second feature of Zacher's case was his patient's addiction to joking, which was evident even during his better periods. Zacher concluded by making two points: first, that Witzelsucht is a symptom of focal diagnostic significance; second, that his patient did not show the gross personality changes associated with prefrontal disease that had been described by Welt. On the other hand, Quensel (1914) reported a patient with prefrontal traumatic injury who showed no demonstrable intellectual impairment on either clinical observation or a comprehensive battery of psychologic tests. Yet he was impulsive and aggressive and showed grossly inappropriate conduct. In Quensel's view, the clinical picture presented by his patient was quite comparable to that of Welt's patient.

Both Schuster (1902) and Bernhardt (Bernhardt and Borchardt, 1909) discussed at some length the question of whether the childishness, moria, and Witzelsucht shown by some tumor patients were in fact a specific sign of frontal lobe disease. They agreed that, while the syndrome was seen in patients with tumors in other locations, it was shown with considerably greater frequency by those with frontal lobe tumors. Hence, in the absence of other symptoms indicative of a lesion in other locations, the appearance of these curious behavioral features was suggestive of frontal lobe disease. Bernhardt also noted that patients with right frontal involvement showed these features more frequently than did those with left frontal disease but, pointing out that aphasic disorder in left-hemisphere–damaged patients might mask the symptoms, he declined to draw a firm conclusion.

World War I produced thousands of cases of penetrating brain injuries including many with wounds more or less restricted to the frontal lobes. The carnage afforded ample opportunity for postwar study of these patients, and attempts were made to formulate a cogent definition of the "frontal lobe syndrome" as well as to relate different types of impairment to specific areas of the prefrontal region.

Feuchtwanger (1923) devoted a comprehensive monograph to his findings and interpretations of the behavioral changes seen in patients with prefrontal injuries. A comparison of frontal and nonfrontal cases showed contrasting patterns of performance. As compared to nonfrontal patients, mood disorders, apathy, attentional disturbance, impulsivity, and Witzelsucht were more frequently manifested, while sensorimotor defects, speech disorders, and memory impairment were less frequently manifested by the frontal patients. Individual patients showed distinctive clinical pictures, e.g., some were depressed or apathetic, others were euphoric, and still others "psychopathic" or "hysteroid." Feuchtwanger ascribed great importance to the patient's premorbid personality as a determinant of his clinical picture. No important differences between predominantly left and predominantly right prefrontal patients were apparent and Witzelsucht was not a frequent occurrence. Feuchtwanger saw his findings as indicating that, although basic cognitive functions such as perceptual capacity, memory, and ideation are not impaired in frontal patients, they show profound disturbances of affect and of the capacity to control or integrate behavior, which he considered to be a change in the total personality. His more detailed theoretic interpretation, fraught with unfamiliar terms and vague concepts, is difficult to understand. Nevertheless his contribution was of considerable value in showing the variety of changes that can follow prefrontal damage and in his demonstration that a simplistic concept of a single "frontal lobe syndrome" is quite untenable.

In the 1920s Kurt Goldstein (1927, 1936a,b, 1944, 1948; Goldstein and Katz, 1937) advanced a theory of neuropsychologic function that was based on his conception of the "abstract attitude." This extremely broad concept incorporated not only the capacity for abstract reasoning but also a variety of other behavioral functions such as initiative, foresight, resistance to suggestion, self-awareness, flexibility in behavior, and the capacity to analyze a complex situation into its constituent components. In fact, his specifications could well serve as a broad definition of "general intelligence." Goldstein interpreted the diverse behavioral defects shown by patients with brain disease, and particularly those with prefrontal injury, as expressions of this single capacity. Given the breadth of the concept, it was easy enough to demonstrate that every patient was defective in one or another aspect of the abstract attitude. In the 1930s and 1940s the approach was widely adopted by clinical psychologists who were searching for signs of prefrontal dysfunction. In due course, however, this "single principle" approach lost popularity as it became evident that the concept of the abstract attitude was too broad and multifaceted to be useful.

Goldstein's more valuable contribution was his insightful interpretation of certain symptoms as defensive reactions on the part of the patient to protect him from failure, confusion, and loss of self-esteem. Thus, at least under some circumstances, the patient who shows apathy, rigidity, lack of concern, or facetiousness may be exhibiting these behaviors in order to cope with his disabilities and avoid painful awareness of his mental incompetence. This approach to the understanding of some of the peculiar behaviors encountered in brain-damaged patients, especially those with frontal lobe disease, was also adopted by Golla (1931) and Brickner (1936).

In a monograph of over 1,000 pages, Karl Kleist (1934) reported his findings on some hundreds of patients who had sustained penetrating brain wounds during World War I. An old-fashioned localizationist who did not hesitate to infer functions from symptoms, he developed a detailed map of the brain in which diverse capacities were assigned to specific cortical areas (see; Benton, 1976, p. 39; Kleist, 1934, pp. 1365–6). However, Kleist was also a careful examiner and a cautious interpreter who compared his findings with earlier observations. He laid great stress on the lack of drive or initiative (Antrieb) associated with orbital lesions and on the personality changes seen in prefrontally injured patients, which he related to deficiencies in self-perception. He also described impoverishment of verbal ideation and expression in the absence of frank aphasic disorder in patients with left prefrontal involvement, an observation that was amply confirmed in later decades (see Benton, 1968; Milner, 1964; Zangwill, 1966). Moreover, he was perhaps the first clinician to emphasize the significance of the close connections between the prefrontal orbital area and structures of the limbic system and to regard them as a neural network subserving self-perception and "ego-functions" (Kleist, 1931). His ideas, in contrast to those of Goldstein, had little influence outside of Germany, probably because his monumental volume was not translated into English or French.

Brickner's (1934, 1936) case report of a patient with practically total excision of the prefrontal region in the course of removal of a large meningioma aroused great interest because of its detailed and vivid account of the patient's social behavior and intellectual and personality characteristics over the course of several years. This 42-year-old businessman of high average intelligence first came under observation 1 year after surgery. During casual interactions of short duration he could appear to be entirely normal even to professional observers. His everyday behavior was quite different. He was obstinate, verbally aggressive, boastful, abusive to his caretakers, and addicted to poor joking. At times he was capable of simple abstract reasoning but usually was unable to maintain or follow a logical train of thought. Psychologic testing yielded IQs of 95–100, indicating a significant decline from premorbid "general intelligence." His Rorschach test performance reflected extreme ideational impoverishment with a predominance of color-naming responses. Brickner viewed his patient's behavior as an exaggerated expression of certain premorbid personality traits rather than as representing a qualitative personality change. Almost echoing Bianchi, he thought that the fundamental disability was a defect in the synthesis of essentially intact cognitive processes that rendered the patient incapable of engaging in complex or temporally integrated conduct.

Ackerly (1937) described unusual findings in a 37-year-old woman in whom the mesial sector of the left prefrontal region had been destroyed by the growth of a large meningioma and the entire right prefrontal region had been amputated in the course of removal of the tumor. Psychometric testing gave no indication of a decline in "general intelligence" or of diminished energy in carrying out household duties or engaging in social fucntions. Moreover, relatives and friends found her to be the same sociable, likable, kindhearted person that she was before her illness. Nevertheless there were some striking changes in her behavior. For example, once having begun a task (e.g., house cleaning or preparing a meal) she should not be made to abandon it, even momentarily, until it was completed. There were other conspicuous findings in this patient. She actually showed an increased capacity for work and physical exercise and she made remarkable progress in speaking and reading English, which was her second language. Ackerly interpreted his patient's behavior as reflecting an abnormal "lack of distractibility" that was based on an inability to handle more than one environmental event at the same time. The case once again illustrated the diversity of behavioral changes that are encountered in patients with prefrontal disease and in addition offered promising clues to the understanding of frontal lobe function.

A radically different note was sounded by the neurosurgeon Clovis Vincent (1936); on the basis of his clinical experience, he insisted that partial or even complete removal of the prefrontal region was not accompanied by the diverse mental symptoms traditionally associated with frontal lobe disease. Vincent pointed out that the prefrontal region is neither a simple nor an autonomous structure. Its activity is regulated by the other parts of the brain with which it is connected and hence pathologic alteration of these parts could disrupt prefrontal functioning.

Vincent presented his paper in the same symposium on the frontal lobes at the 1935 London International Neurological Congress in which Fulton and Jacobsen reported their findings on chimpanzees. With its emphasis on the lack of any major disruptive effects of prefrontal removals in human patients, Vincent's presentation may well have had a more significant effect on the thinking of Egas Moniz than did the Fulton-Jacobsen report, which dealt in the main with the cognitive defects produced by prefrontal lobotomy. However, Moniz himself denied that either presentation had had any such influence (see Valenstein, 1986).

The same theme was taken up in greater detail by Hebb (1945), who attacked the "almost universal belief that surgical removals from this area (the frontal lobes) must produce serious psychologic defects." The impetus for the critique was his study of a patient (Hebb and Penfield, 1940) who at the age of 16 had sustained a severe head injury that had injured both frontal poles. A 10-year period of convulsive disorder, violent behavior, and impairment of memory led to surgical intervention in which a large part of both prefrontal regions (almost all of Brodmann areas 9–12 and 46–47) was excised in the course of removal of scar tissue. Recovery fiollowing the operation was remarkable. He was considered by his relatives and friends to have once again become his old self, i.e., before the head injury. He served successfully in the Canadian army during World War II. The only "prefrontal" trait that he showed was a rather happy-go-lucky attitude with a penchant for changing jobs every few months and with no concern about the future. His test performance improved to a normal level from a preoperative subnormal level.

From the findings in this case, as well a critical review of the literature and an analysis of the methodologic difficulties in interpreting the symptoms of frontal lobe disease, Hebb argued that uncomplicated loss of prefrontal tissue did not have the major deleterious consequences encountered in cases of tumor, atrophy, or trauma where in all probability dysfunction of other parts of the brain was present. His trenchant critique aroused considerable discussion and no doubt encouraged surgical interventions including frontal leukotomy.

SUMMARY

As a perusal of the list of references will show, not a single contribution before 1947 contained the adjective "prefrontal" in its title. Early investigators of the prefrontal region invariably employed the term "frontal" to indicate their field of study. This usage persists in large part today along with the more limiting designations, "prefrontal cortex" and "frontal granular cortex." In any case, the content of these early contributions leaves no doubt that they were dealing specifically with the prefrontal region.

A major achievement of the first three decades of the twentieth century was the description of the distinctive cellular composition of the prefrontal region and its parcellation into architectonic areas. Brodmann's maps, in common use as topographic landmarks today, are a lasting legacy of this monumental effort. Campbell, Brodmann, the Vogts, and Economo produced maps that differed from one another in not unimportant details, a circumstance that inevitably raised questions about their reliability. The negative findings of replicative studies reinforced this skepticism, particularly in regard to the cortical areas delimited by Brodmann. Nevertheless, the fundamental fact of areal cellular differentiation in the prefrontal region, as in other regions of the brain, was firmly established and provided the basis for the more searching studies of Sanides and Fleischhauer.

Of greater significance were the investigations of the connections between the prefrontal region and other parts of the brain that were instituted in the late nineteenth century and continued through the early decades of the twentieth. The most important afferent and efferent connections were determined to be with the dorsomedial nucleus of the thalamus. As Walker and others demonstrated, the connections followed a definite spatial arrangement with the magnocellular sector of the nucleus projecting to the orbital and the parvocellular sector to the dorsolateral area of the prefrontal region. Other connections of the prefrontal region that were brought to light involved the basal ganglia, midbrain, and pons. It was an awareness of these multiple connections that would lead Vincent to the conclusion that prefrontal symptomatology reflected a disruption in the interrelations of the region with other centers rather than a mere loss of tissue.

Animal experimentation, exemplified by the studies of Bianchi and Jacobsen, indicated that prefrontally injured monkeys and dogs did indeed exhibit distinctive cognitive defects and peculiar alterations of personality that an experienced observer could readily detect but which were not easily described. Diverse verbal labels, e.g., "apathy," "agitation," "partial dementia," were employed to characterize the behavioral changes, and tentative hypotheses such as the incapacity to "serialize groups of impressions" and impairment in "recent memory" were advanced to explain them. But neither the behavioral descriptions nor the explanations that were proposed to account for them were felt to be altogether satisfactory and none received wide acceptance.

By 1947 a vast array of diverse behavior deficits of a cognitive, affective, and interpersonal nature had been described in association with disease of the prefrontal region. This mixture of deficits was far too variegated to permit the formulation of a satisfactory description in terms of one or two basic disabilities. Nevertheless, the term "frontal lobe syndrome" was adopted to refer to this aggregation of deficits, perhaps as much as a convenient label as from any conviction that it represented a true syndrome, i.e., a conjunction of inherently related symptoms.

Descriptions of the consequences of prefrontal disease and surgical removals ranged from thoroughgoing dementia to the absence of observable deficits. Between the extremes were reports of highly specific deficits and personality changes that more often than not seriously impaired overall behavioral competence. Still other reports, such as that of Ackerly, described pronounced personality changes that complicated but did not have a devastating effect on a patient's life adjustment. A number of observers related personality changes specifically to orbital-mesial injury, and a few raised the question of whether right hemisphere involvement might be a particularly important factor. The frequent descriptions of personality change in the direction of equanimity, lack of concern, and diminution of anxiety provided some rationale for surgical intervention to alleviate agitation, depression, and anxiety in psychiatric patients.

Thus in 1950 researchers were presented with an embarrassment of riches. They faced a number of formidable challenges. They had to sort out the diverse deficits that had been associated with lesions of the prefrontal region to determine which were primary and which were secondary or adventitious. They had to gain insight into the nature of the primary deficits as derangements of normal neuropsychologic functioning. Mindful of the fact that the prefrontal region is simply a topographic landmark encompassing a number of distinctive anatomic–functional areas, they had to identify the neural mechanisms that mediated the behavioral operations of each of these areas.

While everyone would agree that current factual knowledge is still incomplete and conceptual formulations still not entirely satisfying, researchers have achieved notable success in meeting these challenges at every level—anatomic, physiologic, and behavioral. Indeed the advances in understanding that have been made since 1950 (and particularly since 1970) are so radical and far-reaching as to justify the designation of developments up to 1950 as "early history." The results of this impressive recent progress are epitomized in the contributions to this volume.

ACKNOWLEDGMENTS

I am indebted to Ms. Jan Carter for her help in the preparation of the manuscript.

REFERENCES

Ackerly S. Instinctive, emotional and mental changes following prefrontal lobe extirpation. American Journal of Psychiatry 92:717–729, 1937.
Ajuriaguerra J, Hécaen H. Le cortex cérébral. Paris: Masson, 1949.

Akert K, Hammond HP. Emanuel Swedenborg and his contribution to neurology. Medical History 6:255–256, 1962.

Andral G. Clinique Médicale. Paris: Fortin Masson, 1823–1827.

Arnold F. Bemerkungen über den Bau des Hirns und Rückenmarks. Zurich: S. Hohr, 1838 (cited by Clarke and Dewhurst, 1972).

Baker F. The two Sylviuses: an historical study. Bulletin of the Johns Hopkins Hospital 20:329–339, 1909.

Beck E, McLardy T, Meyer A. Anatomical comments on psychosurgical procedures. Journal of Mental Science 96:157–167, 1950.

Beevor CE, Horsley V. On the pallio-tectal or cortico-mesencepalic system of fibres. Brain 25:436–443, 1902.

Benton AL. Contributions to aphasia before Broca. Cortex: 314–327, 1964.

Benton AL. Differential behavioral effects on frontal lobe disease. Neuropsychologia 6:53–60, 1968.

Benton AL. Historical development of the concept of hemispheric cerebral dominance. In Spicker SF, Engelhardt HT (eds), Philosophical Dimensions of the Neuromedical Sciences. Dordrecht, The Netherlands: Reidel, 1976.

Benton AL. The interplay of experimental and clinical approaches in brain lesion research. In Finger S (ed), Recovery from Brain Damage: Research and Theory. New York: Plenum Press, 1978, pp. 49–68.

Benton AL. Focal brain damage and the concept of localization. In Loeb C (ed), Studies in Cerebrovascular Disease. Milano: Masson Italia Editore, 1981.

Bernhardt M, Borchardt M. Zur Klinik der Stirnhirntumoren nebst Bemerkungen über Hirnpunktion. Berliner Klinische Wochenschrift 46:1341–1347, 1909.

Bianchi L. The functions of the frontal lobes. Brain 18:497–522, 1895.

Bianchi L. La Meccanica del Cervello e la Funzione dei Lobi Frontali. Turin: Bocca, 1920; English translation by JH Macdonald. The Mechanisms of the Brain and the Functions of the Frontal Lobes. Edinburgh: Livingstone, 1922.

Bigelow HJ. Dr. Harlow's case of recovery from the passage of an iron bar through the head. American Journal of the Medical Sciences 39:13–22, 1850.

Bouillaud J-B. Traité clinique et physiologique de l'encéphalite. Paris: Baillière, 1825.

Brickner RM. An interpretation of frontal lobe function based upon the study of a case of partial bilateral frontal lobectomy. In Orton ST, Fulton JF, Davis TK (eds), Localization of Function in the Cerebral Cortex. Baltimore: Williams & Wilkins, 1934, pp. 259–351.

Brickner RM. The Intellectual Functions of the Frontal Lobes. New York: Macmillan, 1936.

Brodmann K. Vergleichende Lokalisationslehre der Grosshirnrinde. Leipzig: Barth, 1909.

Campbell AW. Histological Studies on the Localisation of Cerebral Function. Cambridge: Cambridge University Press, 1905.

Campbell D, Störungen der Merkfähigkeit und fehlendes Krankheitsgefühl bei einem Fall von Stirnhirntumor. Monatsschrift für Psychiatrie 26:33–41, 1909.

Chaussier F. Exposition Sommaire de la Structure et des Différentes Parties de l'Encéphale ou Cerveau. Paris: Théophile Barrois, 1807 (cited by McHenry, 1969 and Meyer, 1971).

Clarke E, Dewhurst K. An Illustrated History of Brain Function. Berkeley: University of California Press, 1972.

Clarke E, Jacyna LS. Nineteenth-Century Origins of Neuroscientific Concepts. Berkeley: University of California Press, 1987.

Clarke E, O'Malley CD. The Human Brain and Spinal Cord. Berkeley: University of California Press, 1968.

Crawford MP, Fulton JF, Jacobsen CF, Wolfe SB. Frontal lobe ablation in chimpanzee: a résumé of 'Becky' and 'Lucy.' Research Publications Association for Nervous and Mental Disease 27:3–58, 1948.

Dejerine J, Dejerine-Klumpke A. Anatomie des Centres Nerveux. Paris: Rueff, 1895–1901.

Ecker A. Die Hirnwindungen des Menschen nach eigenen Untersuchungen. Braunschweig: Vieweg 1869.

Ecker A. The Cerebral Convolutions of Man Represented According to Original Observations. Translated by RT Edes. New York: Appleton, 1873.

Economo C, Koskinas GN. Die Cytoarchitektonik der Hirnrinde des Erwachsenen Menschen. Vienna: Springer, 1925.

Ferrier D. The Functions of the Brain. London: Smith, Elder, 1876; 2nd ed., 1886.

Ferrier D. The Localisation of Cerebral Disease. London: Smith, Elder, 1878.

Feuchtwanger E. Die Funktionen des Stirnhirns. Berlin: Springer, 1923.

Finan JL. Effects of frontal lobe lesions on temporally organized behavior in monkeys. Journal of Neurophysiology 2:208–226, 1939.

Fleischhauer K. Cortical architectonics: the last 50 years and some problems of today. In Brazier MA and Petsche H (eds), Architectonics of the Cerebral Cortex. New York: Raven Press, 1978.

Franz SI. On the functions of the cerebrum. American Journal of Physiology 8:1–22, 1902.

Franz SI. On the functions of the cerebrum: The frontal lobes. Archives of Psychology 1:1–64, 1907.

Franz SI. New phrenology. Science 35:321–328, 1912.

Fulton JF, Jacobsen CF. The functions of the frontal lobes: a comparative study in monkeys, chimpanzees and man. Abstracts, International Second Neurological Congress, Vol. 2, 70–71. London, 1935.

Fuster JM. The Prefrontal Cortex: Anatomy, Physiology and Neuropsychology of The Frontal Lobe. New York: Raven Press, 1980, 2nd ed., 1989.

Gall FJ, Spurzheim G. Recherches sur le système nerveux en général, et sur celui de cerveau en particulier. Paris: F. Schoell, 1809. (Reprint, Amsterdam: Bonsel, 1967).

Gibson WC. Pioneers in localization in the brain. JAMA 180:944–957, 1962.

Glockstein M. Ferrier's mistake. Trends in Neurosciences 8:341–344, 1985.

Goldstein K. Die Lokalisation in der Grosshirnrinde. In Bethe A (ed), Handbuch der Normalen und Pathologischen Physiologie, vol. 10. pp. 600–842. Berlin: Springer, 1927.

Goldstein K. The significance of the frontal lobes for mental performance. Journal of Neurology and Psychopathology 17:27–40, 1936a.

Goldstein K. The modifications of behavior consequent to cerebral lesions. Psychiatric Quarterly 10:586–610, 1936b.

Goldstein K. The mental changes due to frontal lobe damage. Journal of Psychology 17:187–208, 1944.

Goldstein K. Language and Language Disturbances. New York: Grune & Stratton, 1948.

Goldstein K, Katz S. The psychopathology of Pick's disease. Archives of Neurology and Psychiatry 38:473–490, 1937.

Golla F. Discussion on the mental symptoms associated with cerebral tumours. Proceedings of the Royal Society of Medicine 24:1000–1001, 1931.

Goltz F. Über die Verrichtungen des Grosshirns. Pfüger's Archiv für die gesamte Physiologie 42:419–467, 1888. Translation by Von Bonin G. On the Functions of the Hemispheres. In Von Bonin G. (ed), Some Papers on the Cerebral Cortex. Springfield, IL, CC Thomas, 1960, pp. 118–158.

Goltz F. Der Hund ohne Grosshirn: Siebente Abteilung über die Verrichtungen des Grosshirns. Pfuger's Archiv für die gesamte Physiologie 51:570–614, 1892,

Gratiolet P. Note sur les expansions des racines cérébrales du nerf optique et sur leur terminaison dan une région determinée de l'écorce des hémisphères. Comptes Rendus de l'Académie des Sciences, Paris 29:274–278, 1854.

Grünthal E. Geschichte der makroskopischen Morphologie des menschlichen Grosshirnsreliefs nebst Beiträgen zur Entwicklung der Idee einer Lokalisierung psychischer Funktionen. Bibliotheca Psychiatrica et Neurologica, Fasc. 100: 94–128, 1957.

Gudden B. Experimental untersuchungen uber das peripherische und centrale Nervensystem. Archiv für Psychiatrie 2:693–723, 1870.

Harlow HF, Settlage PH. Effect of extirpation of frontal areas upon learning performance of monkeys. Research Publications Association for Research in Nervous and Mental Disorder 27:446–459, 1948.

Harlow JM. Passage of an iron bar through the head. Boston Medical and Surgical Journal 39:389–393, 1848.

Harlow JM. Recovery from the passage of an iron bar through the head. Publications of the Massachusetts Medical Society 2:327–347, 1868.

Hebb DO. Man's frontal lobes: a critical review. Archives of Neurology and Psychiatry 54:10–24, 1945.

Hebb DO, Penfield W. Human behavior after extensive bilateral removal from the frontal lobes. Archives of Neurology and Psychiatry 44:421–438, 1940.

Jacobsen CF. A study of cerebral function in learning: The frontal lobes. Journal of Comparative Neurology 52:271–340, 1931.

Jacobsen CF. Functions of frontal association areas in primates. Archives of Neurology and Psychiatry 33:558–569, 1935.

Jacobsen CF, Nissen HW. Studies of cerebral function in primates. IV. The effects of frontal lobe lesions on the delayed alternation habit in monkeys. Journal of Comparative and Physiological Psychology 23:101–112, 1937.

Jacobsen CF, Wolfe JB, Jackson TA. An experimental analysis of the functions of the frontal association areas in primates. Journal of Nervous and Mental Disease 82:1–14, 1935.

Jastrowitz M. Beiträge zur Localisation im Grosshirn und über deren praktische Verwerthung. Deutsche Medizinische Wochenschrift 14:81–83, 108–112, 125–128, 151–153, 172–175, 188–192, 209–211, 1888.

Kleist K. Die Störungen der Ich-Leistungen und ihre Lokalisation im Orbital-Innen und Zwischenhirn. Monatsschrift für Psychiatrie 71:338–350, 1931.

Kleist K. Gehirnpathologie. Leipzig: Barth, 1934.

Krech D. Cortical localization of function. In Postman L (ed), Psychology in the Making: Histories of Selected Research Problems. New York: Knopf, 1964.

Lashley KS, Clark G. The cytoarchitecture of the cerebral cortex of Ateles: a critical examination of architectonic studies. Journal of Comparative Neurology 85:223–305, 1946.

Levin PM. The efferent fibers of the frontal lobe of the monkey, macaca mulatta. Journal of Comparative Neurology 63:369–419, 1936.

Lewy FH. Historical introduction: the basal ganglia and their diseases. In Putnam TJ, Frantz AM, Ranson SW (eds), The Diseases of the Basal Ganglia. Baltimore: Williams & Wilkins, 1942, pp. 1–20.

Liepmann H. Das Krankheitsbild der Apraxie. Berlin: Karger, 1900.

Loeb J. Die elementaren Störungen einfacher Funktionen nach oberflächlicher, umschriebene Verletzung des Grosshirns. Pflüger's Archiv für die gesamte Physiologie 37:51–56, 1885.

Loeb J. Beiträge zur Physiologie des Grosshirns. Pflüger's Archiv für die gesamte Physiologie 39:265–346, 1886.

Loeb J. Comparative Physiology of the Brain and Comparative Psychology. New York: Putnam, 1902.

Macmillan MB. A wonderful journey through skull and brains: the travels of Mr. Gage's tamping iron. Brain and Cognition 5:67–102, 1986.

Malmo RB. Interference factors in delayed response in monkeys after removal of frontal lobes. Journal of Neurophysiology 5:295–308, 1942.

McLardy T. Thalamic projection to frontal cortex in man. Journal of Neurology, Neurosurgery and Psychiatry 13:198–202, 1950.

Meyer A. Historical Aspects of Cerebral Anatomy. New York: Oxford University Press, 1971.

Meyer A, Beck E, McLardy T. Prefrontal leucotomy: a neuro-anatomical report. Brain 70:18–49, 1947.

Meynert T. Der Bau der Gross-Hirnrinde und seine Örtlichen Verschiedenheiten. Vierteljahresschrift für Psychiatrie 1:77–93; 198–217, 1867 (cited by Clarke and O'Malley, 1968).

Meynert T. Beiträge zur Kenntnis der centralen Projection der Sinnesoberflächen. Sitzungsberichte der Kaiserlichen Akademie der Wissenschaften, Mathematisch-Naturwissenschaftliche Classe, Wien 60:547–566, 1869.

Meynert, T. Die Windungen der Convexen Oberfläche des Vorderhirns bei Menschen, Affen und Raubtieren. Archiv für Psychiatrie und Nervenkrankheiten 7:275–286, 1877.

Meynert T. Psychiatrie: Klinik der Erkrankungen des Vorderhirns. Vienna, Braunmüller, 1884 (Translation by Sachs B. Psychiatry: A Clinical Treatise on Diseases of the Fore-Brain. New York: Putnam, 1885; Reprinted, New York: Hafner, 1968).

Milner B. Some effects of frontal lobectomy in man. In Warren JM, Akert K (eds), The Frontal Granular Cortex and Behavior. New York: McGraw-Hill, 1964, pp. 313–331.

Minkowski M. Etude sur les connexions anatomiques des circonvolutions rolandiques, pariétales et frontales. Schweizer Archiv für Neurologie und Psychiatrie 12:71–104, 227–268, 1923; 14:255–278, 1924; 15:97–132, 1924.

Monakow C. Ueber einige durch circumscripter Hirdrindenregion bedingte Entwickelungshemmungen des Kaninchengehirns. Archiv für Psychiatrie 12:141–156, 1882.

Monakow C. Experimentelle und pathologisch-anatomische Untersuchungen über die Haubenregion, den Sehhügel und die Region subthalamica. Archiv für Psychiatrie 27:1–128, 386–479, 1895.

Morgan CL. Animal Behavior. London: Scott, 1990.

Munk H. Weitere Mittheilungen zur Physiologie der Grosshirnrinde. Archiv für Anatomie und Physiologie 2:162–178, 1878.

Munk H. Weiteres zur Physiologie der Sehsphäre der Grosshirnrinde. Archiv für Anatomie und Physiologie 3:581–592, 1879.

Munk H. Über die Functionen der Grosshirnrinde. Berlin: Hirschwald, 1890.

Neuburger M. Historische Entwicklung der Experimentellen Gehirn- und Rückenmarks physiologie vor Flourens. Stuttgart: Enke, 1897; Englisn translation and edition by E Clarke. The Historical Development of Experimental Brain and Spinal Cord Physiology before Flourens. Baltimore: Johns Hopkins Press, 1981.

Oppenheim H. Zur Pathologie der Gehirngeschwulste. Archiv für Psychiatrie 21:560–578, 705–745, 1890; 22:27–72.

Panizza B. Osservazioni sul nervo ottico. Giornale, Istituto Lombardo di Scienze e Lettere 7:237–252, 1855.

Pfeiffer RA. Myelogenetisch-anatomische Untersuchungen über den zentralen Abschnitt der Taststrahlung, der Pyramidenbahn, der Hirnnerven und zusätzlicher motorischer Bahnen. Nova Acta Leopoldina 1:341–473, 1934.

Quensel F. Stirnhirnverletzung mit Charakterveränderung. Muenchener Medizinische Wochenschrift 61:1761–1763, 1914.

Riese W, Hoff EC. A history of the doctrine of cerebral localization. Journal of the History of Medicine 5:50–71, 1950.

Rolando L. Della struttura degli emisferi cerebrali. Memorie della Reale Academia di Scienze di Torino 35:103–146, 1831 (cited by Meyer, 1971).

Romberg MH. Lehrbuch der Nervenkrankheiten des Menschen. Berlin: Duncker, 1840–1846. English translation by Sieveking EH. A Manual of the Nervous Diseases of Man. London: The New Sydenham Society, 1853.

Rylander G. Personality Changes after Operations on the Frontal Lobes. Copenhagen: Munksgaard, 1939.

Sandes F. Die Architektonik des Menschlichen Stirnhirns. Berlin: Springer, 1962.

Schäfer EA. Experiments on special sense localisation in the cortex cerebri of the monkey. Brain 10:362–380, 1888.

Schiller F. The rise of the 'enteroid process' in the 19th century: some landmarks in cerebral nomenclature. Bulletin of the History of Medicine 39:326–338, 1965.

Schuster P. Psychische Störungen bei Hirntumoren. Stuttgart: Enke, 1902.

Soury J. Le système nerveux central. Paris: Carré et Naud, 1899.

Spillane JD. The Doctrine of the Nerves: Chapters in the History of Neurology. New York: Oxford University Press, 1981.

Starr MA. The visual area in the brain determined by a study of hemianopsia. American Journal of Medical Sciences 87:65–83, 1884.

Steegman AT. Dr. Harlow's famous case: the "impossible" accident of Phineas P. Gage. Surgery 52:952–958, 1962.

Stookey B. A note on the early history of cerebral localization. Bulletin of the New York Academy of Medicine 30:559–578, 1954.

Swazey JP. Action propre and action commune: the localization of cerebral function. Journal of History of Biology 3:213–234, 1970.

Thorndike EL. Animal Intelligence. Psychological Review Monographs, Supplement No. 8, 1898.

Valenstein ES. Great and Desperate Cures. New York: Basic Books, 1986.

Varolio C. De Nervis Opticis. Padua: Meitti, 1573 (cited by Clarke and O'Malley, 1968; Meyer, 1971).

Varolio C. Anatomiae sive de Resolutione Corporis Humani. Frankfurt: Wechel and Fischer, 1591 (cited by Clarke and O'Malley, 1968; Meyer, 1971).

Vincent C. Neurochirurgische Betrachtungen über die Funktionen des Frontallappens. Deutsche Medizinische Wochenschrift 62:41–45, 1936.

Vogt O, Vogt C. Allgemeine Ergebnisse unserer Hirnforschung. Journal für Psychologie und Neurologie 25:273–462, 1919.

Walker AE. The retrograde cell degeneration in the thalamus of macacus rhesus following hemidecortication. Journal of Comparative Neurology 62:407–419, 1935.

Walker AE. The Primate Thalamus. Chicago: University of Chicago Press, 1938.

Walker AE. The development of the concept of cerebral localization in the nineteenth century. Bulletin of the History of Medicine 31:99–121, 1957.

Welt L. Über Charakterveranderungen des Menschen infolge von Läsionen des Stirnhirns. Deutsche Archiv für Klinische Medizin 42:339–390, 1888.

Wernicke C. Der aphasische Symptomenkomplex. Breslau: Cohn und Weigert, 1874.

Willis T. Cerebri Anatome. London: Martyn & Allestry, 1664. Translation by Pordage S. On the Anatomy of the Brain. London: Dring, 1681. Feindel W (ed) Thomas Willis, The Anatomy of the Brain and Nerves. Montreal: McGill University Press, 1965.

Zacher W. Ueber ein Fall von doppelseitigem, symmetrisch gelegenem Erweichungsherd im Stirnhirn und Neuritis optica. Neurologisches Zentralblatt 20:1074–1083, 1901.

Zangwill OL. Psychological deficits associated with frontal lobe lesions. International Journal of Neurology 5:395–402, 1966.

II
Neuroanatomic Organization, Experimental Models, and Neuroimaging in Animals

2

Patterns of Connections of the Prefrontal Cortex in the Rhesus Monkey Associated with Cortical Architecture

HELEN BARBAS
AND DEEPAK N. PANDYA

The prefrontal cortex in the rhesus monkey is situated rostral to the premotor cortex and extends from the arcuate sulcus to the frontal pole on the lateral surface, anterior to the supplementary motor cortex on the medial surface, and rostral to the temporal pole and the anterior insula on the basal surface. It is a heterogeneous region composed of several anatomic and functional subdivisions. On the basis of behavioral studies, different functional attributes have been ascribed to orbital, medial, periprincipalis, and periarcuate prefrontal regions (see Fuster, 1980; Rosenkilde, 1979; Stuss and Benson, 1986 for reviews). The orbital and medial cortices have strong links with limbic structures. Damage to orbital areas results in deficits in tasks requiring withholding of responses to negative stimuli, and in emotional processes including reduced aggression, increased aversive reactions to external stimuli, and changes in activity patterns (Bowden et al., 1971; Butter and Snyder, 1972). There is comparatively less information on the behavioral correlates of the medial prefrontal region. However, the association of this cortex with emotional processes is supported by evidence that medial areas in close proximity to the corpus callosum are associated with vocalization emitted in response to emotional stimuli (MacLean, 1985; for review: Bogt and Barbas, 1988). In addition to these processes affiliated with the limbic system, orbital and medial areas are also involved in a series of cognitive and mnemonic processes. On the lateral surface, areas around the central and caudal parts of the principal sulcus have been associated with delayed response tasks that seem to be dependent on both spatial and mnemonic factors (Bauer and Fuster, 1976; Butters and Pandya, 1969; Jacobsen, 1936; for review: Goldman-Rakic, 1988). The periarcuate cortex has been implicated in compound discrimination and associative tasks (Goldman and Rosvold, 1970; Milner et al., 1978; Petrides and Iversen, 1978; Stamm, 1973; Van Hoesen et al., 1980). The multiplicity of functional processes associated with the prefrontal cortex suggests that each of the preceding prefrontal subdivisions receives a different set of inputs from intrinsic sources, as well as from distant cortical and subcortical structures. In this chapter we will explore some of the anatomic features that seem to be important to the organization of the prefrontal cortex.

The prefrontal cortex has been subdivided architectonically by a number of investigators in the past. There is, however, considerable disagreement regarding the boundaries of its subdivisions (von Bonin and Bailey, 1947; Brodmann, 1905; Vogt and Vogt, 1919; Walker, 1940). In all of these studies, areal boundaries were drawn on the basis of morphologic criteria only. These included cytoarchitectonic features, which rely on the gross characteristics of cells and their arrangement in cortical layers, or myeloarchitectonic characteristics, which focus on the pattern and distribution of myelin within the cortical mantle. While both procedures are useful in the study of cortical architecture, particularly when used in conjunction with each other, they individually have drawbacks. For example, cytoarchitectonic criteria are rather subtle at times and they may not be recognizable easily by all investigators. At the other extreme, myeloarchitectonic criteria are rather crude and thus subtle regional differences may be missed. The inherent difficulties of architectonic methods may be obviated if the study of cerebral architecture is considered within a theoretic framework of progressive cortical laminar organization as has been proposed by Sanides (1972). According to Sanides, the cerebral cortex evolved from two primordial moieties: The hippocampal archicortex on the medial surface, and the olfactory paleocortex on the basal surface. This hypothesis initiated a reevaluation of the architecture of the cortex, and led to the observation of a stepwise increase in the number of cortical layers and their delineation, which can be traced from the limbic cortices to the most architectonically differentiated isocortices in all cortical systems (Pandya et al., 1988).

PROGRESSIVE ARCHITECTONIC ORGANIZATION OF THE PREFRONTAL CORTEX

Our analysis of the architecture of the prefrontal cortex in the rhesus monkey was guided by the hypothesis that the prefrontal cortex can be viewed as a series of areas showing gradual increases in architectonic organization within two major cortical lines (Barbas and Pandya, 1989; Figs. 2–1, 2–2). Each line may be traced from a periallocortical area, characterized by an incipient laminar organization. In the basoventral line the periallocortex is situated in the caudal orbitofrontal region around the olfactory allocortex, and in the mediodorsal line it is found around the rostral tip of the corpus callosum. Within each line neighboring regions exhibit a gradual increase in laminar delineation, spreading radially first to proisocortical, and then to isocortical areas (Figs. 2–1, 2–2).

Our study of the architecture of the prefrontal cortex was conducted also in the context of recent methodologic advances in neuronal pathway tracing procedures that have enhanced our ability to appreciate the cerebral cortex architectonically. The usefulness of tracing procedures in the study of cortical archi-

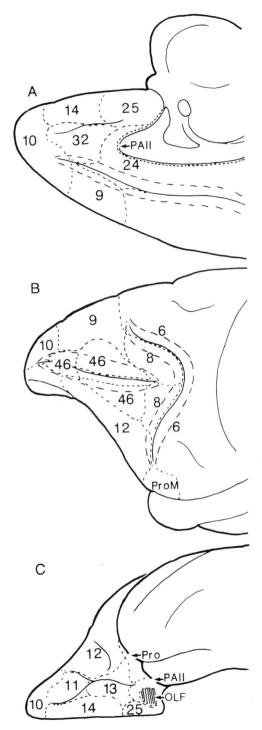

Figure 2–1 The architectonic subdivisions of the prefrontal cortex, based on architectonic criteria are shown on the medial **(A)**, lateral **(B)**, and basal **(C)** surfaces of the hemisphere. Abbreviations: OLF, olfactory area; PAll, periallocortex; Pro, proisocortex; ProM, proisocortical motor area. (From Barbas and Pandya, 1989, with permission.)

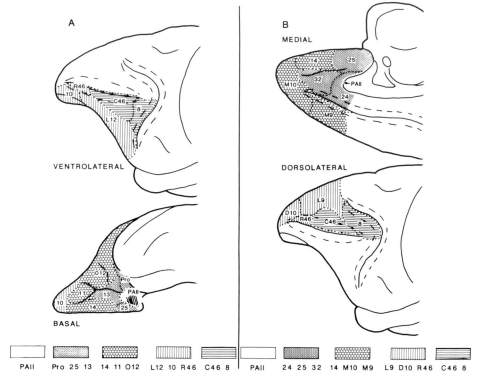

Figure 2–2 Diagrams showing the architectonic stages within the basoventral **(A)**, and mediodorsal **(B)** prefrontal cortices. Within each group of cortices stepwise increases in laminar organization proceed in a direction from the periallocortex (PAll) to area 8, which represents the most architectonically differentiated cortex within the prefrontal region. Letters before numbers designating architectonic areas refer to: C, caudal; D, dorsal; L, lateral; M, medial; O, orbital; R, rostral. (From Barbas and Pandya, 1989, with permission.)

tecture is based on observations that projections emanate from and terminate within the confines of distinct architectonic boundaries (Jones and Powell, 1970; for review: Pandya et al., 1988; Seltzer and Pandya, 1978). We therefore explored the hypothesis that architecture is correlated with connectional features by studying the interconnections of prefrontal subareas with the aid of antero-grade and retrograde tracing procedures.

Using architectonic criteria we noted several consistent features within the prefrontal cortex. Architectonic differentiation is characterized by the aggregation of cells into cortical layers, giving a laminated appearance in progressively more differentiated areas. The process of architectonic differentiation within the prefrontal cortex includes a change in several features that may be observed in the Nissl preparation. For example, the deep layers (V and VI) gradually lose their prominence, and the upper layers increase their cell density in a direction from the limbic to isocortical areas. Another prominently changing feature

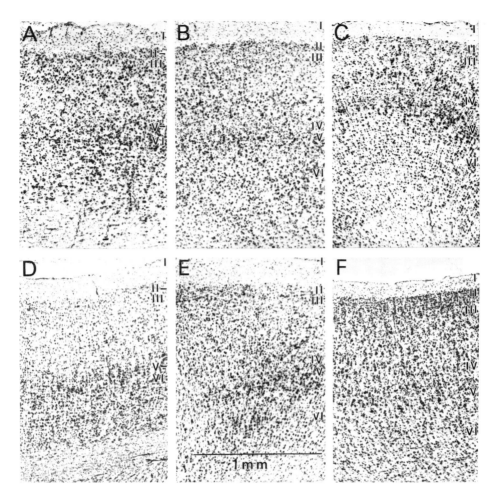

Figure 2-3   Brightfield photomicrographs of some cytoarchitectonic divisions of the prefrontal cortex. Basoventral areas are shown on the top, and mediodorsal on the bottom. **A:** Orbital periallocortex. **B:** Orbital area 12. **C:** Ventral area 8. **D:** Medial Area 25. **E:** Medial area 9. **F:** Dorsal area 8. Cortices depicted in A and D lack a granular layer IV. Gradual increases in laminar organization proceed in a direction from A to C for basoventral areas, and from D to F for mediodorsal cortices. Dash between layer designations indicates indistinct laminar borders. Celloidin embedded tissue, cresyl violet stain. Scale bar = 1 mm.

involves layer IV, which is virtually absent in the periallocortices and proisocortices, and appears to increase gradually and become prominent in the more architectonically differentiated isocortical areas. In addition, the pyramidal cells in the deep and upper layers are small in the limbic cortices, such as the periallocortex and proisocortex, but appear larger and more prominent in layer III in the most architectonically differentiated isocortices such as areas 46 and 8 (Fig. 2-3).

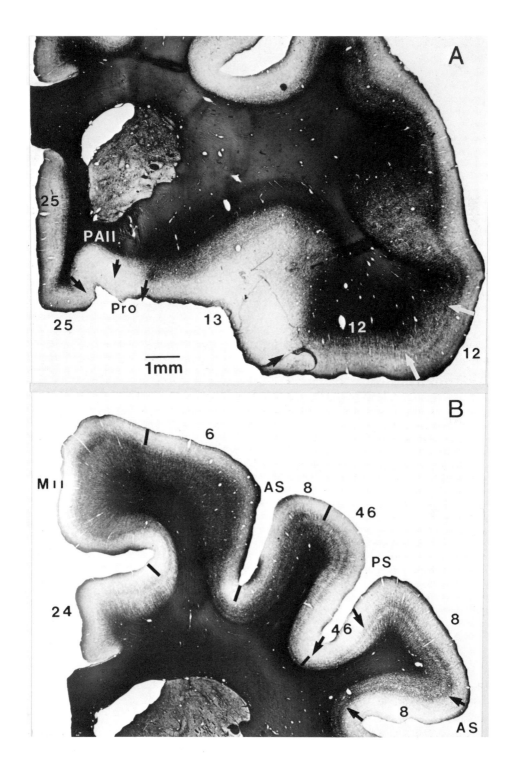

A pattern of gradual architectonic differentiation may be observed also in material stained for myelin (Fig. 2–4). The periallocortices are poorly myelinated. The adjacent proisocortices have a diffuse myelin content confined to the deep layers. Further myeloarchitectonic changes in the prefrontal cortex seem to proceed with the emergence of, first one, and then two, Baillarger bands. The more architectonically differentiated isocortices generally have both inner and outer Baillarger bands. Moreover, according to our observations, mediodorsal cortices generally have a more prominent vertical plexus when compared with basoventral areas. A similar observation was made for the vertical plexus of the dorsal and ventral premotor area (Barbas and Pandya, 1987).

Based on both cytoarchitectonic and myeloarchitectonic criteria, gradual increases in the number of layers and their delineation proceed in a radial direction within the basoventral and mediodorsal prefrontal regions. Within the basoventral line the least architectonically differentiated area is the periallocortex in the caudal orbitofrontal region adjacent to the olfactory allocortex (see Figs. 2–1, 2–2). It is characterized by prominent deep layers, and lacks a granular layer IV (Fig. 2–3A). The periallocortex is bounded medially, laterally, and rostrally by the slightly more differentiated proisocortex, which is also characterized by prominent deep layers, although not as prominent as in the periallocortex. The progression of laminar organization proceeds to the rostrally adjacent area 13, which borders the proisocortex. It is distinguished from proisocortex by the presence of an incipient layer IV composed of occasional granular cells. Area 13 is bounded by isocortical orbital area 12 laterally (Fig. 2–3**B**), 11 rostrally, and 14 medially. Compared to area 13 these areas show a somewhat better laminar delineation and constitute the next stage of architectonic organization (see Fig. 2–2). These areas, however, retain the prominence of the deep layers. Further laminar definition is seen in the adjoining area 10, the lateral portion of area 12, and the rostral part of ventral area 46. At this stage the supragranular and infragranular cell density appears approximately equal. The architectonic progression can be traced further to caudal area 46 and finally to ventral area 8 (Fig. 2–3C). In the latter two areas the supragranular layers become progressively more prominent, and layer IV reaches the peak of its development within the prefrontal cortex. In addition, the pyramidal cells, particularly in layer III, but also in layer V, are larger than in other prefrontal cortices.

The mediodorsal line proceeds from the periallocortex, which surrounds the genu of the corpus callosum, to the proisocortical areas 24 dorsally, 25 ventrally (Fig. 2–3**D**), and 32 rostrally characterized by prominent deep layers and a virtual absence of layer IV. The progression of laminar differentiation proceeds to

←_____

Figure 2–4 Brightfield photomicrographs showing the distribution of myelin within some prefrontal subareas. The least architectonically differentiated medial and orbital prefrontal areas have a low myelin content (**A**). In contrast, the most architectonically organized prefrontal cortices, such as area 8, have a higher myelin content aggregated into distinct Baillarger bands (**B**). Abbreviations: AS, arcuate sulcus; MII, supplementary motor area; PAll, periallocortex; Pro, proisocortex; PS, principal sulcus.

the isocortical areas 14 ventrally, medial 9 dorsally (Fig. 2–3E), and medial 10 rostrally characterized by the emergence of layer IV neurons. The next stage of laminar organization includes the lateral portion of area 9, dorsal area 10, and the rostral part of dorsal area 46. At this stage the supragranular and infragranular cell densities are approximately equal. The architectonic progression is traced further to caudal area 46, and finally to dorsal area 8 (Fig. 2–3F). In the latter two areas the supragranular cell density appears higher than the infragranular, layer IV is well developed, and the pyramidal cells in layers III and V are prominent, as observed also in the basoventral line.

INTERCONNECTIONS OF PREFRONTAL SUBAREAS

The progressive delineation of layers in prefrontal areas is reflected in their intrinsic connections. Within each line a given area projects to and receives input from cortices in two directions: These include more architectonically differentiated areas, on the one hand, and regions with lesser laminar definition, on the other (Fig. 2–5). In each direction more than one region is involved in this connectional system. For example, the orbital proisocortex projects to its architectonic precursor (orbital periallocortex), on one hand, and to areas 13, 11, 12, 14, and 10, its architectonic successors, on the other (Fig. 2–5, **left panel**). Likewise, in the mediodorsal line, rostral area 46 projects to the precursor areas 24, 9, and 10, on one hand, and to caudal areas 46 and 8, which are its architectonic successors, on the other. Thus the multiple connections of each area seem to reflect the radial nature of the stepwise changes in laminar organization, and this is observed within both basoventral and mediodorsal prefrontal regions (Barbas, 1988a; Barbas and Pandya, 1989) (Fig. 2–5).

The intrinsic connections of the prefrontal cortex have several other consistent features. For example, the most architectonically differentiated areas, such as area 8, have restricted connections, whereas the least differentiated areas, such as the limbic, have widespread intrinsic connections (Barbas, 1988a; Barbas and Pandya, 1989). Thus, the connections of area 8 are largely confined to a few neighboring regions on the lateral surface of the hemisphere (Fig. 2–5, **right panel**). On the other hand, both orbital and medial proisocortices, which have a low degree of laminar organization, have extensive connections that span the orbital, medial, and lateral surfaces of the hemisphere (Fig. 2–5, **left panel**). This pattern of connections thus suggests that a low degree of laminar organization is associated with widespread connections, whereas a high degree of laminar differentiation is associated with restricted connections. The widespread connections of the proisocortices are not randomly distributed. They seem rather to respect the observed architectonic progression, projecting to several successive architectonic stages, but avoiding areas exhibiting a high degree of laminar organization (Fig. 2–5, **left panel**).

Most connections are observed between areas within one architectonic line. However, there are some interconnections between the lines that seem to link areas that are at a similar architectonic stage within their respective line of architectonic organization. For example, there are connections between the orbital

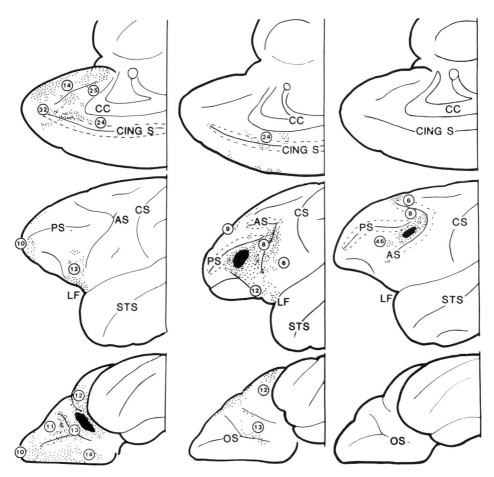

Figure 2-5 The distribution of labeled grains (represented by dots) following isotope injection (represented by black area) in the orbital proisocortex **(left panel),** in ventral area 46 **(central panel),** and in ventral area 8 **(right panel)** is shown on the medial (top), lateral (center), and basal surfaces of the frontal lobe (bottom). The dashed lines represent the cortex buried in sulci. The circled numbers represent architectonic areas. Abbreviations: AS, arcuate sulcus; CC, corpus callosum; CING S, cingulate sulcus; CS, central sulcus; LF, lateral fissure; OS, orbital sulcus; PS, principal sulcus; STS, superior temporal sulcus. (Adapted from Barbas and Pandya, 1989, with permission.)

and medial proisocortices (Fig. 2-5, **left panel**), or area 12 and area 9, and between dorsal and ventral area 8 (Fig. 2-5, **right panel**).

TOPOGRAPHY OF COMMISSURAL FIBERS OF THE PREFRONTAL CORTEX

The hypothesis that architecture is correlated with the system of connections, supported by the connectional pattern observed within the prefrontal cortex, can be tested also for other cortical pathways such as the callosal. The position of

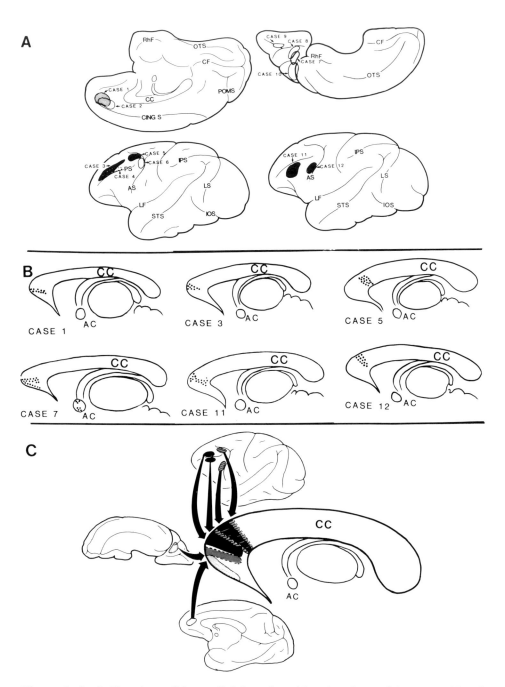

Figure 2–6 **A:** Drawings of the medial, lateral, and basal surfaces of the cerebral hemisphere of the rhesus monkey showing the location of isotope injections in the prefrontal cortex in 12 animals. **B:** Drawings of midsagittal sections of the corpus callosum and anterior commisure in six representative cases, showing the location of labeled callosal fibers (represented by dots). **C:** Summary diagram showing the overlap of fibers within the corpus callosum arising from medial and orbital prefrontal areas, periprincipalis

fibers from the frontal lobe through the commissures was studied in rhesus monkeys using classic ablation-degeneration procedures. Those studies indicate that fibers originating in the frontal lobe course through the rostral part of the corpus callosum and are topographically organized (Pandya et al., 1971; Sunderland, 1940). The autoradiographic procedure, developed subsequent to the ablation-degeneration methods, allows for a more precise delineation of efferent fiber pathways. This procedure was used to describe the topography of commissural fibers originating in various architectonic subareas from the basoventral and mediodorsal regions of the prefrontal cortex (Barbas and Pandya, 1984). The results indicate that fibers from rostromedial and adjacent dorsolateral prefrontal areas respectively occupy the ventral and dorsal parts of the genu of the corpus callosum. The dorsal arcuate region sends fibers through the rostral part of the body of the corpus callosum (Fig. 2–6**A**, left, **B** top). Fibers from orbitofrontal and adjacent ventrolateral prefrontal regions respectively traverse the ventral and dorsal sectors of the genu, and those from the ventral arcuate region course at the border of the genu and the body of the corpus callosum (Fig. 2–6**A**, right, **B** bottom). The anterior commissure contains some interhemispheric fibers originating exclusively from the caudal orbitofrontal region (Fig. 2–6, case 7).

The relative rostrocaudal position of fibers within the corpus callosum seems to be correlated with the relative architectonic organization of their prefrontal cortical region of origin. Thus, fibers originating in limbic periallocortices and proisocortices are situated rostrally and ventrally in the genu of the corpus callosum; fibers from progressively more architectonically differentiated areas are represented in successively more caudal sectors of the corpus callosum. This evidence suggests that neither the relative dorsoventral, nor the rostrocaudal location of a prefrontal cortical region, but rather its relative degree of architectonic organization, determines the site of passage of its fibers through the corpus callosum.

Fibers emanating from sites that are at approximately the same stage of laminar organization within the two lines overlap to some extent within the corpus callosum (Fig. 2–6**C**). For example, fibers from two proisocortical areas, one situated on the medial and the other on the orbital surface, are found in the rostral portion of the corpus callosum. Similarly, regions above and below the principal sulcus have a common callosal site, as do dorsal and ventral arcuate regions (Fig. 2–6**C**). This evidence suggests that commissural fibers originating in regions that are at the same stage of laminar organization in the two prefrontal architectonic lines share a common place within the corpus callosum. This applies for regions that are located at a distance from one another, as well as for regions that are

←——

regions, and areas within the concavity of the arcuate sulcus. Abbreviations: AC, anterior commisure; AS, arcuate sulcus; CC, corpus callosum; CF, calcarine fissure; CING S, cingulate sulcus; IOS, inferior occipital sulcus; IPS, intraparietal sulcus; LF, lateral fissure; LS, lunate sulcus; OTS, occipitotemporal sulcus; POMS, medial parietooccipital sulcus; PS, principal sulcus; RhF, rhinal fissure; STS, superior temporal sulcus (From Barbas and Pandya, 1984, with permission.)

closely apposed. It is possible that this is because regions with similar architectonic features may have developed at the same time. These data suggest that the position of fibers from the prefrontal cortex within the corpus callosum parallels the trend of architectonic changes observed within the prefrontal cortex.

TOPOGRAPHY OF PROJECTIONS FROM POST-ROLANDIC CORTICES DIRECTED TO PREFRONTAL REGIONS

The preceding evidence suggests that prefrontal interconnections and the course of prefrontal fibers through the corpus callosum are correlated with the laminar differentiation of the cortices involved in these pathways. The question arises as to whether architecture is associated also with the pattern of connections between the prefrontal and other cortices. Post-rolandic areas associated with one sensory modality are connected with several sites within the prefrontal cortex in a specific manner. For example, the limbic orbitofrontal and medial prefrontal cortices receive the majority of their auditory projections from the rostral part of the superior temporal gyrus, which has the least architectonically differentiated laminar pattern within the cortical auditory system (Galaburda and Pandya, 1983). Regions around the principal sulcus receive their auditory projections from the midportion of the superior temporal gyrus, characterized by better delineated cortical layers. Periarcuate sites receive their auditory projections from caudal regions of the superior temporal gyrus, which have the highest degree of laminar definition within the auditory cortical system (Barbas, 1988a; Barbas and Mesulam 1981; 1985; Chavis and Pandya, 1976; Jones and Powell, 1970; Petrides and Pandya, 1988) (Fig. 2–7).

A similar pattern is seen in the connections between prefrontal and visual cortices. Within the basoventral group of prefrontal cortices, the orbitofrontal regions receive visual input from the anterior part of the inferior temporal cortex (Barbas, 1988a,b; Chavis and Pandya, 1976) (Fig. 2–8); the latter forms the first step in the caudally directed axis of architectonic organization of the visual cortical system (Rosene and Pandya, 1983). The more architectonically differentiated areas below the principal sulcus receive projections primarily from caudal inferior temporal areas. Periarcuate areas receive their cortical visual projections from caudal visual cortices. Within the mediodorsal architectonic line limbic area 32 receives visual input from rostromedial preoccipital regions. On the other hand, area 8 receives projections from posterior visual cortices, which have better delineated layers than rostral visual areas (Barbas, 1988a,b; Barbas and Mesulam, 1981; Chavis and Pandya, 1976) (Fig. 2–8). Similar observations were made for the premotor to prefrontal, and for the somatosensory to prefrontal projections. For example, orbital area 12 receives somatosensory projections from rostral areas 1 and 2 within the frontal operculum, and from the anterior insula. On the other hand, the much better architectonically differentiated ventral area 46 receives most of its somatosensory projections from more caudal and better laminated portions of the somatosensory cortex (Barbas, 1988a; Barbas and Mesulam, 1985; Petrides and Pandya, 1984; Preuss and Goldman-Rakic, 1989).

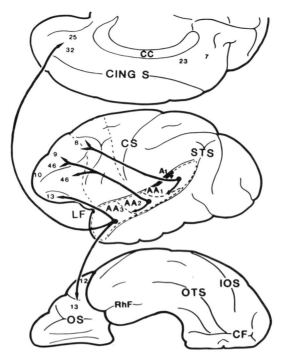

Figure 2-7 Summary diagram showing the pattern of connections from auditory cortices to the prefrontal cortex. This is an example of cortico-cortical connections occurring between areas that are at approximately the same stage of laminar organization. (Abbreviations for sulci are as in Figures 2-5 and 2-6.)

There are several other differences in the connectional organization of prefrontal subareas, which seem to be correlated with their stage of architectonic organization as well. The proisocortical limbic prefrontal regions show little specificity in their cortico-cortical connections, receiving input from more than one modality. Moreover, they receive a substantial proportion of their projections from other limbic cortices such as the cingulate and the parahippocampal gyrus (Baleydier and Mauguiere, 1980; Barbas, 1988a,b; Pandya et al., 1981; Van Hoesen, 1982). On the other hand, prefrontal areas that have more, and better delineated, layers receive most of their sensory-related projections from cortices associated with one modality. For example, within the basoventral architectonic line, the orbital periallocortex receives input from visual, auditory, somatosensory, gustatory, polymodal, and, to a large extent, from limbic areas (Barbas, 1988b). On the other hand, isocortical areas, such as area 46, show modality specificity in their distant connections and have only a few connections with limbic cortices (Barbas, 1988a). A similar pattern is observed for mediodorsal cortices. Thus limbic area 32 receives substantial projections from auditory, polymodal, and limbic cortices, and some projections from visual areas. On the other hand, the considerably more architectonically differentiated area 8 receives projections predominantly from visual and visuomotor cortices and has

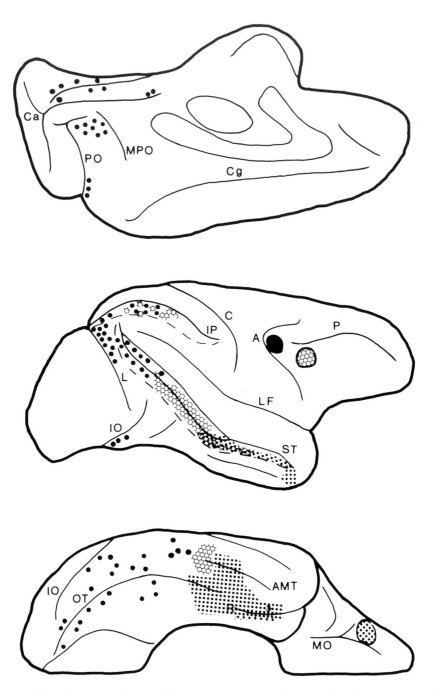

Figure 2–8 Summary diagram showing the pattern of connections from visual cortices to some prefrontal subareas (circled areas). This diagram is another example showing that cortico-cortical connections occur between areas that are at approximately the same stage of laminar organization. Abbreviations: A, arcuate sulcus; AMT, anterior middle temporal dimple; C, central sulcus; Ca, calcarine fissure; Cg, cingulate sulcus; IO, inferior occipital sulcus; IP, intraparietal sulcus; L, lunate sulcus; LF, lateral fissure; MO, medial orbital sulcus; MPO, medial parietooccipital sulcus; OT, occipitotemporal sulcus; P, principal sulcus; PO, parietooccipital sulcus; R, rhinal fissure; ST, superior temporal sulcus.

very few connections with the limbic system (Barbas, 1988a; Barbas and Mesulam, 1981). Thus the specific links of prefrontal areas with other cortices are associated with stages of architectonic organization. The same pattern is observed for the intrinsic connections of prefrontal subareas. Thus, while medial and orbital proisocortices have widespread intrinsic connections, area 8, which lies at the opposite pole of laminar organization within the prefrontal cortex, has restricted connections (Barbas and Pandya, 1989) (see Fig. 2–5).

LAMINAR RELATIONSHIPS OF CONNECTIONS

Architectonic differentiation seems to be associated with the laminar origin and termination of connections as well. For example, the terminations of efferent intrinsic connections from one prefrontal region to another show a pattern that is correlated with the laminar organization of the cortex of origin and its relation to the site of termination (Barbas and Pandya, 1989). Efferent terminations from one prefrontal region to another fall into three different patterns. In one pattern efferent fibers terminate into columns that span the entire width of the cortex. In another pattern fibers terminate into columns as well, but the label in layer I is denser than in the other layers. In a third pattern efferent fibers terminate within layer I only. The incidence of each pattern within the prefrontal cortex seems to depend on the architectonic relationship of the cortices that are interconnected. For example, when fibers originate in a prefrontal region that has a better laminar organization than the site of termination, the fibers terminate mostly into columns and are less likely to project selectively to layer I (Fig. 2–9). In contrast, when the site of origin has a lower degree of laminar organization

Figure 2–9 Histogram showing the incidence of each of three laminar patterns of termination of projections into three cortical categories. Category 1 represents all terminations in cortices with fewer delineated laminae than the areas giving rise to the projections; 0 represents all terminations in areas whose laminar organization is at approximately the same stage as that of the sites of origin; +1 represents all terminations in cortices that have more delineated laminae than the regions of origin of the projections. The three bars in each cortical category add up to 100%. (From Barbas and Pandya, 1989, with permission.)

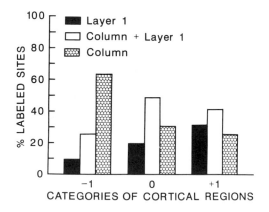

than the site of termination, fibers are more likely to terminate in layer I than in a columnar pattern. When the site of origin and termination are at approximately the same stage of laminar organization, the pattern of efferent connections falls in between the preceding two extremes (Fig. 2–9).

The laminar origin of afferent projections to the frontal cortex from both nearby and distant cortices varies in accordance with the laminar organization of the cortical regions that give rise to such projections (Barbas, 1986). Thus, when the least architectonically differentiated limbic areas project to the frontal cortex, the cells of origin are found mainly in layers V and VI. Projections from regions with increasing laminar organization arise progressively from the supragranular layers. This pattern is observed for projections originating along the axis of architectonic differentiation of the visual, somatosensory, auditory, motor, and prefrontal cortical systems (Fig. 2–10). Thus, as the cortical architecture within each system changes from limbic areas toward the primary cortices, the origin of frontally directed projections shifts from predominantly infragranular to predominantly supragranular layers.

TOPOGRAPHY OF PROJECTIONS TO BASOVENTRAL AND MEDIODORSAL PREFRONTAL CORTICES

The preceding observations suggest that the connections of the prefrontal cortex with distant sensory areas and the premotor cortex show an orderly pattern that seems to be correlated with the architectonic organization of the regions involved in each set of connections. Moreover, the origin of projections directed to basoventral and to mediodorsal cortices differs. Thus, for the most part, basoventral prefrontal regions are connected with other prefrontal, premotor, somatosensory, and visual areas situated on the ventrolateral surface, whereas mediodorsal prefrontal cortices are connected with premotor, somatosensory, and visual cortices situated on the dorsolateral and dorsomedial aspects of the cerebral hemisphere (Barbas, 1988a,b; Barbas and Pandya, 1987, 1989; Chavis and Pandya, 1976; Jones and Powell, 1970; Petrides and Pandya, 1984).

Figure 2–10   The laminar distribution of ipsilateral frontally directed neurons originating in the least architectonically differentiated, or limbic cortical regions (1, left), and in cortices with progressively higher degrees of laminar organization (5, right). Categories 1–5 in each system (A–E) represent groups of architectonic regions delineated with the aid of matched sections stained for the visualization of cell bodies, myelin, or acetylcholinesterase, based on descriptions of classic and, where available, recent studies describing cortical boundaries. The black (lamina III) and white (laminae V and VI) bars in each category (left) add up to 100%. Outlines of the boundaries or regions 1–5 are shown on the dorsolateral (DL), ventromedial (VM), medial (M), and ventral (V) surfaces of the brain (right). The primary cortices are shown by arrows. Abbreviations for sulci are as in Figure 2–8. (From Barbas, 1986, with permission.)

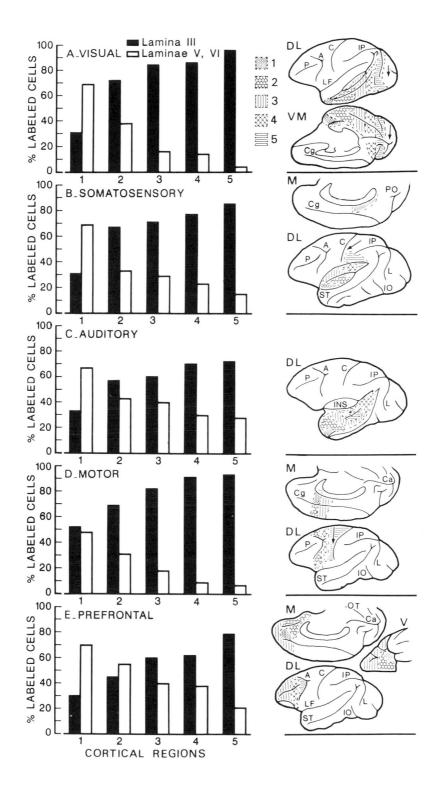

Physiologic, behavioral, and anatomic studies suggest that the visual input to basoventral and to mediodorsal prefrontal areas may be functionally as well as topographically segregated (see Barbas, 1988a). Thus basoventral prefrontal regions receive projections from the inferior temporal cortex, where neurons respond to stimuli associated with pattern and feature analysis (Desimone and Gross, 1979; Fuster and Jervey, 1981; Gross and Bender, 1969). In fact, damage to the inferior prefrontal convexity, which includes area 12 and parts of area 11 results in deficits in pattern discrimination, in delayed matching to sample, and in visual recognition, which are reminiscent of tasks supported by the inferior temporal cortex (Bachevalier and Mishkin, 1986; Gaffan et al., 1986; Gaffan and Harrison, 1986; Horel et al., 1987; Mishkin and Manning, 1978; Passingham, 1975; Voytko, 1985; 1986).

In contrast, mediodorsal prefrontal sites receive most of their visual cortical projections from dorsomedial and dorsolateral extrastriate cortices (Barbas, 1988a). For example, medial area 32 receives projections from area PO of Covey et al. (1982) and from the rostral part of medial area V2. These cortices lie along a line of regions associated with visual spatial tasks (Mishkin et al., 1982; Ungerleider and Mishkin, 1982). Moreover, they both contain a representation of the peripheral portion of the visual field (Covey et al., 1982; Gattass et al., 1981), which is not suited for pattern discrimination, but is suited well for the analysis of motion and space (McKee and Nakayama, 1984; Motter and Mountcastle, 1981).

Another mediodorsal prefrontal site, dorsal area 8, receives the majority of its cortical visual projections from areas MST and MT in the depths of the superior temporal sulcus (Barbas, 1988a), where neurons are particularly sensitive to moving stimuli (Albright et al., 1984; Desimone and Ungerleider, 1986; Maunsell and Van Essen, 1983; Zeki, 1974). In addition, area 8 receives projections from dorsal visual areas V3A and V3. In these regions neurons show little selectivity for color but respond to stimulus orientation, direction, or speed (Baizer, 1982; Felleman and Van Essen, 1987; Van Essen and Zeki, 1978; Zeki, 1978a,b). Moreover, most neurons projecting to area 8 are found in areas representing the peripheral portion of the visual field. Taken together, these findings suggest a bias for spatial, rather than pattern or color analysis. This evidence suggests that the dorsal periarcuate cortex may be continuous with a series of dorsal and medial prefrontal cortices that have a role in visual spatial tasks. These regions seem to include dorsal area 8 within and rostral to the anterior bank of the upper limb of the arcuate sulcus, the periprincipalis region, parts of area 9, and medial area 32 (Barbas, 1988a; Barbas and Mesulam, 1981; 1985; Mikami et al., 1982). This view is consistent with physiologic observations indicating that the periarcuate zone, which is linked with the superior colliculus, participates in eye movement tasks involving orienting to sensory stimuli and searching the environment (Goldberg and Bruce, 1985; Goldberg and Bushnell, 1981; Latto, 1978a,b; Rizzolatti et al., 1981; Schiller et al., 1979a,b; Wurtz and Mohler, 1976). Ventrolateral visual cortices, associated with pattern recognition and discrimination, on the other hand, seem to have an increasing influence on ventrolateral and basal prefrontal cortices.

In addition to receiving projections from visual cortices associated with spatial tasks, some dorsal prefrontal areas also receive preferential projections from the ventral bank of the intraparietal cortex, an area associated with visuomotor functions (for reviews: Hyvärinen, 1982; Lynch, 1980). This visuomotor cortex projects primarily to area 8, followed by the caudal portion of area 46 (Andersen et al., 1985; Barbas, 1988a; Barbas and Mesulam, 1981; 1985; Divac et al., 1977; Mesulam et al., 1977; Schwartz and Goldman-Rakic, 1984). The lateral portion of area 12 receives only a few projections from the parietal visuomotor region, and the rest of the prefrontal cortex does not seem to have direct links with the ventral intraparietal cortex (Barbas, 1988a). Besides differences in the preponderance of input from the visuomotor cortex, the origin of projections within the ventral bank of the intraparietal sulcus directed to dorsolateral periarcuate and ventrolateral periprincipalis areas differs to some extent. The periarcuate sites receive a considerable proportion of their intraparietal projections from the depths of the sulcus, whereas the ventral periprincipalis regions receive projections from more superficial portions of the ventral intraparietal bank (Barbas, 1988a). In this context it should be noted that only the deep part of the ventral intraparietal bank receives projections from area MT, an area associated with motion analysis (Blatt et al., 1990; Ungerleider and Desimone, 1986). This evidence suggests that the intraparietal visuomotor cortex may have distinct functional as well as architectonic subdivisions (Seltzer and Pandya, 1980).

The origin of projections from other cortices to basoventral and to mediodorsal regions also differs. For example, mediodorsal prefrontal areas receive most of their superior temporal projections from area TPO of Seltzer and Pandya (1978) situated in the upper bank of the superior temporal sulcus, whereas basoventral prefrontal regions receive projections from areas PGa and IPa as well within the depths of the superior temporal sulcus (Barbas, 1988a). In addition, mediodorsal areas receive projections primarily from the dorsal portions of the premotor and somatosensory cortices, and basoventral areas from the ventral sectors of these regions (Barbas and Pandya, 1987; Godschalk et al., 1984; Petrides and Pandya, 1984).

The functional significance of the segregated input to the two prefrontal lines from parietotemporal, premotor, and visuomotor cortices is difficult to address, and the answer will ultimately lie in the realm of physiology. The dorsal and ventral premotor regions have different architecture and frontal connections (Barbas and Pandya, 1987). The dorsal premotor area, which contains a representation of the trunk and the lower limb, may have a role in postural mechanisms. On the other hand, the ventral premotor region, which contains a representation of the head may be involved with movement of the head in orienting to sensory stimuli. By analogy with the visual and motor systems, it may be expected that mediodorsal prefrontal areas are involved in the localization of auditory and somatosensory stimuli, whereas basoventral prefrontal areas may be involved in the identification of stimulus characteristics within these modalities. In fact, this hypothesis is consistent with behavioral and physiologic data supporting a discriminative role for ventral, and a spatial role for dorsal prefrontal areas (Bachevalier and Mishkin, 1986; Mishkin and Manning, 1978; Vaadia et al., 1986; Voytko, 1985).

MULTIPLE REPRESENTATIONS OF SENSORY MODALITIES WITHIN THE PREFRONTAL CORTEX

The preceding discussion suggests that the two prefrontal cortical lines may have different functions. However, it is not clear why there are so many regions within one line that receive projections from cortices associated with one modality. The gradual architectonic changes observed within the prefrontal system suggest that cortical areas may have been added during evolution, perhaps in response to different postural and/or environmental demands imposed on the organism. The least architectonically differentiated areas, which show little modality specificity in their cortico-cortical connections and have strong connections with the limbic cortices, may have been among the first to develop during evolution. These cortices may have a global but integral role in the processing of sensory information. With regard to visual input in the prefrontal cortex, the orbitofrontal and anterior inferior temporal cortex, which are linked with cortico-cortical connections, thus may form the first step in the analysis of visual form. Similarly, the medial prefrontal and rostromedial visual cortices may represent the first step in the analysis of motion and space. The most architectonically differentiated areas within both mediodorsal and basoventral prefrontal lines show rather high modality specificity in their cortico-cortical connections. These areas, which have few connections with limbic cortices, may have a more specific role in the processing of sensory information.

The preceding discussion suggests that the connections of the prefrontal cortices seem to be organized according to the particular line they belong to, to the degree of the laminar organization of each subarea, and to the architectonic organization of the cortex as a whole. Thus, input from sensory, motor, and polymodal cortices reaches basoventral and mediodorsal prefrontal regions largely via parallel anatomic and perhaps functionally distinct pathways. Most interconnections of prefrontal subareas are confined within one architectonic line. The two prefrontal lines are interconnected only at some points, linking areas that are at approximately the same stage of laminar organization. Moreover, both the number and direction of interconnections of prefrontal subareas, the site of fibers from distinct prefrontal sites within the commissures, as well as the topography and laminar origin and termination of cortico-cortical connections seem to be correlated with cortical architecture.

ACKNOWLEDGMENTS

We thank Mr. Brian Butler and Ms. Michelle Richmond Kalajian for excellent technical assistance. This work was supported by NIH grant NS24760, NSF grant BNS 8315411 (H.B.), the E.N.R.M. Veterans Administration Hospital, Bedford MA, and NIH grant 16841 (D.N.P.)

REFERENCES

Albright TD, Desimone R, Gross CG. Columnar organization of directionally selective cells in visual area MT of the macaque. J Neurophysiol 51:16–31, 1984.

Andersen RA, Asanuma C, Cowan WM. Callosal and prefrontal associational projecting cell populations in area 7a of the macaque monkey: A study using retrogradely transported fluorescent dyes. J Comp Neurol 232:443–455, 1985.

Bachevalier JB, Mishkin M. Visual recognition impairment follows ventromedial but not dorsolateral prefrontal lesions in monkeys. Behav Brain Res 20:249–261, 1986.

Baizer J. Receptive field properties of V3 neurons in monkey. Invest Ophthal Vis Sci 23:87–95, 1982.

Baleydier C, Mauguiere F. The duality of the cingulate gyrus in monkey; neuroanatomical study and functional hypothesis. Brain 103:525–559, 1980.

Barbas H. Pattern in the laminar origin of corticocortical connections. J Comp Neurol 252:415–422, 1986.

Barbas H. Anatomic organization of basoventral and mediodorsal visual recipient prefrontal regions in the rhesus monkey. J Comp Neurol 276:313–342, 1988a.

Barbas H. Cortical projections to orbitofrontal limbic cortices in the rhesus monkey. Neurosci Abstr 14:373–376, 1988b.

Barbas H, Mesulam M-M. Organization of afferent input to subdivisions of area 8 in the rhesus monkey. J Comp Neurol 200:407–431, 1981.

Barbas H, Mesulam M-M. Cortical afferent input to the principalis region of the rhesus monkey. Neuroscience 15:619–637, 1985.

Barbas H, Pandya DN. Topography of commissural fibers of the prefrontal cortex in the rhesus monkey. Exp Brain Res 55:187–191, 1984.

Barbas H, Pandya DN. Architecture and frontal cortical connections of the premotor cortex (area 6) in the rhesus monkey. J Comp Neurol 256:211–218, 1987.

Barbas H, Pandya DN. Architecture and intrinsic connections of the prefrontal cortex in the rhesus monkey. J Comp Neurol 286:353–375, 1989.

Bauer RH, Fuster JM. Delayed-matching and delayed-response deficit from cooling dorsolateral prefrontal cortex in monkeys. J Comp Physiol Psychol 90:293–302, 1976.

Blatt GJ, Anderson RA, Stoner GR. Visual receptive field organization and cortico-cortical connections of the lateral intraparietal area (area LIP) in the macaque. J Comp Neurol 299:421–445, 1990.

Bowden DM, Goldman PS, Rosvold HE. Free behavior of rhesus monkeys following lesions of the dorsolateral and orbital prefrontal cortex in infancy. Exp Brain Res 12:265–274, 1971.

Brodmann K. Beitrage zur histologischen localisation der Grosshirnrinde. III. Mitteilung: Die Rindenfelder der niederen Affen. J Psychol Neurol 4:177–266, 1905.

Butter CM, Snyder DR. Alterations in aversive and aggressive behaviors following orbital frontal lesions in rhesus monkeys. Acta Neurobiol Exp 32:525–565, 1972.

Butters N, Pandya DN. Retention of delayed-alternation: Effect of selective lesion of sulcus principalis. Science 165:1271–1273, 1969.

Chavis DA, Pandya DN. Further observations on corticofrontal connections in the rhesus monkey. Brain Res 117:369–386, 1976.

Covey E, Gattass R, Gross CG. A new visual area in the parieto occipital sulcus of the macaque. Neurosci Abstr 8:681, 1982.

Desimone R, Gross CG. Visual areas in the temporal cortex of the macaque. Brain Res. 178:363–380, 1979.

Desimone R, Ungerleider LG. Multiple visual areas in the caudal superior temporal sulcus of the macaque. J Comp Neurol 248:164–189, 1986.

Divac I, LaVail JH, Rakic P, Winston KR. Heterogeneous afferents to the inferior parietal lobe of the rhesus monkey revealed by the retrograde transport method. Brain Res 123:197–207, 1977.

Felleman DJ, Van Essen DC. Receptive field properties of neurons in area V3 of macaque monkey extrastriate cortex. J Neurophys 57:889–920, 1987.

Fuster JM. The Prefrontal Cortex. Raven Press, New York, 1980.

Fuster JM, Jervey JP. Inferotemporal neurons distinguish and retain behaviorally relevant features of visual stimuli. Science 212:952–955, 1981.

Gaffan EA, Harrison S. Visual identification following inferotemporal ablation in the monkey. Q J Exp Psych 38:5–30, 1986.

Gaffan EA, Harrison S, Gaffan D. Single and concurrent discrimination learning by monkeys after lesion by inferotemporal cortex. Q J Exp Psychol 38:31–51, 1986.

Galaburda AM, Pandya DN. The intrinsic, architectonic and connectional organization of the superior temporal region of the rhesus monkey. J Comp Neurol 221:169–184, 1983.

Gattass R, Gross CG, Sandell JH. Visual topography of V2 in the macaque. J Comp Neurol 201:519–539, 1981.

Godschalk M, Lemon RN, Kuypers HGJM, Ronday HK. Cortical afferents and efferents of monkey postarcuate area: An anatomical and electrophysiological study. Exp Brain Res 56:410–424, 1984.

Goldberg ME, Bruce CJ. Cerebral cortical activity associated with the orientation of visual attention in the rhesus monkey. Vision Res 25:471–481, 1985.

Goldberg ME, Bushnell MC. Behavioral enhancement of visual responses in monkey cerebral cortex. II. Modulation in frontal eye fields specifically related to saccades. J Neurophys 46:773–787, 1981.

Goldman PS, Rosvold E. Localization of function within the dorsolateral prefrontal cortex of the rhesus monkey. Exp Neurol 27:291–304, 1970.

Goldman-Rakic PS. Topography of cognition: Parallel distributed networks in primate association cortex. Ann Rev Neurosci 11:137–156, 1988.

Gross CG, Bender DB. Visual receptive fields of neurons in inferotemporal cortex of the monkey. Science 166:1303–1306, 1969.

Horel JA, Pytko-Joiner DE, Voytko ML, Satabury K. The performance of visual tasks while segments of the inferotemporal cortex are suppressed by cold. Behav Brain Res 23:29–42, 1987.

Hyvärinen J. Posterior parietal lobe of the primate brain. Physiol Rev 62:1060–1129, 1982.

Jacobsen CF. Studies of cerebral function in primates: I. The functions of the frontal association area in monkeys. Comp Psychol Monogr 13:3–60, 1936.

Jones EG, Powell TPS. An anatomical study of converging sensory pathways within the cerebral cortex. Brain 93:793–820, 1970.

Latto R. The effects of bilateral frontal eye-field, posterior parietal or superior collicular lesions on visual search in the rhesus monkey. Brain Res 146:35–50, 1978a.

Latto R. The effects of bilateral frontal eye-field lesions on the learning of a visual search task by rhesus monkeys. Brain Res 147:370–376, 1978b.

Lynch JC. The functional organization of posterior parietal association cortex. Behav Brain Sci 3:485–534, 1980.

MacLean PD. Brain evolution relating to family, play, and the separation call. Arch Gen Psych 42:405, 1985.

Maunsell JHR, Van Essen DC. Functional properties of neurons in middle temporal visual area of the macaque monkey. I. Selectivity for stimulus direction, speed, and orientation. J Neurophysiol 49:1127–1147, 1983.

McKee SP, Nakayama K. The detection of motion in the peripheral visual field. Vision Res 24:25–32, 1984.

Mesulam M-M, Van Hoesen GW, Pandya DN, Geschwind N. Limbic sensory connections of the inferior parietal lobule (area PG) in the rhesus monkey: A study with a new method for horseradish peroxidase histochemistry. Brain Res 136:393–414, 1977.

Mikami A, Ito S, Kubota K. Visual response properties of dorsolateral prefrontal neurons during visual fixation task. J Neurophysiol 47:593–605, 1982.

Milner AD, Foreman NP, Goodale MA. Go-left go-right discrimination performance and distractibility following lesions of prefrontal cortex or superior colliculus in stumptail macaque. Neuropsychologia 16:381–390, 1978.

Mishkin M, Lewis ME, Ungerleider LG. Equivalence of parietopreoccipital subareas for visuospatial ability in monkeys. Behav Brain Res 6:41–55, 1982.

Mishkin M, Manning FJ. Non-spatial memory after selective prefrontal lesions in monkeys. Brain Res 143:313–323, 1978.

Motter BC, Mountcastle VB. The functional properties of the posterior parietal cortex studied in waking monkeys: Foveal sparing and opponent vector organization. J Neurosci 1:3–26, 1981.

Pandya DN, Karol EA, Heilbronn D. The topographic distribution of interhemispheric projections in the corpus callosum of the rhesus monkey. Brain Res 32:31–43, 1971.

Pandya DN, Seltzer B, Barbas H. Input-output organization of the primate cerebral cortex in the rhesus monkey. In Comparative Primate Biology, Vol 4: Neurosciences, Steklis HD, ed. Alan R. Liss, New York, 1988, pp. 39–80.

Pandya DN, Van Hoesen GW, Mesulam M-M. Efferent connections of the cingulate gyrus in the rhesus monkey. Exp Brain Res 42:319–330, 1981.

Passingham R: Delayed matching after selective prefrontal lesions in monkeys (Macaca mulatta). Brain Res 92:89–102, 1975.

Petrides M, Iversen S. The effect of selective anterior and posterior association cortex lesions in the monkey on performance of a visual-auditory compound discrimination test. Neuropsychologia 16:527–537, 1978.

Petrides M, Pandya DN. Projections to the frontal cortex from the posterior parietal region in the rhesus monkey. J Comp Neurol 228:105–116, 1984.

Petrides M, Pandya DN. Association fiber pathways to the frontal cortex from the superior temporal region in the rhesus monkey. J Comp Neurol 273:52–66, 1988.

Preuss TM, Goldman-Rakic PS. Connections of the ventral granular frontal cortex of macaques with perisylvian premotor and somatosensory areas: Anatomical evidence for somatic representation in primate frontal association cortex. J Comp Neurol 282:293–316, 1989.

Rizzolatti G, Scandolara C, Matelli M, Gentilucci M. Afferent properties of periarcuate neurons in macaque monkeys. II. Visual responses. Behav Brain Res 2:147–163, 1981.

Rosene DL, Pandya DN. Architectonics and connections of the posterior parahippocampal gyrus in the rhesus monkey. Neurosci Abstr 9:222, 1983.

Rosenkilde CE. Functional heterogeneity of the prefrontal cortex in the monkey: A review. Behav Neural Biol 25:301–345, 1979.

Sanides F. Representation in the cerebral cortex and its areal lamination pattern. In The Structure and Function of Nervous Tissue, Vol 5. Bourne GH, ed. Academic Press, New York, 1972, pp. 329–453.

Schiller PH, True SD, Conway JL. Effects of frontal eye field and superior colliculus ablations on eye movements. Science 206:590–592, 1979a.

Schiller PH, True SD, Conway JL. Paired stimulation of the frontal eye fields and superior colliculus of the rhesus monkey. Brain Res 179:162–164, 1979b.

Schwartz ML, Goldman-Rakic PS. Callosal and intrahemispheric connectivity of the prefrontal association cortex in rhesus monkey: Relation between intraparietal and principal sulcal cortices. J Comp Neurol 226:403–420, 1984.

Seltzer B, Pandya DN. Afferent cortical connections and architectonics of the superior temporal sulcus and surrounding cortex in the rhesus monkey. Brain Res 149:1–24, 1978.

Seltzer B, and Pandya DN. Converging visual and somatic cortical input to intraparietal sulcus of the rhesus monkey. Brain Res 192:339–351, 1980.

Stamm JS. Functional dissociation between the inferior and arcuate segments of dorsolateral prefrontal cortex in the monkey. Neuropsychologia 11:181–190, 1973.

Stuss DT, Benson DF. The Frontal Lobes. Raven Press, New York, 1986.

Sunderland S. The distribution of commissural fibers in the corpus callosum in the macaque monkey. J Neurol Psychiat 3:9–18, 1940.

Ungerleider LG, Desimone R. Cortical connections of visual area MT in macaque. J Comp Neurol 248:190–222, 1986.

Ungerleider LG, Mishkin M. Two cortical visual systems. In Analysis of Visual Behavior. Ingle DJ, Goodale MA, Mansfield RJW (eds). MIT Press, Cambridge, 1982, pp. 549–586.

Vaadia E, Benson DA, Hienz RD, Goldstein MH. Unit study of monkey frontal cortex: Active localization of auditory and of visual stimuli. J Neurophysiol 56:934–952, 1986.

Van Essen DC, Zeki SM. The topographic organization of rhesus monkey prestriate cortex. J Physiol (Lond.) 277:193–226, 1978.

Van Hoesen GW. The parahippocampal gyrus: New observations regarding its cortical connections in the monkey. Trends Neurosci 5:345–353, 1982.

Van Hoesen GW, Vogt BA, Pandya DN, McKenna TM. Compound stimulus differentiation behavior in the rhesus monkey following periarcuate ablation. Brain Res 186:365–378, 1980.

Vogt BA, Barbas H. Structure and connections of the cingulate vocalization region in the rhesus monkey. In The Physiological Control of Mammalian Vocalization. Newman JD (ed). Plenum Publishing, New York, 1988.

Vogt C, Vogt O. Allgemeinere Ergebnisse unserer Hirnforschung. J Psychol Neurol 25:279–462, 1919.

von Bonin G, Bailey P. The Neocortex of Macaca Mulatta. The University of Illinois Press, Urbana, 1947.

Voytko ML. Cooling orbital frontal cortex disrupts matching-to-sample and visual discrimination learning in monkeys. Physiol Psychol 13:219–229, 1985.

Voytko ML. Visual learning and retention examined with reversible cold lesions of the anterior temporal lobe. Behav Brain Res 22:25–39, 1986.

Walker C. A cytoarchitectural study of the prefrontal area of the macaque monkey. J Comp Neurol 98:59–86, 1940.

Wurtz RH, Mohler CW. Enhancement of visual responses in monkey striate cortex and frontal eye fields. J Neurophys 39:766–772, 1976.

Zeki SM. Functional organization of a visual area in the posterior bank of the superior temporal sulcus of the rhesus monkey. J Physiol (Lond.) 236:549–573, 1974.

Zeki SM. Functional specialization in the visual cortex of the rhesus monkey. Nature 274:423–428, 1978a.

Zeki SM. The third visual complex of rhesus monkey prestriate cortex. J Physiol (Lond.) 277:245–272, 1978b.

3

Role of Prefrontal Cortex in Delay Tasks: Evidence from Reversible Lesion and Unit Recording in the Monkey

JOAQUIN M. FUSTER

It is a well-established fact that the prefrontal cortex plays a critical role in the temporal organization of behavior, that is, in the order and timing of behavioral acts. It is not clear, however, precisely what that role is. A plausible hypothesis is that it has to do with what I have called the mediation of cross-temporal contingencies (Fuster, 1985), in other words, the integration of behavior in accord with sensory information that is not present at the time of the action: Information that was present in the recent past, or information that is expected to be present in the near future.

Because of the role that it attributes to the prefrontal cortex in the bridging of time between sensation and movement, this hypothesis puts the prefrontal cortex at the highest integrative level of the perception-action cycle (Fig. 3–1). This cycle is the circular pattern of cybernetic influences that flow between sensation and movement in all sequential behavior characterized by deliberation and choice (Arbib, 1981; Fuster, 1989; Weizsacker, 1950). When time is interposed in the cycle, that is, when movement is temporally separated from sensation, I postulate that two basic cognitive functions intervene to mend and close the broken cycle: Short-term memory and preparatory motor set. These two functions are mutually complementary, temporally symmetric—one retrospective, the other prospective—and are represented in dorsolateral prefrontal cortex. Parenthetically, I should note that this is the last part of that cortex to develop, phylogenetically as well as ontogenetically, and perhaps therefore it is a fitting substrate for those higher cognitive functions.

In this chapter, I will summarize the evidence that we have gathered in my laboratory in support of those propositions. Specifically I will present some of the work we have done with reversible cryogenic lesions and recording single-unit activity in behaving monkeys. My collaborators in this work have been G. Alexander, R. Bauer, J. Jervey, K. Posley, J. Quintana, C. Rosenkilde, W.

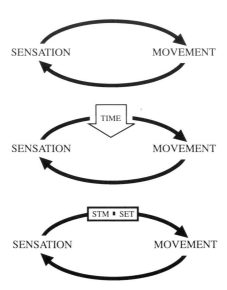

Figure 3–1 The perception-action cycle. Normally, in the course of sequential behavior, regulatory influences flow continuously between the neural structures involved in sensation and those controlling movement. Sensory input leads to movement, movement produces changes in the internal and external environment, those changes produce new sensory input, which leads to further movement, and so on. If the cycle is interrupted and time interposed between sensation and movement, by whatever agent (e.g., the experimenter), then the prefrontal is postulated to come into play to bridge the gap: two temporally reciprocal prefrontal functions, one retrospective (short-term memory, STM) and the other prospective (preparatory motor set), help the organism bridge the time and mend the cycle.

Shindy, and J. Yajeya. The behavioral focus of our research is the performance of a category of behavioral tasks, delay tasks, which epitomize cross-temporal contingencies and the cognitive operations that the animal must exercise to cover those contingencies (Fig. 3–2).

All delay tasks require the performance of behavioral acts in accord with, i.e., contingent upon, events in the recent past. All these tasks are impaired by lesions of dorsolateral prefrontal cortex (Fuster, 1989). All are based on the principle of cross-temporal contingency. The logic of this principle can be simply stated in two sentences: *If now this, then later that; if earlier that, then now this.* It is important to note the universality of this principle. It applies to all behavioral sequences with substantial temporal separations between mutually contingent events. It applies not only to delay tasks but to certain neuropsychologic tests (e.g., the Wisconsin Card Sorting Test) in which decisions are made on the basis of temporally separate and temporally changing information. The principle, of course, applies also to spoken language, which represents the highest form of sensory-motor integration and of the perception-action cycle.

A form of short-term memory, also referred to as "working memory," is the first function that appears necessary to close that cycle. Localized functional

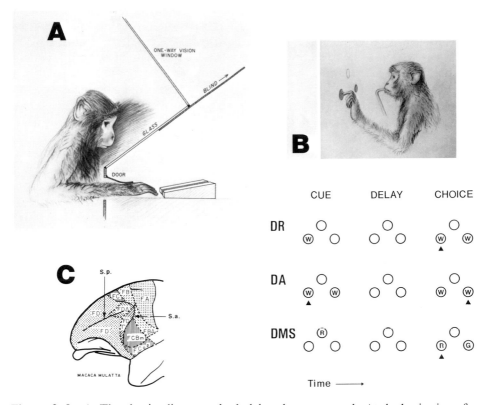

Figure 3–2 **A:** The classic, direct-method, delayed-response task. At the beginning of a trial, a food morsel is placed under one of the two blocks in full view of the animal. The opaque screen (blind) is then lowered. After a delay of a few seconds or minutes, the screen is raised and the animal given the choice of one object. If he choses the correct object (with concealed food), he retrieves the food as reward; if not the trial terminates without reward. Bait position is changed randomly between trials. **B:** Automated, indirect-method, delay tasks. The monkey faces a panel with three stimulus-response buttons. Below is the sequence of events for three different tasks (light stimuli: W, white; G, green; R, red); triangles mark correct response, rewarded by fruit juice. DR: Delayed response. The cue is the brief illumination of one of the lower buttons; after the delay, both lower buttons are lit for the choice; correct response is pressing the button lit before the delay. DA: Delayed alternation. The subject must press one of the two lower buttons when they appear simultaneously lit between delays; the correct button alternates between right and left. DMS: Delayed matching-to-sample. The sample (cue) is the brief colored illumination of the top button. After the delay, two colors appear simultaneously in the lower buttons; correct response is pressing the button with the sample color. The sample color and its position in the lower buttons are changed randomly from one trial to the next. **C:** Cytoarchitectural map of the frontal cortex of the rhesus monkey, from Bonin and Bailey. The prefrontal cortex is labeled FD. Monkeys with dorsolateral prefrontal lesions show deficits in performance of the four tasks depicted above.

depression by cooling is a useful way to test the cortical substrate of that function. The main advantage of the method is its reversibility, and it is for this reason that we have used it extensively in monkeys performing delay tasks. With Richard Bauer (Bauer and Fuster, 1976) we used it in delayed matching-to-sample; both the cooling method and the task served us well to demonstrate that the dorsolateral prefrontal cortex is important for the retention of not only spatially defined information but nonspatial information as well. The task is depicted in Figure 3–2**B**. We observed that prefrontal cooling, unlike parietal cooling, induced a fully reversible deficit in short-term memory for color (Fig. 3–3). It is worth noting that the deficit increased as a function of the delay that was interposed between the presentation of a color and a choice that was contingent on that color. This is a clear indication that the function impaired was indeed short-term memory, which is known to have a temporal decay, in the human as well as in the animal.

More recently, with Posley and Shindy, we have succeeded in further substantiating the supramodal character of the kind of short-term memory supported by the prefrontal cortex. We have shown that, by cooling dorsolateral prefrontal cortex, one can obtain a reversible deficit in performance of haptic delayed matching-to-sample, that is, of short-term memory for somesthetic cues acquired by active touch. The deficit is not only apparent when the animal must recognize by touch a previously touched object, but when he must recognize by sight that previously touched object and vice versa, i.e., recognize by palpation what he has previously seen. Thus, the prefrontal time-bridging function is not only supramodal but cross-modal (Figs. 3–4 and 3–5).

Now let us turn to the electrophysiologic data bearing on the dorsolateral prefrontal functions postulated. The first electrical evidence of the involvement of the prefrontal cortex in cross-temporal contingency was obtained by Walter and his colleagues in Bristol (Walter et al., 1964). It was a slow surface-negative potential, the Contingent Negative Variation (CNV), recorded from the frontal region of human subjects performing a delay task. The potential took place during the delay interval, that is, in the interval of time between a sensory cue and a motor act contingent on it.

It was in part that evidence that prompted us in the late sixties and early seventies to explore with microelectrodes the prefrontal cortex of monkeys performing delay tasks. The first data from this exploration were obtained with the classic delayed-response task (Fuster, 1973; Fuster and Alexander, 1971). Several types of units were observed; each type differed from the others by its pattern of discharge during the delayed-response trial (Fig. 3–6). The most striking discovery was the presence of large contingents of prefrontal units that underwent sustained activation during the delay period, namely, during the period of retention of the cue before the animal was required to respond to it. The phenomenon was tentatively interpreted as a manifestation of the involvement of those neurons in short-term memory.

It was only later, however, with more sophisticated behavioral methods, including better control of the sensory cues, that the phenomenon of delay activation could be definitely ascribed to short-term memory. The evidence for this interpretation was clear to us in the case of prefrontal units that, during the delay

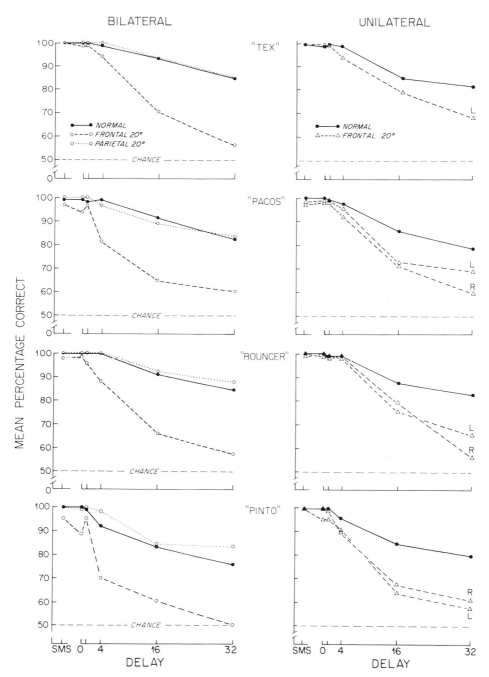

Figure 3–3 Performance curves from four monkeys in delayed matching-to-sample (Fig. 3–2 **B**) at normal temperature and under bilateral or unilateral—L, left; R, right— cooling of dorsolateral or posterior parietal cortex. SMS: simultaneous matching-to-sample; delay in seconds. Note the increasing deficit as the delay is prolonged.

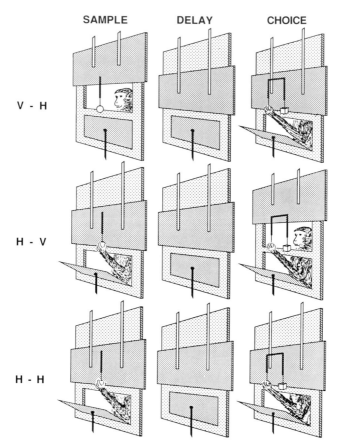

Figure 3–4 Schematic diagram of three haptic (tactile) delayed matching-to-sample tasks. **Top** (V-H, cross-modal): visual cue to haptic choice. **Middle** (H-V, cross-modal): haptic cue to visual choice. **Bottom** (H-H, unimodal): haptic cue to haptic choice. Sample object and its position at the choice are changed in random order from trial to trial.

period, showed a different level of sustained activity depending on the particular cue that the animal had to retain for a correct response (Fuster et al., 1982; Quintana et al., 1988; Rosenkilde et al., 1981). Such delay-differential cells have also been observed by other authors in the dorsolateral prefrontal cortex of monkeys performing a variety of delay tasks (Funahashi et al., 1988; Kubota et al., 1980; Niki, 1974).

Already in our early studies (Fuster, 1973; Fuster et al., 1982), we recognized the existence of a type of prefrontal cells, activated during the delay of delay tasks, that did not conform to a memory hypothesis, either by the time-course of their discharge or the differentiation of cues during that period. At first, however, such units appeared to us to be rare and for this reason they were not represented in the scheme of Figure 3–6. They were characterized by accelerat-

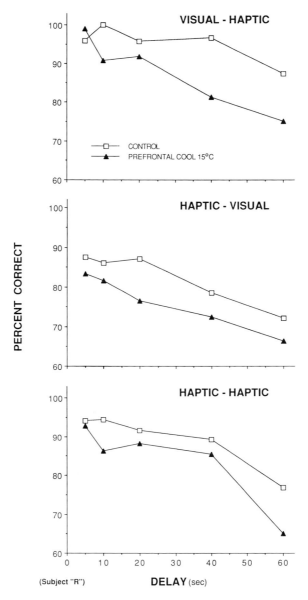

Figure 3–5 Performance curves from one animal in tactile delayed matching tasks, at normal temperature (control) and during bilateral prefrontal cooling.

ing discharge in anticipation of motor responses. They, too, were observed by other investigators (Niki and Watanabe, 1979; Sakai 1974). In delay tasks, they showed increasing activations that practically covered the entirety of the delay period. Again, however, because their activation was in most instances nondifferential, that is, unrelated to any peculiar characteristic of the cue or the

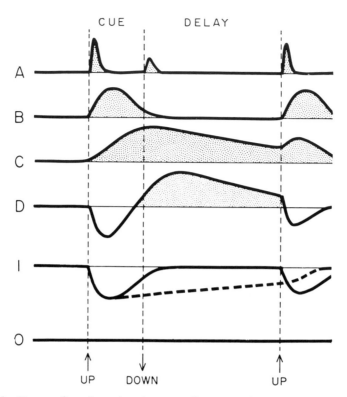

Figure 3–6 Types of prefrontal units according to their pattern of discharge during delayed response (direct method, Fig. 3–2 **A**). Deviations of firing above intertrial base line are marked by shading. "Up" and "down" refer to the movements of the screen (blind). Note the increased firing of types C and D during the delay period.

response, they could not be directly related to either. Besides, "anticipatory" units seemed to be anatomically inseparable from "memory" units. The two types of cells seemed to coexist in close proximity of each other and thoroughly intermixed in dorsolateral prefrontal cortex (Fuster et al., 1982).

Since in most of the delay tasks utilized for single-unit studies the response is predictably in the same site as the cue (delayed response) or unpredictable until the delay is over (delayed matching), it is difficult with such tasks to ascribe "anticipatory units" to the preparation to respond. In order to establish this relationship with some assurance, it is necessary to separate the cue from the response not only temporally, as in all delay tasks, but spatially, as in delayed matching. In addition, it is desirable to allow the animal the possibility to predict with varying degrees of probability the site of response between at least two possible alternatives (e.g., right or left). Quintana and I designed such a task (Quintana and Fuster, 1989). In essence, the sequence of events in one of its trials is as follows: (1) A central visual cue differing from trial to trial only in color and

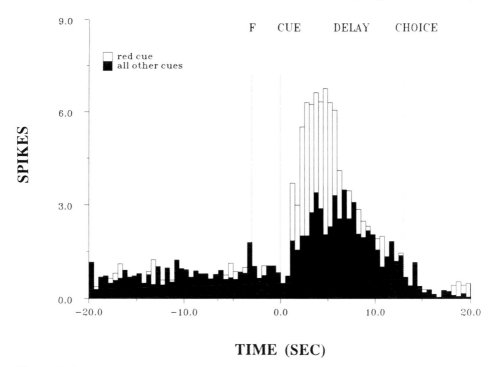

Figure 3–7 Average frequency histograms (0.5-sec bins) from a cell in prefrontal cortex during a delay task with spatial and temporal dissociation of cues and responses. A color cue, preceded by a warning flash (F) determines the direction of the correct choice (right or left) with different degrees of probability: red, 75% to the left; green, 75% to the right; blue, 100% to the left; yellow, 100% to the right. The cell shows a marked activation particularly during the early part of the delay. That activation is significantly higher after red cue than after any of the other cues.

predicting the side of the correct response with either 75 or 100% probability, depending on the color; (2) a period of delay of a few seconds; and (3) a pair of simultaneous and spatially separate choice stimuli that, depending on the anteceding color cue, determine the response to the right or to the left.

Using such a task with temporal and spatial dissociation of cue and response, as well as a symbolic relationship of probability between the two, it has become possible to ascertain the participation of prefrontal neurons in the anticipatory preparation of the response. It is now clear that, in addition to neurons that are tied to the memory of a nonspatially defined feature of the cue, such as color (Fig. 3–7), there are in dorsolateral prefrontal cortex many neurons that, in anticipation of the response, discharge differently in accord with the side of the response that the cue calls for. Furthermore, we have observed that the degree of accelerating and anticipatory activation of some of those cells during the delay is directly related to the predictability and probability of the anticipated response according to the rules of the task (Fig. 3–8). It is plausible to infer that

F   CUE   DELAY   CHOICE

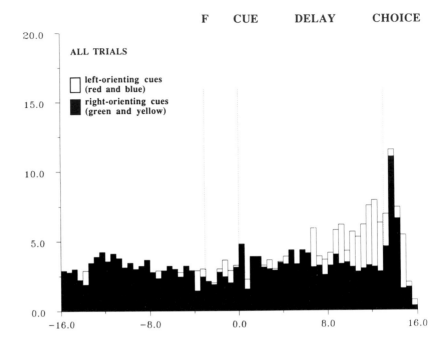

ALL TRIALS

□ left-orienting cues
(red and blue)
■ right-orienting cues
(green and yellow)

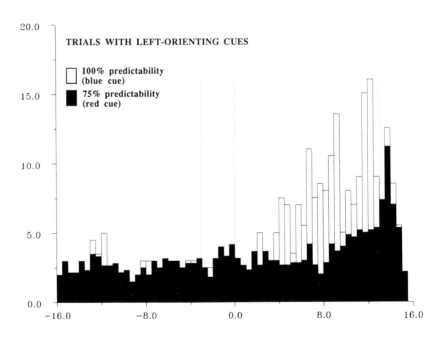

TRIALS WITH LEFT-ORIENTING CUES

□ 100% predictability
(blue cue)
■ 75% predictability
(red cue)

SPIKES

TIME (SEC)

all these delay-differential and response-related neurons take part in the neural process of preparation for the response, in other words, in preparatory motor set.

CONCLUDING COMMENTS

The results of the research studies that I have reviewed in this chapter allow us to reach the following conclusions:

1. The functional depression of the dorsolateral prefrontal cortex induces a reversible deficit in performance of a variety of delay tasks. The deficit is not circumscribed to tasks in which the cue to be remembered is visual and defined by its position in space. Rather, the deficit extends to delay tasks with visual and nonspatial—i.e., color—cues. The deficit also extends to haptic delay tasks in which the cue to be remembered is an object perceived by active touch. Thus, the deficit appears to be supramodal. Furthermore, the deficit affects the cross-modal (and cross-temporal) transfer from visual memory to haptic recognition, and vice versa. These findings suggest a general role of prefrontal cortex in short-term memory for mediation of cross-temporal contingencies of behavior.

2. Two distinct types of neurons are present in dorsolateral prefrontal cortex. During the delay period of delay tasks, the cells of the first type show a sustained pattern of firing that is attuned to the cue; these cells appear involved in the representation and temporary retention of the sensory information contained in the cue. Cells of the second type, on the other hand, show firing that is attuned to the forthcoming motor response; these cells appear to participate in preparatory motor set.

The mechanisms of short-term memory and preparatory set in which the prefrontal cortex intervenes are unknown. However, what we know about prefrontal connectivity and single-cell properties allows us to infer, indirectly, that, while the animal retains a cue and prepares for the appropriate response to it, there is a transfer of information from memory cells to motor-set cells: in other words, a transfer from the neural network that represents the cue to the neural network that represents the motor response. That transfer probably takes place, in part, within the prefrontal cortex itself. Also in part, the transfer probably involves connections between the prefrontal cortex and other neocortical and subcortical structures that constitute the substrate of the perception-action cycle. This may be the functional foundation of the role of the prefrontal cortex in the syntax of the action—literally the syntax of the action in the case of language— and, therefore, the temporal organization of behavior.

Figure 3–8 Average frequency histograms from a prefrontal cell related to preparation for movement in a delay task with spatial and temporal separation between cues and responses. Upper histograms show the discharge of the cell during trials with left- and right-orienting cues. Note accelerating discharge during the delay in trials with probable left response. Bottom histograms show the breakdown of activity in trials with left-orienting cues: blue and red (unequal numbers of trials). Note that acceleration of firing is greater when left response is 100% predictable than when it is 75% predictable.

SUMMARY

In this chapter, experiments are presented that substantiate the role of the dorsolateral prefrontal cortex in two mutually complementary and cooperant functions mediating cross-temporal contingencies of behavior: short-term memory and preparatory set. The cooling of dorsolateral prefrontal cortex in monkeys induces reversible deficits in performance of visual, tactual, and cross-modal delay tasks. These deficits implicate that cortex in a supramodal form of short-term memory. This inference is supported by electrophysiologic demonstration of prefrontal units that appear involved in the temporary retention of sensory information. Single-unit recording also demonstrates the presence of neurons that, before the manual responses required by delay tasks, exhibit accelerating firing activity patterns dependent on the direction of the expected response of the animal. Such neurons appear engaged in the preparation of that motor response. The two types of prefrontal neurons, one attuned to the sensory cue and the other to the motor response, presumably support the two postulated functions of, respectively, short-term memory and preparatory set, by which the prefrontal cortex mediates temporal discontinuities in the perception-action cycle.

REFERENCES

Arbib MA. Perceptual structures and distributed motor control. *In:* Handbook of Physiology; Nervous System, Vol. II. (VB Brooks, ed.), Am Physiol Soc, Bethesda, 1981, pp. 1448–1480.

Bauer RH, Fuster JM. Delayed-matching and delayed-response deficit from cooling dorsolateral prefrontal cortex in monkeys. J Comp Physiol Psychol 90:293–302, 1976.

Funahashi S, Bruce CJ, Goldman-Rakic PS. Mnemonic coding of visual space in the monkey's dorsolateral prefrontal cortex. J Neurophysiol 61:331–34, 1989.

Fuster JM. Unit activity in prefrontal cortex during delayed-response performance: Neuronal correlates of transient memory. J Neurophysiol 36:61–78, 1973.

Fuster JM. The prefrontal cortex, mediator of cross-temporal contingencies. Hum Neurobiol 4:169–179, 1985.

Fuster JM. The Prefrontal Cortex, 2nd ed. Raven Press, New York, 1989.

Fuster, JM, Alexander GE. Neuron activity related to short-term memory. Science 173:652–654, 1971.

Fuster JM, Bauer RH, Jervey JP. Cellular discharge in the dorsolateral prefrontal cortex of the monkey in cognitive tasks. Exp Neurol 77:679–694, 1982.

Kubota K, Tonoike M, Mikami A. Neuronal activity in the monkey dorsolateral prefrontal cortex during a discrimination task with delay. Brain Res 183:29–42, 1980.

Niki H. Differential activity of prefrontal units during right and left delayed response trials. Brain Res 70:346–349, 1974.

Niki H, Watanabe M. Prefrontal and cingulate unit activity during timing behavior in the monkey. Brain Res 171:213–224, 1979.

Quintana, J, Fuster JM. Reciprocal temporal trends of sensory- and motor-coupling in prefrontal units during visual delay tasks. Soc Neurosci Abstr 15:78, 1989.

Quintana J, Yajeya J, Fuster JM. Prefrontal representation of stimulus attributes during delay tasks. I. Unit activity in cross-temporal integration of sensory and sensory-motor information. Brain Res 474:211–22, 1988.

Rosenkilde CE, Bauer RH, Fuster JM. Single cell activity in ventral prefrontal cortex of behaving monkeys. Brain Res 209:375–394, 1981.

Sakai M. Prefrontal unit activity during visually guided lever pressing reaction in the monkey. Brain Res 81:297–309, 1974.

Walter W, Cooper R, Aldridge V, McCallum W, Winter A. Contingent negative variation: an electric sign of sensori-motor association and expectancy in the human brain. Nature 203:380–384, 1964.

Weizsaecker V. Der Gestaltkreis. Thieme, Stuttgart, 1950.

4

The Circuitry of Working Memory Revealed by Anatomy and Metabolic Imaging

PATRICIA S. GOLDMAN-RAKIC
AND HARRIET R. FRIEDMAN

Recent advances in anatomical, behavioral, and physiological techniques have produced new information about the nature of prefrontal function, its cellular basis, and its anatomical underpinnings. A major advance in our understanding of prefrontal function is the recognition that prefrontal subdivisions such as the principal sulcus (Walker's area 46) are embedded in a complex but delimited network involving a large number of other cortical areas and subcortical structures (Fig. 4–1) (Goldman-Rakic, 1988; Selemon and Goldman-Rakic, 1988). Certain questions concerning the operation of a distributed neural network need to be addressed. Among these is the question of whether an anatomically defined network is functionally unified and, if so, what the nature of the contribution of each node is to the overall function of the network. A related issue is whether there is one central executive system or multiple special purpose transient memory systems. The answers to each of these questions will not come from any one method but will require a number of different strategies and approaches.

We have begun to address some of these issues with the 2-deoxyglucose (2DG) method (Sokoloff et al., 1977) for labeling functional pathways during performance on relevant behavioral tasks. This method has the advantage of allowing examination of any and all structures of interest to a given behavior in a single animal. If plasma samples are obtained during the test session, the evaluation of local cerebral glucose metabolism is quantitative, and rigorous comparisons can be made not only across structures within the same animal but across animals that perform different tests. As part of a wider study on the contributions of each part of a spatial cognition network to behavior (see later), we have begun with studies of components of the hippocampal formation and also nuclei of the medial thalamus. In this chapter, we will review the anatomical background and functional analysis of thalamic and hippocampal subdivisions that are connected with the prefrontal cortex. The approach used in these initial studies can be applied to other areas, and studies of the posterior parietal, medial temporal, and prefrontal cortical areas, for example, are currently in progress. We begin with a brief review of working memory followed by a description of the anatomical network(s) that we believe mediate this process in the visuospatial domain.

WORKING MEMORY: DISSOCIATION FROM ASSOCIATIVE MEMORY

The concept that memory is divisible into several forms represents a major contribution to the study of memory from the field of cognitive psychology. The historical development of this field and the empiric evidence derived from cognitive studies in normal and brain-damaged individuals is well documented (for review: Baddeley, 1986). Working memory is the term applied by cognitive psychologists and theorists to the type of memory which is a limited capacity memorandum that is active and relevant for only a short period of time, usually on the scale of seconds. A common simple example of working memory is keeping in mind a newly read phone number until it is dialed and then immediately forgotten. Working memory has been referred to as "scratch-pad" memory (Baddeley, 1983). The criterion—relevant only transiently—distinguishes working memory from the process that has been termed reference memory (Olton et al., 1979), semantic memory (Tulving, 1972), and procedural memory (Squire and Cohen, 1984)—all of which have in common that their contents are always true and, in principle, remain stable over time, e.g., someone's name, the color of one's eyes, the shape of an apple. Each of these forms of memory are associative in the traditional sense, i.e., based on the repetition of association between stimuli and responses and/or consequences. By contrast, working memory is short-lived, dynamic, and ever changing. Hence, the brain's working memory function, i.e., the ability to bring to mind information and hold it "on line" in the absence of direct stimulation, may be its inherently most flexible mechanism and its evolutionarily most significant achievement. It confers the ability to guide behavior by representations of the outside world rather than by immediate stimulation and thus to base behavior on ideas and thoughts. For example, the fundamental ability to understand that an object exists when it is *out of view* depends on the capacity to keep events in mind beyond the direct experience of those events (Piaget, 1954). Working memory has been implicated as a cardinal process in the highest functions of language, perception, and logic (Baddeley, 1986; Shallice, 1990).

SPATIAL COGNITION NETWORKS

The idea that cortical functions are carried out through "networks" of cortical areas is not a new concept and, indeed, it is rather obvious that this must be the case. However, it is one matter to believe in neural networks, in general, and another matter to specify the dimensions and nodes of a particular neuronal ensemble for the purpose of a specific function. Anatomical tracing studies in our laboratory have elucidated the blueprint of two major networks involving the caudal principal sulcus. One of these networks is characterized by rich corticocortical interconnectivity. It involves, in addition to the principal sulcus, the posterior parietal cortex, areas of limbic cortex such as the anterior and posterior cingulate cortex and parahippocampal gyrus, and a number of other regions within the frontal, parietal, and temporal lobes (Selemon and Goldman-Rakic, 1988). The evidence for this specific constellation comes from the analysis of double anterograde tracing studies in which one anterograde tracer was injected into the caudal principal sulcus and a second anterograde tracer was injected into the posterior parietal cortex, which we know to be interconnected with the principal sulcus (Cavada and Goldman-Rakic, 1989; Leichnitz, 1980; Petrides and Pandya, 1984; Schwartz and Goldman-Rakic, 1984). We have proposed that this distributed network of areas, which interconnects the principal sulcus and posterior parietal cortex, is dedicated to the general domain of spatial cognition (Goldman-Rakic, 1987; 1988).

The particular role of the caudal principal sulcus in spatial cognition is well documented. This region of prefrontal cortex is essential for behavioral performance when it is guided by *remembered* spatial locations rather than by external cues in the environment and when such memoranda are constantly changing (for review: Fuster, 1989 and Goldman-Rakic, 1987, but also Passingham, 1985). Thus, the caudal principal sulcus may be the focus for working memory of visuospatial cues. On the other hand, the posterior parietal cortex is widely regarded as the brain's center for spatial or motion vision, i.e., the perception and representation of spatial relations among body parts and external objects (e.g., Mountcastle et al., 1984). This region is thought to be the source of the visuospatial information that drives neurons in the principal sulcus (Goldman-Rakic, 1987).

The behavioral contribution of other cortico-cortical components of the network defined in anatomical studies are much less obvious and more difficult to infer, as many cortical areas have not yet been studied with respect to delayed-response behavior. However, some functional information is available for subcortical structures. Thus, delay-enhanced discharge during delayed-response tasks has been reported in several key structures with which the principal sulcus is connected, e.g., the hippocampus (Watanabe and Niki, 1985), the head of the caudate nucleus (Hikosaka et al., 1989) and the mediodorsal nucleus of the thalamus (Fuster and Alexander, 1971; 1973), though not from the cholinergic system of basal forebrain nuclei (Richardson and DeLong, 1986). The evidence from these physiology studies is consistent with the supposition of a richly interconnected system of neural structures engaged in spatial information processing. In such systems, integrative functions may emerge from the dynamics of the entire network and from its interactions with similarly constructed networks rather than from linear computations performed at each nodal point in the circuit.

Thus, in addition to cortico-cortical circuits, the principal sulcus is a part of a cortico-subcortical circuit involving, in sequence, the neostriatum, the substantia nigra and globus pallidus, and the mediodorsal nucleus (MD) of the thalamus (Giguere and Goldman-Rakic, 1988; Goldman and Nauta, 1977; Goldman-Rakic and Porrino, 1985; Ilinsky et al., 1985). This circuit can be considered a positive feedback loop in that its activation is thought to trigger specific motor actions by disinhibition of thalamo-cortical neurons. Therefore, the thalamus is an important link through which the principal sulcus can influence motor responses. The studies described later focus on the mediodorsal nucleus, a key node in this circuit.

ANATOMICAL ORGANIZATION OF THE THALAMO-CORTICAL PROJECTIONS

The mediodorsal nucleus of the diencephalon provides the major thalamic innervation to the prefrontal cortex and is a major component of the cortico-striato-thalamo-cortical circuit mentioned before. An important feature of the thalamic innervation of the prefrontal cortex is that it is topographically organized. The dorsolateral parvocellular portion of the MD projects to the dorsal bank of the principal sulcus (Fig. 4–1A, 1B), the ventromedial magnocellular nucleus projects to the inferior convexity cortex adjacent to the principal sulcus (Fig. 4–1C) and the dorsomedial magnocellular subdivision projects to the ventral and more posterior areas of prefrontal cortex (Fig. 4–1D), i.e., the orbital regions (Goldman-Rakic and Porrino, 1985).

In addition to its innervation by the mediodorsal nucleus, the principal sulcus has been shown to have additional thalamic inputs, for example, from the anteromedial and anteroventral thalamus as shown in Figure 4–2, and from the medial pulvinar nuclei (Baleydier and Mauguiere, 1985; Goldman-Rakic and Porrino, 1985; Kievet and Kuypers, 1977; Preuss and Goldman-Rakic, 1987). The nature of interaction between these converging thalamo-cortical fiber systems in the primate brain awaits further analysis. However, it seems clear that convergence of multiple thalamic inputs to a given cytoarchitectonic area redefines the prefrontal areas by a unique *set* of thalamic inputs rather than by a relationship with a single thalamic nucleus. Of course, each thalamic input could be expected to have a distinctive role in cortical function, and multiple thalamic innervation does not rule out that one nucleus could prove most essential, as the lateral geniculate nucleus is to striate visual cortex, for example.

LESIONS OF THALAMIC NUCLEI IN NONHUMAN PRIMATES

The role of the medial thalamus in mnemonic processes has been a subject of intense interest but little consensus since the seminal observation of Victor and colleagues (1971) that the mediodorsal nucleus was degenerated in Wernicke-Korsakoff disease. Studies of nonhuman primates with discrete lesions of the mediodorsal nucleus have been few and mostly with negative or inconclusive results. An early study by Schulman had provided evidence of profound impairments on delayed-response tasks in monkeys with large lesions of the thalamus produced by implanting radioactive pellets into the thalamus (Schulman, 1964).

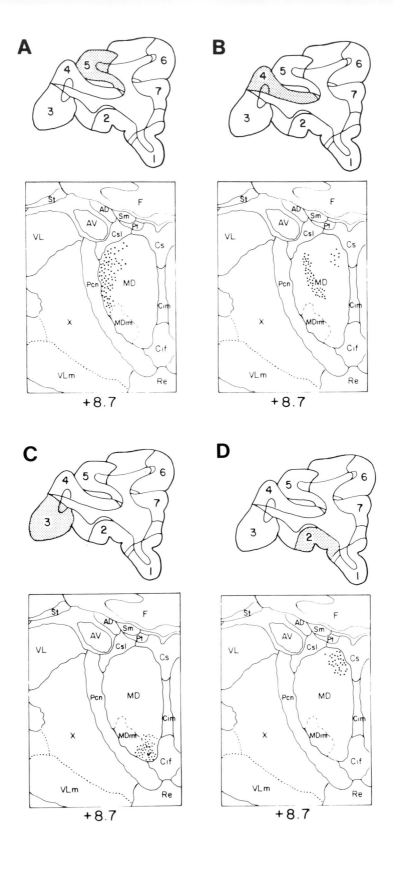

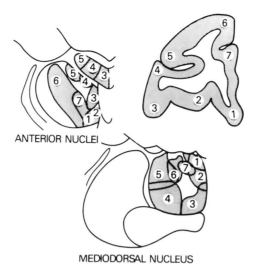

ANTERIOR NUCLEI

MEDIODORSAL NUCLEUS

Figure 4–2 Summary of topographic relationships between the anterior thalamic nuclei (labeled 3, 4, and 5 in the upper left diagram), the mediodorsal thalamus (lower right diagram), and selected cytoarchitectonic subdivisions of the prefrontal cortex (upper right diagram). The diagram shows that each subdivision of these major thalamic nuclei projects to one and only one cytoarchitectonic area of cortex and correspondingly, that each cortical area receives unique, though multiple, thalamic inputs. (Adapted from Goldman-Rakic and Porrino, 1985.)

However, this procedure produced lesions that encompassed the entire thalamus and therefore precluded attribution of the deficit to a single nucleus or nuclear grouping. We reinvestigated this issue in the late seventies with radiofrequency lesions (Isseroff et al., 1982). The lesions produced in our study were partial and neither MD nor any other thalamic nucleus was entirely damaged nor, on the other hand, was damage ever confined strictly to the mediodorsal nucleus. Nevertheless, we were able to demonstrate that lesions of sufficient extent in the mediodorsal nucleus produced an impairment on delayed-response performance and the impairments were more profound on a spatial alternation task (Isseroff et al., 1982). Like monkeys with principal sulcus lesions (Goldman and Rosvold,

←

Figure 4–1 Summary of topographic relationships between the mediodorsal thalamus (MD) and selected regions of the prefrontal cortex derived from anatomic tracing studies of retrogradely labeled cells in the thalamus after HRP injections were made to circumscribed regions of the prefrontal cortex. **A** and **B:** HRP injections were made to, respectively, the dorsal and ventral bank of the principal sulcus. In both cases, cells were labeled in the lateral, parvocellular MD. **C:** The injection was made in the inferior convexity prefrontal cortex and cells were labeled in the ventromedial MD. **D:** The injection was made in the orbital prefrontal cortex, and here the labeled cells were located within the medial, magnocellular division of MD. (Adapted from Goldman-Rakic and Porrino, 1985.)

1970), the animals with thalamic damage were unimpaired on an associative learning task, e.g., a visual pattern discrimination. Similar results were subsequently obtained with delayed nonmatching-to-sample paradigms (Aggleton and Mishkin, 1983a,b; Zola-Morgan and Squire, 1985a). We have argued that these paradigms are working memory tests for nonspatial features of objects in that the information important for a correct response is relevant only transiently and must be updated on a trial-by-trial basis (Friedman et al., 1990; Goldman-Rakic, 1987). The lack of effect of mediodorsal lesions on visual discrimination habits in these studies supports the idea that working memory and associative memory depend on different neuronal circuits and substrates.

METABOLIC STUDIES OF THE THALAMUS IN WORKING MEMORY TASKS

Given the common streams of evidence from anatomical, lesion, and electrophysiological studies that clearly implicate the mediodorsal thalamus and, to a lesser extent, the anterior thalamic nuclei as important neural elements of a system dedicated to working memory processing, the 2DG method was used to assess whether metabolic activity in these areas substantiates and extends this association (Friedman et al., 1990). Indeed, the basic issue that these studies addressed was whether metabolic activity in the thalamus is differently or preferentially influenced when monkeys perform tasks that demand working memory processing as compared to the pattern of functional activity underlying a monkey's performance on behavioral paradigms that instead draw exclusively on well-learned stimulus-response associations.

Two groups of monkeys were trained to perform either a working memory task or an associative memory task and then were given ^{14}C-2-DG for a final testing session following the procedures of a typical 2DG experiment (Sokoloff et al., 1977). The monkeys of the working memory group were trained to perform one of three tests (Fig. 4–3). Two of these were the classic tests of spatial working memory; the spatial delayed-response task and the delayed spatial alternation task. In these spatial memory tests, the monkey was required to remember the spatial location of a reward, but because the relevance of this information was short-lived, spatial position changed for each trial. This information must be updated on a trial by trial basis in order for a correct response to occur. In the third working memory task, delayed object alternation, features of objects rather than spatial position, was the preeminent guide for performance. But this task, like the spatial working memory paradigms, preferentially engaged working memory because each object (one of two) covered the reward on alternate trials and, therefore, the monkey was required to keep a flexible record of this information in order to obtain the reward. Thus, while these tasks differed both with respect to the spatial versus object features of their stimulus components and with respect to the exact nature of the information presented on each trial, all three tests were similar in their reliance on working memory processes. The data for this group of monkeys performing working memory tasks were compared with the metabolic activity data for a control group of monkeys that performed either a sensory-motor control task that had no explicit memory component or

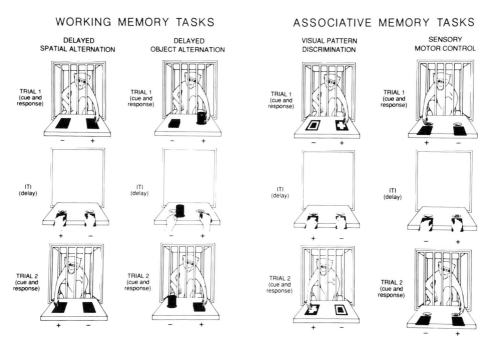

Figure 4–3 Working memory and associative memory control tasks that monkeys performed during the 2DG experiments. In delayed spatial alternation, the placement of the reward alternated on each trial; in the delayed object alternation task, one of two objects alternately covered the reward on each trial. (Not shown is the delayed spatial response task.) Therefore, the information guiding a correct response changed from trial to trial, and the monkey was required to update this information in order to achieve the reward. By contrast, on both the visual pattern discrimination and the sensory motor control tasks, there was an invariant relationship between stimuli and the correct response. In the discrimination task, the "plus sign" always covered the reward, and in the sensory motor task, there was no implicit mnemonic requirement as the monkey always was able to retrieve a reward from under the plaques. (Adapted from Friedman and Goldman-Rakic, 1988.)

a visual pattern discrimination task in which the correct stimulus-response association was invariant across all trials and all test sessions (Fig. 4–3). Therefore, in contrast to the working memory tasks, where performance was guided by internalized representations of preceding events, on the control tasks, performance was guided by external cues that reliably indicated the correct response.

One interesting finding that has been common through much of our 2DG studies of functionally complex regions of the thalamus, cortex, and elsewhere, is that for monkeys performing cognitive tasks, a differential pattern of activation in the brain is not readily apparent simply by viewing the autoradiography film records of metabolic labeling. Understanding the relationship of brain metabolic activity and *psychological* processing requires quantitative measurements and comparisons across groups of monkeys. For example, the mediodorsal thalamus, particularly the parvocellular component, was darkly labeled in the

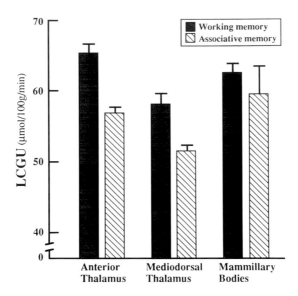

Figure 4–4 Local cerebral glucose utilization (LCGU) in the anterior thalamic nuclei, mediodorsal thalamus, and the mammillary bodies in monkeys performing working memory and associative memory tasks. The mean LCGU in both thalamic areas was significantly enhanced for the monkeys performing working memory tasks. By contrast, in the mammillary bodies, there were no significant differences in mean LCGU between these two groups. (Adapted from Friedman et al., 1990)

majority of monkeys irrespective of the behavioral task they performed. Indeed, both the anterior thalamic nuclei and the mediodorsal nuclei were outlined in the autoradiography films: these regions were darker and more distinct than adjacent thalamic regions. However, differences in metabolic activity as a function of behavioral performance were revealed by analysis of the local cerebral glucose utilization rates (LCGU) measured in each of these nuclei (Fig. 4–4). LCGU rates were significantly enhanced in the group of monkeys performing the working memory tasks relative to monkeys performing the control tasks. Overall, in the animals performing working memory tasks, LCGU was significantly enhanced by 12–16% in the ventral and medial nuclei of the anterior thalamus and in the magnocellular and parvocellular components of the mediodorsal thalamus. Of interest was a subtle difference between two aspects (dorsal and ventral) of the magnocellular mediodorsal thalamus because group differences were greatest in the ventral component. This distinction is anatomically meaningful, because, as summarized in Figure 4–2, the parvocellular and ventral magnocellular components of the mediodorsal thalamus are reciprocally connected to adjacent regions of the dorsolateral prefrontal cortex (Goldman-Rakic and Porrino, 1985).

Perhaps the relevance of these data is best seen in the context of our examination of LCGU in the mammillary bodies of these same monkeys. Like the the thalamic regions that were studied, the mammillary bodies also have a long history of association with memory function in both clinical and experimental reports, but there is yet no wholly consistent view of the importance of these nuclei for cognitive performance in the monkey (e.g., Aggleton and Mishkin, 1985; Holmes et al., 1983; Zola-Morgan et al., 1989). The results of this 2DG study showed that glucose utilization in the mammillary bodies was not preferentially enhanced by performance on working memory tasks (Fig. 4–4). These results are consonant with a report showing that lesions of the mammillary bodies do not greatly impair the performance of monkeys in behavioral paradigms that ostensively engage working memory processing (Zola-Morgan et al., 1989). While the mammillary bodies and the anterior and mediodorsal thalamus share some anatomic features, most notably their common membership in an enlarged limbic circuit (for review: Amaral, 1987), an important difference lies in the cortical connectivity of these diencephalic regions. Whereas the anterior and mediodorsal nuclei maintain extensive connections with the prefrontal cortex, the cortical connectivity of the mammillary bodies is quite restricted (Jacobson et al., 1978; Veazy et al., 1982; for review: Amaral, 1987). We have proposed that this feature may be a defining characteristic for participation in the neural circuit underlying working memory processing. In this light, it is interesting that our initial studies of the posterior thalamus similarly indicate that working memory processing does not produce a general enhancement of metabolic activity in the lateral pulvinar or lateral posterior thalamic nucleus (Friedman and Goldman-Rakic, unpublished data); these regions do not project to or receive extensive prefrontal cortical projections (Goldman-Rakic and Porrino, 1985, Selemon and Goldman-Rakic, 1988).

PREFRONTAL CONNECTIONS WITH HIPPOCAMPAL FORMATION

A major contribution of anatomical studies of neural pathways has been the elucidation of complex cortico-cortical networks. In the context of working memory, the relationship between the principal sulcus and the limbic system has been of great interest. Our studies (Goldman-Rakic et al., 1984; Selemon and Goldman-Rakic, 1988) have revealed that the dorsolateral prefrontal cortex is connected with a number of limbic areas including the anterior cingulate cortex (Brodmann's area 24), the posterior cingulate cortex (area 23), as well as the orbital prefrontal cortex (area 11). Whereas traditional views held that dorsolateral prefrontal cortex connections with the cortex of the parahippocampal gyrus were indirect, more recent work from this laboratory (Goldman-Rakic et al., 1984) has shown that these indirect routes are supplemented by two pathways that directly interconnect the dorsolateral prefrontal cortex and the presubicular, entorhinal, and parahippocampal cortices (area TF; see Fig. 4–5). Interestingly, the majority of these projections are bidirectional. However, the subicular cortex projects to but does not receive dorsolateral prefrontal cortex afferents. Thus, which prefrontal cortical information may influence the processing of information through the hippocampal formation, because the entorhinal cortex is the principal gateway into the hippocampal circuit and the subicular cortices represent a common final path for hippocampo-cortical projections (for review: Rosene and Van Hoesen, 1987).

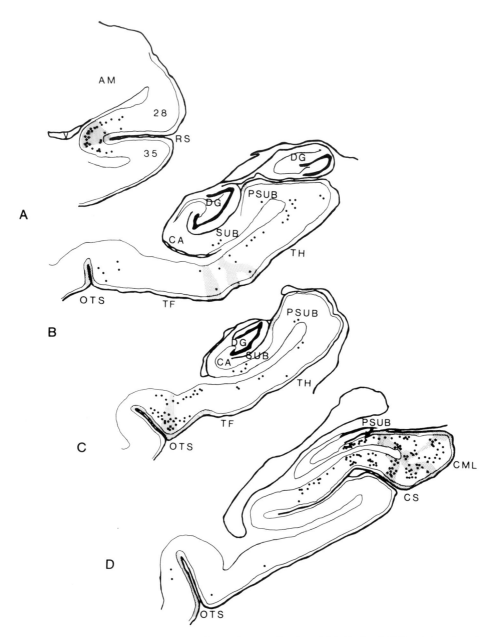

Figure 4–5 The results of anatomic tracing studies in which WGA-HRP, tritiated aminoacids, or fluorescent dyes were injected in the dorsolateral prefrontal cortex and anterograde and retrograde labeling was examined in the parahippocampal cortex. Crosshatched regions represent terminal areas, i.e., areas receiving prefrontal cortical afferents, whereas cells of the parahippocampal region that project to the prefrontal cortex are indicated as dots. Note that in **A**, labeling is quite marked in the depths of the entorhinal cortex (area 28) and in **D**, cell and terminal labeling in the caudomedial lobule (CML) is dense. Abbreviations: AM, amygdala; CA, ammonic fields of the hippocampus; CS, cingulate sulcus; DG, dentate gyrus; OTS, occipitotemporal sulcus; PSub, presubiculum; Sub, subiculum. (Adapted from Goldman-Rakic et al., 1984.)

CAUDOMEDIAL LOBULE

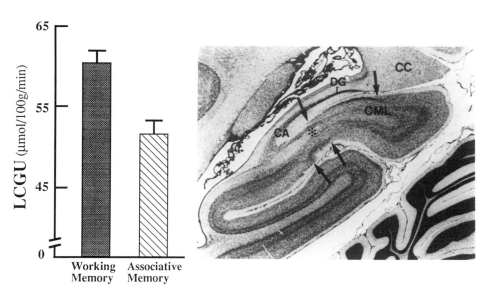

Figure 4-6 Local cerebral glucose utilization (LCGU) in the caudomedial lobule in monkeys performing working memory and associative memory tasks. **Left:** Mean LCGU in the caudomedial lobule was significantly enhanced in monkeys performing the working memory tasks relative to the associative memory control tasks. **Right:** A cresyl violet-stained section showing the caudomedial lobule and posterior parahippocampal cortex in the monkey. Abbreviations: CC, corpus callosum; and as in Figure 4-5.

The anatomical data, therefore, support the close association of prefrontal cortical and hippocampal function and provide a neural basis for functional similarities between these structures that have been reported. For example, while other aspects of their behavioral profile are not identical, monkeys sustaining damage to either the hippocampal formation (Zola-Morgan and Squire, 1985b) or dorsolateral prefrontal cortex show impaired performance on spatial memory tasks (Goldman and Rosvold, 1970; for review: Goldman-Rakic, 1987); and memory-task delay-related activity, such as has been recorded from neurons in the prefrontal cortex (e.g., Funahashi et al., 1989; Fuster and Alexander, 1971) also can be demonstrated in cells of the hippocampal formation in monkeys performing delay response type tasks (Watanabe and Niki, 1985).

Another facet of these anatomical tracing studies is that they revealed a prominent reciprocal projection of the prefrontal cortex and a little-studied region of the caudal parahippocampal gyrus (Fig. 4-5D and Fig. 4-6, **right**), termed the caudomedial lobule (Goldman-Rakic et al., 1984). Apart from its prefrontal connectivity, little else of functional significance is known about this region, and yet this prominent anatomic association would suggest some commonalities of function with the prefrontal cortex. On this basis, it was suggested that the caudomedial lobule is likely to be related more to the hippocampal formation (from which it appears to be a caudal extension) than to the subadjacent ventromedial occipital cortex, which it appears to resemble on cytoarchitectonic grounds (Goldman-Rakic et al., 1984). The complementary results obtained in our 2DG studies of the caudomedial lobule and the hippocampus and dentate gyrus buttress this association, as detailed below.

METABOLIC STUDIES OF HIPPOCAMPAL FORMATION DURING WORKING MEMORY

To provide a first functional analysis of the caudomedial lobule, metabolic activity in this caudal extension of the parahippocampal gyrus was measured in monkeys performing working memory and associative memory tasks. Because the 2DG method effectively provides a profile of metabolic activity for the entire brain in each subject, we were able to pose the question of whether functional activity in the caudomedial lobule is differentially influenced by working memory processing in the very same monkeys that had been examined in the context of our studies of the thalamus above and hippocampal formation (see below).

Caudomedial Lobule

Metabolic activity was measured through the full anterior-posterior extent of the caudomedial lobule, and the mean data (Friedman and Goldman-Rakic, unpublished data) showed that glucose utilization was significantly enhanced by 18% in monkeys performing working memory tasks relative to monkeys performing the associative memory tasks (Fig. 4–6). These findings comprise a significant addition to the body of evidence implicating this little-studied region as an important node in the neural circuit underlying working memory processing; the caudomedial lobule is an intriguing focus for further lesion and electrophysiological studies.

Hippocampus and Dentate Gyrus

By contrast with the caudomedial lobule, the circuitry of the hippocampus and dentate gyrus is well studied. Indeed, the rather precise anatomic geometry of the dentate gyrus and the CA1 and CA3 fields of the hippocampus proper provides an opportunity to relate metabolic activity to separate functional pathways (for review: Rosene and Van Hoesen, 1987). While the circuitry is more complex than indicated here, it is basically the case that cortical afferent information is relayed to the hippocampus proper via entorhinal cortical afferents to the dentate gyrus. At the other end, hippocampal efferents are relayed to cortical targets via projections from the CA1 sector of the hippocampus to the subiculum. At the juncture, the CA3 sector of the hippocampus is both the recipient of information from the dentate gyrus and gives rise to collaterals that synapse in CA1. The data from our 2DG studies (Friedman and Goldman-Rakic, 1988) indicated that metabolic activity was highest in the two components, the dentate gyrus and CA1 field of the hippocampus, that are most closely related to cortical information processing (Fig. 4–7). And, as was the case for the caudomedial lobule, glucose utilization was significantly enhanced by nearly 20% in monkeys per-

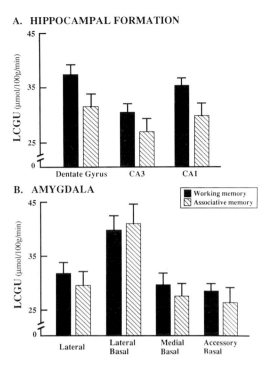

Figure 4–7 Local cerebral glucose utilization (LCGU) in the hippocampus, dentate gyrus, and the amygdala of monkeys performing working memory and associative memory tasks. (Adapted from Friedman and Goldman-Rakic, 1988.) **A:** Mean LCGU was significantly enhanced in the dentate gyrus and CA1 field of the hippocampus in monkeys performing working memory tasks relative to monkeys performing associative memory control tasks. No group differences in mean LCGU were evident in the CA3 field of the hippocampus. **B:** Mean LCGU in the basal and lateral nuclei of the amygdala was similar for the group of monkeys performing working memory tasks and the group of monkeys performing associative memory tasks. The results for three additional nuclei: the cortical, medial, and central nuclei of the amygdala (not shown) also revealed no group differences in LCGU.

forming the working memory tasks relative to monkeys performing the associative memory control tasks. By contrast, metabolic activity in the CA3 sector, though higher in the former than in the latter group, was not significantly different across the two groups of monkeys.

Amygdala

In the initial report of these data (Friedman and Goldman-Rakic, 1988), metabolic activity in the dentate gyrus and hippocampus was also compared with metabolic activity in the amygdala. Like the hippocampal formation, the role of the amygdala in memory processing also has been a topic of much research (for review: Sarter and Markowitsch, 1985), and the functional contribution of these structures has not yet been fully dissociated. The results of these 2DG studies, however, indicated that unlike the hippocampus and dentate gyrus, metabolic activity in the amygdala of the rhesus monkey does not differentiate between performance on working memory tasks and performance on associative memory tasks. For the four large nuclei of the basal-lateral amygdala (Fig. 4–7), mean LCGU differed by less than 10% across the two groups of monkeys; the results were similar for three additional nuclei (central, medial, and cortical nuclei) that were also measured (not shown in Fig. 4–7). These results suggest that the amygdala is not preferentially engaged by working memory processing in the monkey—a suggestion that is consonant with evidence showing that discrete lesions of the amygdala do not impair the performance of monkeys on spatial and recognition memory tasks or on discrimination problems (Zola-Morgan et al., 1989). Instead, the amygdala may play a common role in both the associative memory control tasks and the working memory tasks. Indeed, features of both the working memory and control tasks were similar with respect to their reward and motivational content, and many previous studies have emphasized the importance of the amygdala for encoding stimuli that have reward and motivational significance (e.g., Gaffan et al., 1989).

These data also underscore the proposal that prefrontal cortical connectivity is a hallmark of the neural circuit underlying spatial working memory processing. The sectors of the hippocampus and dentate gyrus that were most notably influenced by working memory performance are also most closely related to the flow of dorsolateral prefrontal cortical information. However, the anatomic connections of the amygdala are more closely related to orbital prefrontal and anterior cingulate cortex (Porrino et al., 1981; for review: Amaral, 1987).

FUTURE DIRECTIONS: CORTICAL CONTRIBUTION TO WORKING MEMORY

The special purpose network for cognition that we have proposed is made up of cortico-cortical connections to a large degree, and we are most interested in and are currently analyzing these cortical components. Some preliminary results have been obtained. For example, our early studies provided evidence that metabolic activity in prefrontal cortex is increased when monkeys are performing delayed-response tasks (Bugbee and Goldman-Rakic, 1981). And our preliminary analysis of the parietal cortex (Friedman and Goldman-Rakic, unpublished data) indicates as well that metabolic activity is preferentially enhanced in monkeys performing working memory tasks. However, it is well known that the metabolic activity in prefrontal cortex is not homogeneously distributed but rather takes the form of alternating patches of high and low metabolic activity. Therefore, we have decided that the best way to analyze the contribution of cortical areas is to examine specific cortical columns or territories in the same animal. To accomplish this goal, we have developed a powerful double-label 2DG method (Friedman et al., 1987; 1989) and are currently employing this technique for analysis of cortical circuitry.

A related goal is to more fully explore the potentially different contribution of spatial versus nonspatial working memory processing to brain metabolic activity. In our single-label 2DG studies, no profound differences in metabolic activity in the thalamus and in the components of the hippocampal formation could be attributed to the spatial versus nonspatial components of the three working memory tasks that were used (Friedman and Goldman-Rakic, 1988; Friedman et al., 1990). In part, these findings may be related to the nature of the nonspatial working memory task, delayed object alternation, that was tested. Although in this task the memory of object features was the relevant guide for performance, monkeys were quick to revert to a spatial strategy when the contingencies of the task were made more difficult (for discussion see: Friedman et al., 1990). Thus, one latent characteristic of this "nonspatial" task may be that it requires the successful inhibition of competing, *spatial* performance strategies; this capacity to suppress prepotent, but inappropriate, spatial response patterns has been linked to prefrontal cortical function (for review: Goldman-Rakic, 1987). Therefore, further studies using a behavioral paradigm that is more completely devoid of spatial attributes are warranted.

PARALLEL DISTRIBUTED NETWORKS FOR HIGHER CORTICAL FUNCTION

This chapter has reviewed recent data about the anatomical organization of two major connections of the principal sulcus—the thalamo-cortical and cortico-limbic. We have shown that these areas that are interconnected anatomically are also functionally related. They are all driven by tasks that require working memory, i.e., constant updating of information, relative to tasks that depend either on associative processes or tasks that require only sensorimotor performance. Furthermore, structures that are not connected directly with the principal sulcus do not exhibit the same dissociation of function. Thus, neither the amygdala nor the mammillary bodies were activated more by the working memory tasks than the control tasks. These findings indicate both a high degree of anatomic and functional specificity and tend to support our concept of a neural network dedicated to mnemonic processing of a particular type.

This view of parallel distributed circuitry emerging from our anatomical and metabolic studies is somewhat different from older models of cortical function, according to which sensory signals are progressively elaborated in sensory association cortices and information flow is thought of as mainly unidirectional, i.e., from sensory through associational to motor cortices. In these serial models, some sort of convergence occurs and increases at each stage along a hierarchy of areas such that integration of the different sensory inputs takes place in key polymodal areas like the posterior parietal (Mesulam et al., 1977; Seltzer and Pandya, 1980), the superior temporal polysensory area (Bruce et al., 1981), and/or prefrontal cortex (Barbas and Mesulam, 1985; Bignall and Imbert, 1969; Nauta, 1971; Pandya and Kuypers, 1969). In this scheme, the areas furthest removed from sensory receptors receive the information from a variety of modalities or sources and hence are considered as integrative centers.

The considerations discussed in the present chapter, however, lead toward a view that instead focuses on the distribution of function in parallel distributed systems. If this is so, the structures that compose a circuit should be coactivated during spatial working memory tasks; and other structures not embedded in the circuit should be no more engaged by spatial performance than in control conditions. So far, the evidence in nonhuman primates supports this view. But also, clinical and neuropsychological studies in humans concur. For example, studies of cerebral blood flow in normal humans show that different constellations of cortical areas are activated when subjects perform different types of psychological tasks. Tasks that demand "spatial thinking" by requiring subjects to perform internal route-finding operations activate several zones within the prefrontal cortex as well as components of the parietal, temporal, and occipital cortex (Roland and Friberg, 1985; Roland et al., 1987). This network of cortical areas may well represent the same circuit of interconnected cortico-cortical and thalamo-cortical regions that has been described in the nonhuman primate. By contrast, mathematical thinking (Roland and Friberg, 1985) or linguistic thinking (Petersen et al., 1988; Roland and Friberg, 1985) involves a similarly organized but differently distributed circuit, because blood flow studies show that these tasks activate distinctive sets of cortical areas. These findings emphasize that whereas the traditional ideas of hierarchic processing may apply to sensory processing within some systems, higher cortical functions in human and nonhuman primates appear to engage a finite number of dedicated parallel arrangements of reciprocally interconnected areas.

REFERENCES

Aggleton JP, Mishkin M. Visual recognition impairment following medial thalamic lesions in monkeys. Neuropsychologia 21:189–197, 1983a.

Aggleton JP, Mishkin M. Memory impairments following restricted medial thalamic lesions in monkeys. Exp Brain Res 52:199–209, 1983b.

Aggleton JP, Mishkin M. Mammillary-body lesions and visual recognition in monkeys. Exp Brain Res 58:190–197, 1985.

Amaral DG. Memory: anatomical organization of candidate brain regions. In F Plum (ed), Handbook of Physiology: The Nervous System, Vol 5, Bethesda, MD: American Physiological Society, 1987, pp. 211–294.

Baddeley AD. Working memory. Proc Trans R Soc Lond B 302:311–324, 1983.

Baddeley A. Working Memory. Oxford: Clarendon Press, 1986.

Baleydier C, Mauguiere F. Anatomical evidence for medial pulvinar connections with the posterior cingulate cortex, the retrosplenial area, and the posterior parahippocampal gyrus in monkeys. J Comp Neurol 232:219–228, 1985.

Barbas H, Mesulam M-M. Cortical afferent input to the principalis region of the rhesus monkey. Neuroscience 15:619–637, 1985.

Bignall KE, Imbert M. Polysensory and cortico-cortical projections to frontal lobe of squirrel and rhesus monkey. Electroencephologr Clin Neurophysiol 26:206–215, 1969.

Bruce CJ, Desimone R, Gross CG. Visual properties of neurons in a polysensory area in superior temporal sulcus of the macaque. J Neurophysiol 46:369–384, 1981.

Bugbee NM, Goldman-Rakic PS. Functional 2-deoxyglucose mapping in association cortex: Prefrontal activation in monkeys performing a cognitive task. Soc Neurosci Abstr 7:416, 1981.

Cavada C, Goldman-Rakic PS. Posterior parietal cortex in rhesus monkey: II. Evidence for segregated corticocortical networks linking sensory and limbic areas with the frontal lobe. J Comp Neurol 287:422–445, 1989.

Friedman HR, Bruce CJ, Goldman-Rakic PS. A sequential double-label ^{14}C and ^{3}H-2-DG technique: validation by double-dissociation of functional states. Exp Brain Res 66:543–554, 1987.

Friedman HR, Bruce CJ, Goldman-Rakic PS. Resolution of metabolic columns by a double-label 2-DG technique: Interdigitation and coincidence in visual cortical areas of the same monkey. J Neurosci 9:4111–4121, 1989.

Friedman HR, Goldman-Rakic PS. Activation of the hippocampus and dentate gyrus by working memory: A 2-deoxyglucose study of behaving rhesus monkeys. J Neurosci 8:4693–4706, 1988.

Friedman HR, Janas J, Goldman-Rakic PS. Enhancement of metabolic activity in the diencephalon of monkeys performing working memory tasks: A 2-deoxyglucose study in behaving rhesus monkeys. J Cognitive Neurosci 2:18–31, 1990.

Funahashi S, Bruce CJ, Goldman-Rakic PS. Mnemonic coding of visual space in the monkey's dorsolateral prefrontal cortex. J Neurophysiol 61:331–349, 1989.

Fuster JM. The Prefrontal Cortex. New York: Raven Press, 1989.

Fuster JM, Alexander GE. Neuron activity related to short-term memory. Science 173:652–654, 1971.

Fuster JM, Alexander GE. Firing changes in cells of the nucleus medialis dorsalis associated with delayed response behavior. Brain Res 61:79–91, 1973.

Gaffan D, Gaffan EA, Harrison S. Visual-visual associative learning and reward-association learning in monkeys: The role of the amygdala. J Neurosci 9:558–564, 1989.

Giguere M, Goldman-Rakic PS. Mediodorsal nucleus: Areal, laminar, and tangential distribution of afferents and efferents in the frontal lobe of rhesus monkeys. J Compar Neurol 277:195–213, 1988.

Goldman PS, Nauta WJH. An intricately patterned prefronto-caudate projection in the rhesus monkey. J Comp Neurol 171:369–386, 1977.

Goldman PS, Rosvold HE. Localization of function within the dorsolateral prefrontal cortex of the rhesus monkey. Exp Neurol 27:291–304, 1970.

Goldman-Rakic PS. Circuitry of primate prefrontal cortex and regulation of behavior by representational memory. *In* F Plum (ed), Handbook of Physiology: The Nervous System. Vol 5. Bethesda, MD: American Physiological Society, 1987, pp. 373–417.

Goldman-Rakic PS. Topography of cognition: Parallel distributed networks in primate association cortex. Annu Rev Neurosci 11:137–156, 1988.

Goldman-Rakic PS, Porrino LJ. The primate mediodorsal (MD) nucleus and its projection to the frontal lobe. J Comp Neurol 242:535–560, 1985.

Goldman-Rakic PS, Selemon LD, Schwartz MS. Dual pathways connecting the dorsolateral prefrontal cortex with the hippocampal formation and parahippocampal cortex in the rhesus monkey. Neuroscience 12:719–743, 1984.

Hikosaka O, Sakamoto M, Usui S. Functional properties of monkey caudate neurons. I. Activities related to saccadic eye movements. J Neurophysiol 61:780–798, 1989.

Holmes EJ, Jacobson S, Stein BM, Butters N. Ablations of the mammillary nuclei in monkeys: Effects on postoperative memory. Exp Neurol 81:97–113, 1983.

Ilinsky IA, Jouandet ML, Goldman-Rakic PS. Organization of the nigrothalamocortical system in the rhesus monkey. J. Comp Neurol 236:315–330, 1985.

Isseroff A, Rosvold HE, Galkin TW, Goldman-Rakic PS. Spatial memory impairments following damage to the mediodorsal nucleus of the thalamus in rhesus monkeys. Brain Res 232:107–113, 1982.

Jacobson S, Butters N, Tovsky NJ. Afferent and efferent subcortical projections of behaviorally defined sectors of prefrontal granular cortex. Brain Res 159:279–296, 1978.

Kievet J, Kuypers HGJM. Organization of the thalamo-cortical connexions to the frontal lobe in the rhesus monkey. Exp Brain Res 29:299–322, 1977.

Leichnitz GR. An interhemispheric columnar projection between two cortical multisensory convergence areas (inferior parietal lobule and prefrontal cortex): An anterograde study in macaque using HRP gel. Neurosci Lett 18:119–124, 1980.

Mesulam M-M, Van Hoesen GW, Pandya DN, Geschwind N. Limbic and sensory connections of the inferior parietal lobule (area PG) in the rhesus monkey: A study with the new method for horseradish peroxidase histochemistry. Brain Res 136:393–414, 1977.

Mountcastle VB, Motter BC Steinmetz MA, Duffy CJ. Looking and seeing: The visual functions of the parietal lobe. In GM Edelman, WE Gall, WM Cowan (eds), Dynamic Aspects of Neocortical Function. New York: John Wiley & Sons, 1984, pp. 159–193.

Nauta WJH. The problem of the frontal lobe: A reinterpretation. J Psychiatr Res 8:167–187, 1971.

Olton DS, Becker JT, Handelmann GE. Hippocampus, space and memory. Behav Brain Sci 2:313–365, 1979.

Pandya DN, Kuypers HGJM. Cortico-cortical connections in the rhesus monkey. Brain Res 13:13–36, 1969.

Passingham RE. Cortical mechanisms and cues for action. Philosophical Transactions Royal Society London B Biological Sciences 308:101–111, 1985.

Petersen SE, Fox PT, Posner MI, Mintun M, Raichle ME. Positron emission tomographic studies of the cortical anatomy of single-word processing. Nature 331:585–589, 1988.

Petrides M, Pandya DN. Projections to the frontal cortex from the posterior parietal region in the rhesus monkey. J Comp Neurol 228:105–116, 1984.

Piaget J. The Construction of Reality in the Child. New York: Basic Books, 1954.

Porrino LJ, Crane AM, Goldman-Rakic PS. Direct and indirect pathways from the amygdala to the frontal lobe in rhesus monkeys. J Comp Neurol 198:121–136, 1981.

Preuss TM, Goldman-Rakic PS. Crossed corticothalamic and thalamocortical connections of macaque prefrontal cortex. J Comp Neurol 257:269–281, 1987.

Richardson RT, DeLong MR. Nucleus basalis of Meynert neuronal activity during a delayed response task in the monkey. Brain Res 399:364–368, 1986.

Roland PE, Eriksson L, Stone-Elander S, Widen L. Does mental activity change the oxidative metabolism of the brain? J Neurosci 7:2373–2389, 1987.

Roland PE, Friberg L. Localization of cortical areas activated by thinking. J Neurophysiol 53:1219–1243, 1985.

Rosene DL, Van Hoesen GW. The hippocampal formation of the primate brain. In EG Jones, A Peters (eds), Cerebral Cortex. New York: Plenum Press, 1987, pp. 345–456.

Sarter M, Markowitsch HJ. Involvement of the amygdala in learning and memory: A critical review with emphasis on anatomical relations. Behav Neurosci 99:342–380, 1985.

Schulman S. Impaired delayed response from thalamic lesions. Arch Neurol 11:477–499, 1964.

Schwartz ML, Goldman-Rakic PS. Callosal and intrahemispheric connectivity of the prefrontal association cortex in rhesus monkey: Relation between intraparietal and principal sulcal cortex. J Comp Neurol 226:403–420, 1984.

Selemon LD, Goldman-Rakic PS. Common cortical and subcortical targets of the dorsolateral prefrontal and posterior parietal cortices in the rhesus monkey: Evidence for a distributed neural network subserving spatially guided behavior. J Neurosci 8:4049–4068, 1988.

Seltzer B, Pandya DN. Converging visual and somatic sensory cortical input to the intraparietal sulcus of the rhesus monkey. Brain Res 192:339–351, 1980.

Shallice T. From Neuropsychology to Mental Structure. Cambridge: Cambridge University Press, 1990.

Sokoloff L, Reivich M, Kennedy C, Des Rosiers MH, Patlak CS, Pettigrew KD, Sakurada O, Shinohara M. The ^{14}C-deoxyglucose method for the measurement of local cerebral glucose utilization: Theory, procedure, and normal values in the conscious and anesthetized albino rat. J Neurochem 28:897–916, 1977.

Squire LR, Cohen NJ. Human memory and amnesia. *In* G Lynch JL McGaugh, NM Weinberg (eds), Neurobiology of Learning and Memory. New York: Guilford, 1984, pp. 3–64.

Tulving E. Episodic and semantic memory. *In* E Tulving, W Donaldson (eds), Organization of Memory. New York: Academic Press, 1972, pp. 381–403.

Veazey RB, Amaral DG, Cowan WM. The morphology and connections of the posterior hypothalamus in the cynomolgus monkey (Macaca fascicularis). II. Efferent connections. J Comp Neurol 207:135–156, 1982.

Victor M, Adams RD, Collins GH. The Wernicke-Korsakoff Syndrome. Philadelphia: FA Davis, 1971.

Watanabe T, Niki H. Hippocampal unit activity and delayed response in the monkey. Brain Res 325:241–254, 1985.

Zola-Morgan S, Squire LR. Amnesia in monkeys after lesions of the mediodorsal nucleus of the thalamus. Ann Neurol 17:558–564, 1985a.

Zola-Morgan S, Squire LR. Medial temporal lesions in monkeys impair memory on a variety of tasks sensitive to human amnesia. Behav Neurosci 99:22–34, 1985b.

Zola-Morgan S, Squire LR, Amaral DG. Lesions of the hippocampal formation but not lesions of the fornix or the mammillary nuclei produce long-lasting memory impairments in monkeys. J Neurosci 9:898–913, 1989.

5

Neuroanatomy of Frontal Lobe in Vivo: A Comment on Methodology

HANNA C. DAMASIO

The technologic progress of the past 15 years has given us neuroimaging methods that permit the reliable in vivo investigation of human brain anatomy. Naturally they have become an invaluable tool in the understanding of the functional role of frontal lobe cortices.

There are two main types of neuroimaging procedures available: *Structural* imaging, such as magnetic resonance imaging (MR) and X-ray computerized tomography (CT); and *dynamic* imaging such as positron (dual photon) emission tomography (PET), and single photon detection (the latter can use either single photon emission computerized tomography (SPECT), or lateral probes). The dynamic imaging methods reveal indexes of functional activity in varied brain regions, rather than their detailed structure. Although both structural and dynamic procedures have contributed to our understanding of frontal lobe function, it should be no surprise that the structural approach is still paying off the best. The dynamic approaches, which are both newer and more complex, are still struggling with many technologic and theoretic problems, although it should be clear that their promise is truly outstanding.

In its most refined version for use in human subjects, MR can resolve brain structures to about 0.5 millimeter. It can deliver, in vivo, a "brain autopsy" at gross anatomy level. It allows for correlation of anatomic findings with the results of neuropsychologic experiments obtained *contemporaneously.* And, in so doing, it permits the use of circumscribed lesions as probes to the state of hypothetic neural systems posited for the human brain in relation to specified cognitive functions.

GENERAL FRONTAL LOBE ANATOMY

In order to take full advantage of MR, a thorough knowledge of anatomy is indispensable. No doubt this is true for any brain region, but it becomes even more so in relation to the frontal lobe because of the paucity of reliable land-marks in this region (see Crosby et al., 1962; Mesulam, 1987; Truex and Car-penter, 1969).

The frontal cortices constitute about half of the entire cerebral mantle. Their posterior limit is the central sulcus. Their mesial border is the corpus cal-losum. The central sulcus runs in the lateral surface of the hemisphere, from approximately the midpoint of the hemisphere circumference, interiorly and anteriorly, toward the temporal lobe. The precentral sulcus lies parallel and ante-rior to the central sulcus. There are two other major sulci to consider in the lateral surface of the frontal lobe: The superior frontal and the inferior frontal. Both have an anteroposterior course starting at the lower, orbital border of the lateral surface of the frontal lobe, and abutting in the precentral sulcus. In the mesial surface the most important sulcus is the cingulate, which runs antero-posteriorly, parallel to the corpus callosum (which is itself separated from the frontal lobe by the pericallosal sulcus).

Several gyral subcomponents need to be considered: (1) The precentral gyrus, which runs parallel to the central sulcus and constitutes the most caudal sector of the frontal lobe; its anterior limit is the precentral sulcus; (2) the first or superior frontal gyrus, which occupies the mesial and most anterior sector of the frontal lobe and is limited by the cingulate sulcus medially, by the superior frontal sulcus laterally, and by the superior sector of the precentral sulcus pos-teriorly; (3) the second or middle frontal gyrus, parallel to the first frontal gyrus and occupying a more lateral and inferior position, between the superior and the inferior frontal sulci; (4) the third or inferior frontal gyrus most of which consti-tutes the frontal operculum; (5) the orbital frontal gyri, which include the gyrus rectus (which runs anteroposteriorly and forms the mesial limit of the orbital sector), and the orbital gyri themselves; (6) the cingulate gyrus, which runs par-allel to the corpus callosum and is separated from the remainder of the mesial frontal area by the cingulate sulcus. This gyrus continues into the region of the mesial parietal lobe. It is the anterior half that may be considered under the area of the frontal lobe. The operculum can be divided in three sections: the pars opercularis (the most posterior sector immediately in front of the inferior seg-ment of the precentral gyrus), the pars triangularis (immediately in front and below the pars opercularis), and the pars orbitalis (the most inferior sector).

The same landmarks that define these gyri in gross anatomic terms must be used to define them in either CT or MR. However, this is easier said than done. If we take an unmarked brain and inspect its lateral surface (Fig. 5–1**A** and **D**) it is not an easy task to decide speedily and unequivocally where the superior, middle, and inferior frontal gyri run. Even the identification of the well-known central sulcus may pose problems. In the lateral surface of the brain, this partic-ular sulcus is sandwiched between the postcentral and precentral gyri, and in its downward course it usually does not reach the sylvian fissure, a fact that can help its identification. In the mesial surface of the hemispheres (Fig. 5–1**B** and **E**) the frontal areas are somewhat more straightforward, e.g., the cingulate sulcus is readily identifiable as the sulcus parallel to the corpus callosum and the peri-callosal sulcus. In its posterior sector it curves upward forming the ascending branch of the cingulate sulcus, which constitutes an important orienting land-

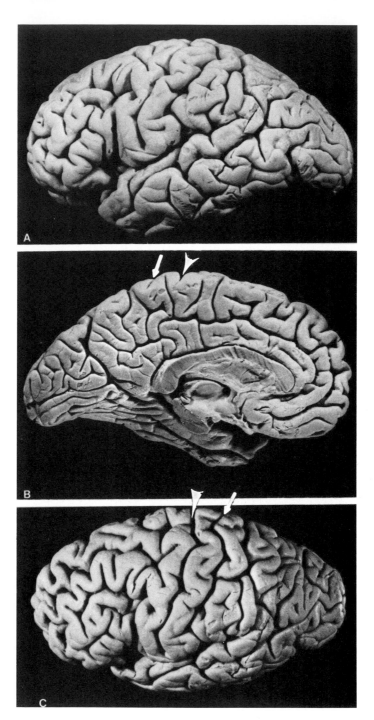

Figure 5–1 Left **(A, B, C)** and right **(D, E, F)** hemispheres of a human brain. Lateral (**A** and **C**), mesial (**B** and **E**), and superior (**C** and **F**) views. In Figures 5–2 and 5–3, which depict the same brain, the main sulci and gyri have been identified. Arrowhead points to central sulcus. Thick arrow points to the precentral sulcus. Thin arrow points to the post-central sulcus.

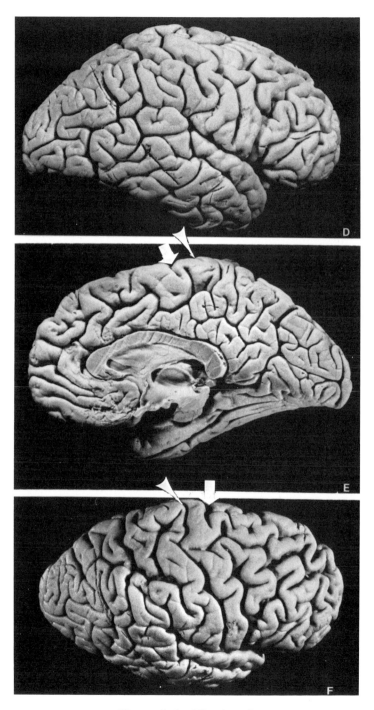

Figure 5–1 (*Continued*)

mark, as will be seen later. Yet, the posterior limit of the mesial frontal region may again pose some problems. The mesial extension of the central sulcus must be identified. It is known that in the mesial surface this sulcus is only seen for a small extension and that it should have an anteroposterior course. But in the brain depicted in Figure 5-1**B** and **E,** there seem to be two candidates for the role (arrows). In order to decide which of the two is the central sulcus, we must look for the ascending branch of the cingulate sulcus mentioned before. The mesial tip of the central sulcus lies immediately anterior to it. In the particular case depicted in Figure 5-1, looking at the two hemispheres from above (Fig. 5-1**C** and **F**) can further help in the decision. In the left hemisphere it can be seen that the postcentral sulcus (thin arrow) is evident in the mesial aspect, pointing to the fact that in the straight mesial view the central sulcus (arrowhead) should be the anterior of the two possible candidates. On the other hand, in the right hemisphere it is the precentral gyrus that is deeper and more evident (Fig. 5-1**F**, thick arrow) and therefore, in the **E** panel it is the posterior depression that corresponds to the central sulcus (arrowhead). For the identification of these anatomic events refer to Figures 5-2 and 5-3.

FURTHER BREAKDOWN OF FRONTAL LOBE ANATOMY

Cytoarchitectonic Fields

From the point of view of neuroimaging analysis, the most complex aspect of frontal lobe anatomy is its cytoarchitectonic structure. The cytoarchitectonic divisions used in our laboratory to generate anatomic "areas of interest" are largely based on the classic Brodmann's maps of cytoarchitectonic fields (Brodmann, 1909; 1925). Because Brodmann did not map the ventral surface of the frontal lobe, we also include the extension that E. Beck introduced in 1949 to deal with the orbital region (Beck, 1949). In addition, we take into consideration the more recent maps of F. Sanides (1964) and Braak (1980).

We consider area 4 to occupy the depth of the central sulcus and reach the dorsolateral surface of the precentral gyrus, at the level of the middle frontal gyrus continuing to expand, in fanlike fashion, to occupy the lateral surface of the precentral gyrus. In the mesial sector, it goes on to occupy the paracentral lobule.

Area 6 constitutes an anteriorly located mantle to area 4, occupying the remainder of the precentral gyrus as well as the superior and posterior sector of the middle frontal gyrus and the posterior segment of the superior frontal gyrus, both in its lateral and mesial surface.

Areas 44, 45, and 47 correspond roughly to the pars opercularis, pars triangularis, and pars orbitalis, respectively.

Area 8 is a relatively narrow band, just in front of area 6, in the superior and middle frontal gyri.

Areas 9 and 10 constitute parallel bands occupying the frontopolar area in the superior and middle frontal gyri with 9 just anterior to 8, and 10 below 9.

Area 46 can be found on the anterior dorsolateral surface, in the inferior portion of the middle frontal gyrus, above the most lateral portion of area 10 and otherwise surrounded by area 9.

In the mesial surface of the frontal lobe, apart from the mesial extensions of areas 4 and 6 that reach the cingulate sulcus, we find the extension of areas 8, 9, and 10 that abut at area 32. This area forms an anterior cap to the cingulate gyrus.

Area 24 corresponds to the anterior cingulate gyrus. In the orbital region area 11 occupies the more lateral sector and area 12 the more mesial one. The most posterior sector corresponds to area 25. Figure 5–4 shows these cytoarchitectonic markings on a left hemisphere.

Functional Regions

From a functional standpoint, the frontal lobe is traditionally divided into motor, premotor, prefrontal, and limbic sectors. Because these four divisions are directly linked to cytoarchitectonic structure, it is not any easier to delineate them, at macroscopic level, than to assign cytoarchitectonic fields. There is not much trouble in defining the posterior border of the motor region, since it coincides with the central sulcus. But that is the extent to which we can come with ease. The separation between motor and premotor is fuzzy, and the border between premotor and prefrontal is worse. It is generally accepted that the transition from motor to premotor cortex occurs with the change from area 4 to area 6. The transition from premotor to prefrontal cortex corresponds to the anterior limit of areas 6 and 44, but since there are no clearly identifiable gross anatomic landmarks, in the absence of cytologic studies, the division is somewhat arbitrary. Figure 5–5* shows the most generally accepted borders (see Fuster, 1989; Mesulam, 1987; Stuss and Benson, 1986). The prefrontal region commonly is subdivided further into dorsolateral prefrontal, mesial prefrontal, and orbital prefrontal. There are no clear limits for these areas either, as might be expected. The limbic component of the frontal lobe includes the anterior cingulate and the posterior sector of the orbital frontal surface.

Vascular Territories

Another important aspect of frontal anatomy that must be considered in imaging studies pertains to the vascular supply. This becomes an especially important issue in instances of stroke, the best type of neuropathologic specimen available for lesion method studies, because the placement of lesions directly reflects the patterns of supply. As shown in Figure 5–6, most of the dorsolateral sector of the frontal lobe, the inferior and middle frontal gyri and the lateral sector of the superior frontal gyrus as well as most of the precentral gyrus, lie in the territory of the anterior branches of the middle cerebral artery (orbitofrontal, prefrontal, precentral, and central branches). The mesial, superior frontal, and cingulate gyri and the mesial extension of the precentral gyrus, the paracentral lobule, and orbital sectors are supplied by the anterior branches of the anterior cerebral

*See color section for Figures 5–5, 5–6, 5–7, 5–8B, 5–9B, 5–10B, 5–11B, and 5–13B.

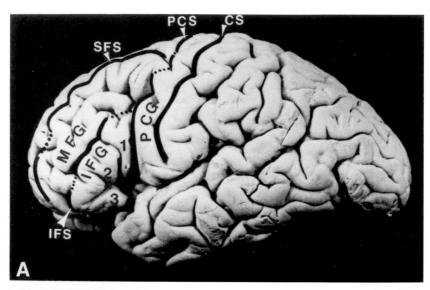

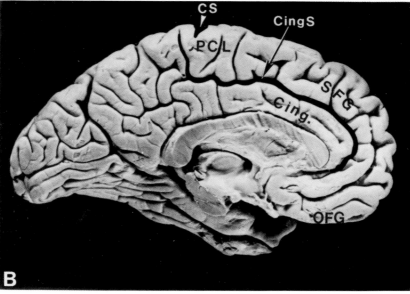

Figure 5–2 **A** and **B** left hemisphere in lateral and mesial views, respectively. **C** and **D** right hemisphere in lateral and mesial views. CS, central sulcus; PCS, precentral sulcus; SFS, superior frontal sulcus; IFS, inferior frontal sulcus; CinS, cingulate sulcus (the posterior sector curved upward is designated the ascending branch); PCG, precentral gyrus; SFG, superior frontal gyrus; MFG, middle frontal gyrus; IFG, inferior frontal gyrus (1, pars opercularis; 2, pars triangularis; 3, pars orbitalis); OFG, orbital frontal gyri; PCL, paracentral lobule; Cing, cingulate gyrus.

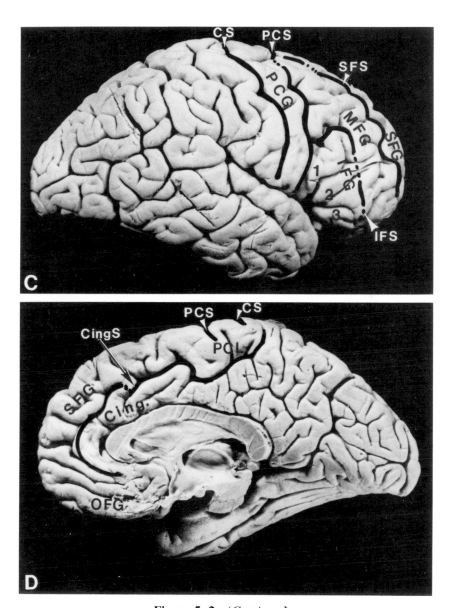

Figure 5–2 (*Continued*)

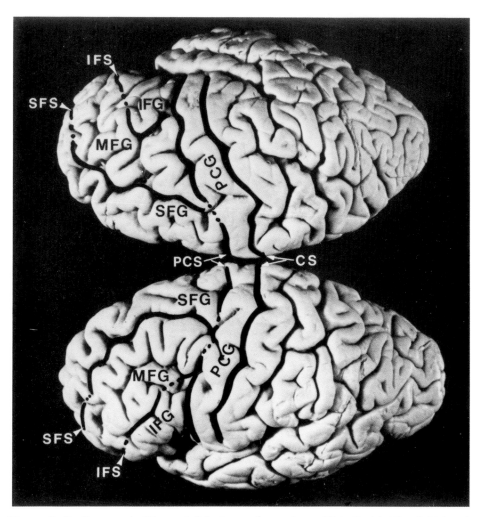

Figure 5–3 Same as in Figure 5–2 but seen from above. Note that in the right hemisphere **(top)** the precentral sulcus is deeper than in the left **(bottom)** when it reaches the mesial surface. Compare with the mesial views of the two hemispheres in Figure 5–2.

artery (orbitofrontal, anterior-middle, and posterior internal frontal and paracentral branches). The two territories overlap creating the anterior watershed or border zone, which covers the lateral sector of the superior frontal gyrus and the mesial sector of the middle frontal gyrus (see Lazorthes et al., 1976; Waddington, 1974).

READING FRONTAL LOBE ANATOMY FROM NEUROIMAGING DATA

Given the problems that frontal lobe anatomy poses, even in a real postmortem specimen, one wonders how different sulci and gyri can ever be identified in CT

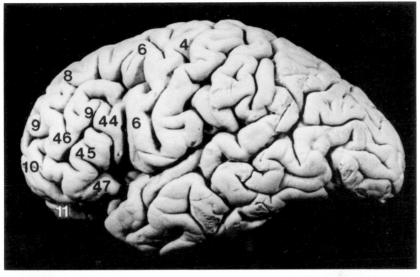

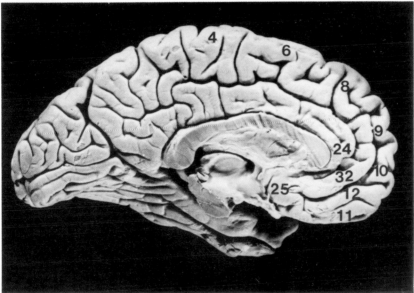

Figure 5–4 Brodmann's major cytoarchitectonic fields depicted in lateral and mesial views of the left hemisphere.

or MR films. The answer is that they can, thanks to the good anatomic detail that MR offers, along with images in three orthogonal planes (transverse, coronal, and parasagittal). MR allows for a good three-dimensional reconstruction and is clearly the method of choice. It permits us to localize precisely any site of damage from a stroke or area of resection within the frontal lobe (Damasio and Damasio, 1989). But even here precision does not come easily. Most often, MR scans that are not performed for research purposes are obtained in one or two

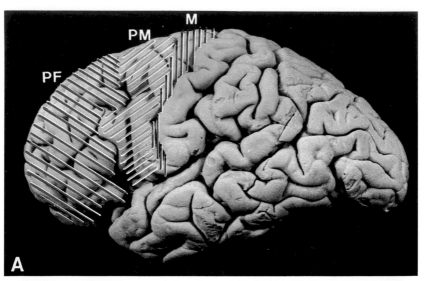

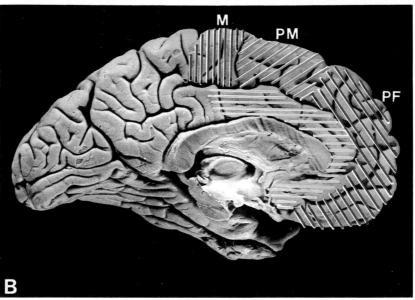

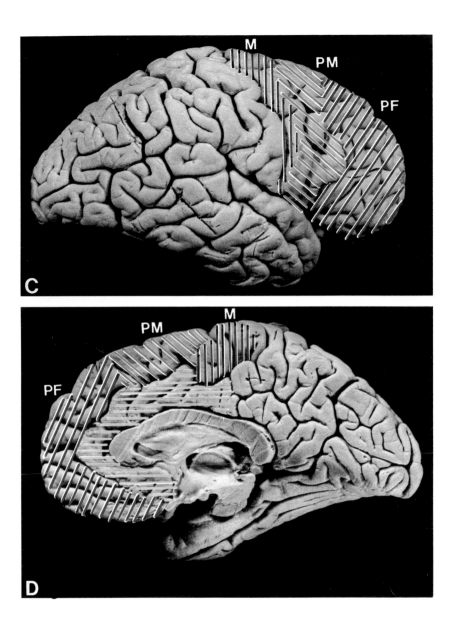

Figure 5–5 Functional regions of the frontal lobe, motor (M blue), premotor (PM green), and prefrontal (PF red) seen in the left hemisphere (**A** lateral, **B** mesial views) and the right hemisphere (**C** lateral, **D** mesial views). The limbic region is marked in yellow.

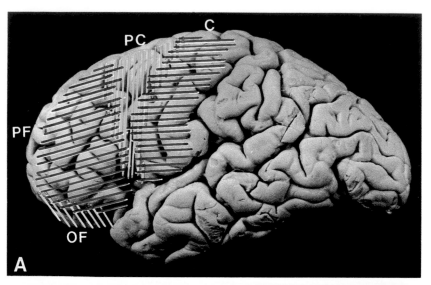

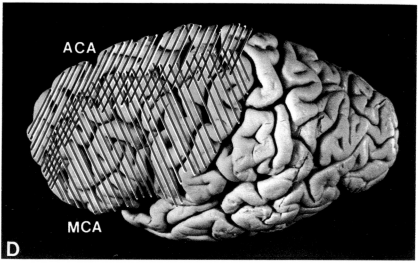

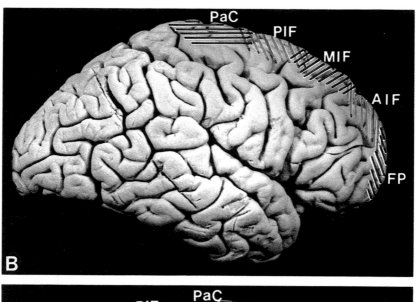

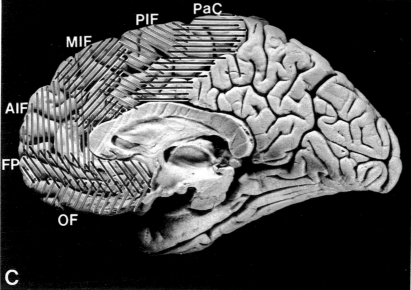

Figure 5–6 **A:** Lateral view of the left hemisphere showing the area supplied by the anterior branches of the middle cerebral artery. **B and C:** Lateral (B) and mesial (C) view of the right hemisphere showing the territory of the anterior cerebral artery. **D:** Left hemisphere seen from above showing the area of overlap of the two vascular territories seen in A and B (the watershed or border zone). ACA, anterior cerebral artery; MCA, middle cerebral artery; OF, orbitofrontal branches (note that both the anterior cerebral artery and the middle cerebral artery have orbitofrontal branches); PF, prefrontal branch; PC, precentral branch; C, central branch; FP, frontopolar branch; AIF, anterior internal frontal branch; MIF, middle internal frontal branch; PIF, posterior internal frontal branch; PaC, paracentral branch.

incidences alone, usually transverse and coronal. As for CTs, they are generally obtained in transverse sections only. In order to interpret such images we must rely on template systems or anatomic atlases to help with anatomic interpretation (Damasio and Damasio, 1989; Matsui and Hirano, 1978; Roberts and Hanaway, 1970). The most reliable way to analyze MR and CT images of frontal lobe damage in order to establish the anatomic placement of lesions relies on the interactive transfer of the contour of the damaged area to an appropriate set of templates, using an X/Y plotting strategy (see Damasio and Damasio, 1989 for a detailed explanation of the method).

The angle of incidence of CT or MR is of paramount importance. The relative position of the different gyri varies significantly if the angulation of the MR/CT cuts varies in relation to the inferior orbitomeatal line. Figure 5–7 shows the left hemisphere in lateral (A) and mesial (B) views. The colored lines indicate the orientation of the cuts seen in Figures 5–8 through 5–13. Figures 5–8 through 5–10 illustrate how the view of the frontal lobe changes in transverse cuts, when the scanning incidence changes from an approximately caudal angle of 10 degrees to the orbitomeatal line, to a negative, rostral angle. Consider the area depicting frontal lobe in these three incidences. In the caudal angulation seen in Figure 5–9, the lower cuts show the *anterior one-fourth* occupied by frontal lobe. In the higher cuts, however, all of the *anterior half* is taken up by the frontal lobe. But in the horizontal cuts of Figure 5–8, the lower sections show only the *anterior one-third* occupied by the frontal lobe, while in the highest sections the frontal lobe occupies most of the cut (the *anterior three-fourths*). In sections obtained with a negative (rostral) tilt (Fig. 5–10), the lower images show the frontal lobe only at the most anterior rim of the cut, while in the two highest sections, the frontal lobe occupies virtually the entire area.

The apparent relation between the three major frontal gyri (the superior, middle, and inferior), and the precentral gyrus also varies with the incidence. In the caudal angulation (Fig. 5–9) the three frontal gyri (superior = blue, middle = red, and inferior = green) are visible simultaneously, immediately above the level of the orbital gyri. The precentral gyrus (yellow) is added in the next section. However, in the horizontal sections (Fig. 5–8) the inferior frontal gyrus is seen first (next to the orbital gyri), and it is only in the section above that the remaining gyri can be detected. In the sections obtained with a negative (rostral) angulation the relations are even more distorted (Fig. 5–9). To begin with, the orbital gyri are seen, from the lower to higher sections, in a caudal-rostral direction. First the most caudal portion is seen, and, only two cuts above, does the rostral tip appear. Moreover, when the rostral orbital sector becomes visible, the most posterior and inferior portion of the middle frontal gyrus is next to it followed by the inferior frontal gyrus and the precentral gyrus.

In Figure 5–10, at first glance the relation between frontal lobe structures and lateral ventricles may seem odd. It is difficult to imagine how the frontal lobe can be seen *anteriorly and posteriorly* to the image of what appears to be the *body of the lateral ventricle* (cuts 5 and 6). However, with the help of line C–C in Figure 5–7, it becomes evident that the ventricular component seen in cut 5 is merely the *frontal horn* and *the very anterior portion* of the body of the lateral ventricle.

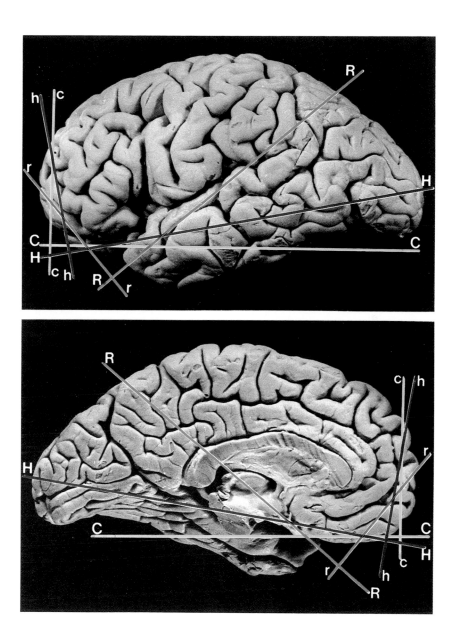

Figure 5–7 Left hemisphere in lateral and mesial views. The different colored lines indicate the orientation of the cuts seen in Figures 5–8 through 5–13. H-H (red), approximate level of the first transverse cut in which the frontal lobe is seen in Figure 5–8. h-h (red), approximate level of the first coronal cut seen in Figure 5–11. C-C and c-c (yellow), same as H-H and h-h but for Figures 5–9 and 5–12, respectively. R-R and r-r (green), same as H-H and h-h but for Figures 5–10 and 5–13, respectively.

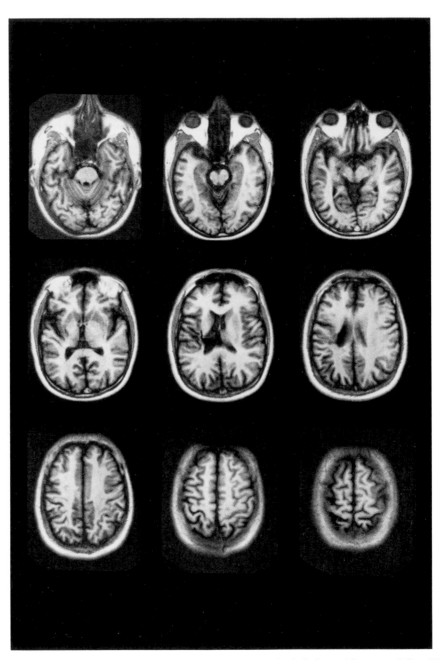

Figure 5–8 A: T₁ weighted MR obtained parallel to the inferior orbitomeatal line (H-H in Figure 5–7).

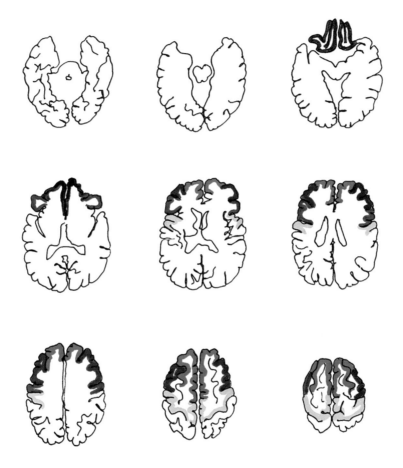

Figure 5–8 B: Line drawing of the sections showing the frontal lobe. The different frontal gyri are depicted in different colors: purple, orbital gyri; blue, superior frontal gyrus; red, middle frontal gyrus; green, inferior frontal gyrus; yellow, precentral gyrus and mesially the paracentral lobule. The cingulate gyrus was left unmarked.

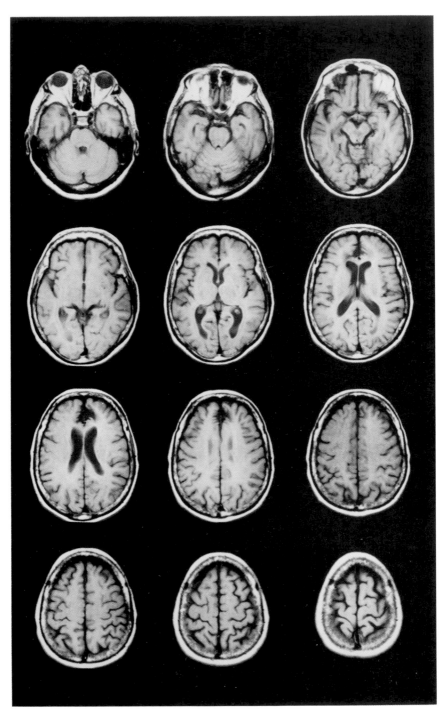

Figure 5–9 **A:** T$_1$ weighted MR obtained at approximately 10 degree caudal angulation to the inferior orbitomeatal line (C-C in Figure 5–7).

110

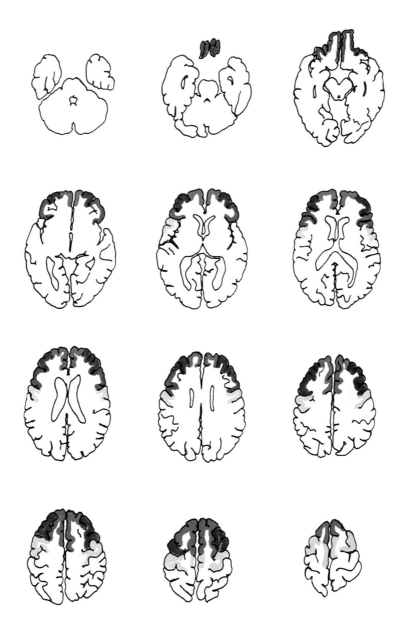

Figure 5-9 B: Line drawing of the cuts in this MR that show the frontal lobe. Color code as in Figure 5-8.

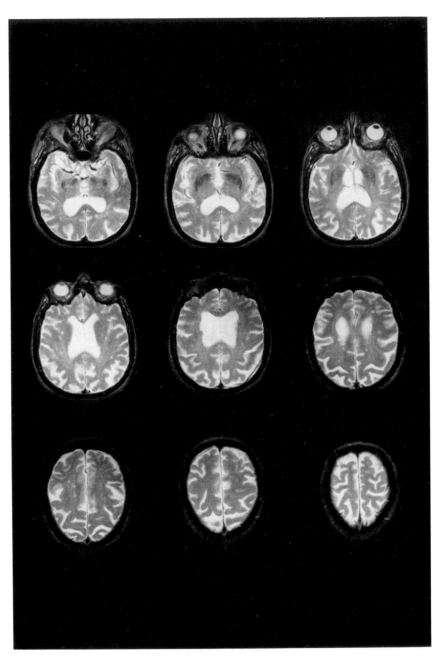

Figure 5–10 **A:** T_2 weighted MR obtained with a negative tilt (rostral tilt) in relation to the inferior orbitomeatal line (R-R in Figure 5–7).

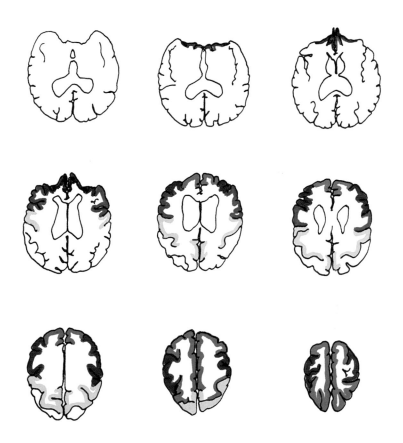

Figure 5–10 **B:** Line drawing of the sections showing the frontal lobe. Color code as in Figure 5–8.

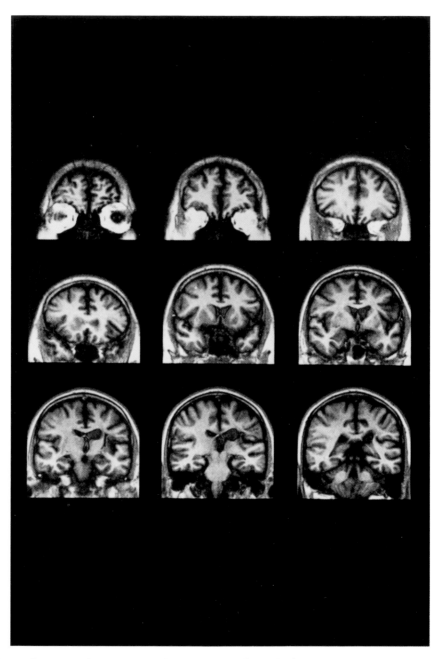

Figure 5–11 **A:** Coronal, T_1 weighted, MR sections obtained at a 90 degree angle to the sections depicted in Figure 5–8 (h-h in Figure 5–7).

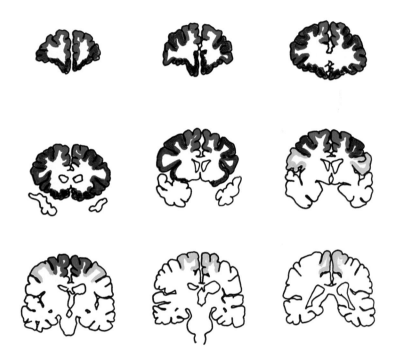

Figure 5–11   B: Line drawing showing the frontal lobe structures. Color code as in Figure 5–8.

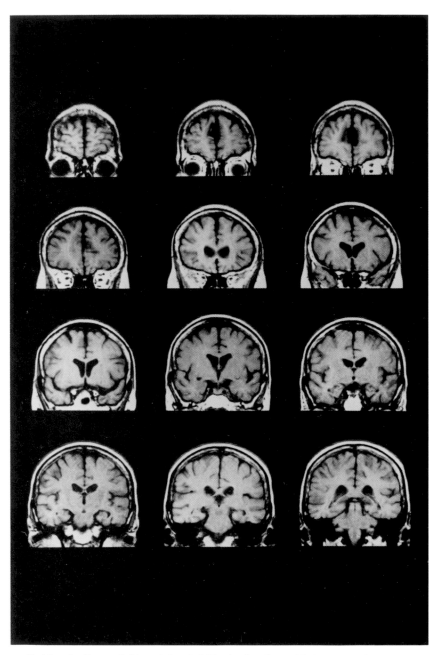

Figure 5–12 **A:** Coronal, T_1 weighted, MR obtained at a 90 degree angle to the sections depicted on Figure 5–9 (c-c in Figure 5–7).

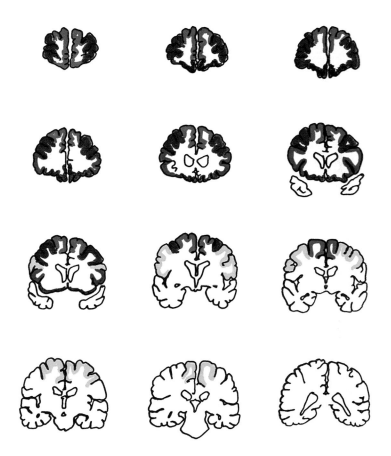

Figure 5–12   B: Line drawing depicting the frontal lobe structures. Color code as in Figure 5–8.

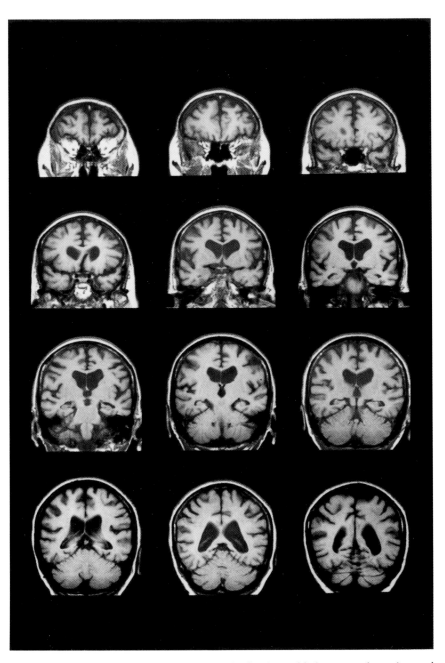

Figure 5–13 **A:** Coronal, T_1 weighted, MR obtained at a 90 degree angle to the sections depicted in Figure 5–10 (r-r in Figure 5–7).

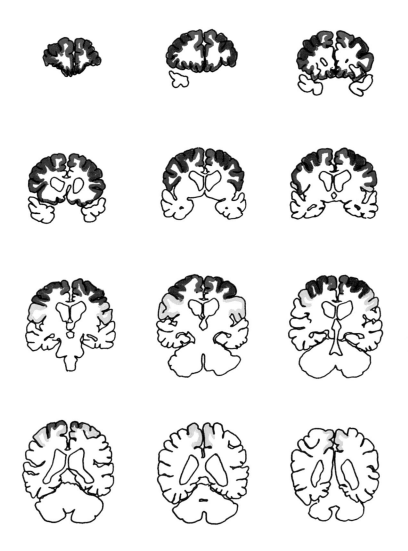

Figure 5–13 **B:** Line drawing depicting the frontal lobe structures. Color code as in Figure 5–8.

It is important to note that when regular coronal cuts are obtained with MR, these are at a 90 degree angle in relation to the plane of the transverse cuts, i.e., when the plane of transverse sections changes, so does the plane of the coronal sections (see Figs. 5–7 and 5–11 through 5–13). This fact will once again change anatomic relations. For instance, coronal sections obtained at a 90 degree angle to the caudally angulated transverse cuts of Figure 5–9 show, in the more anterior section, the superior frontal gyrus located mesially and the middle frontal gyrus located laterally to it. No segment of the orbital gyri can be seen (Fig. 5–12). However, in the coronal cuts of Figure 5–11 and in those of Figure 5–13 (obtained, respectively, at a 90 degree angle to the cuts seen in Figures 5–8 and 5–10), the more anterior sections show orbital frontal lobe and, to a different extent, part of the superior and middle frontal gyrus.

At the more posterior level, the last portion of the frontal lobe to be seen is the posterior segment of the paracentral lobule. In a straight coronal cut this coincides with the image of the splenium (Fig. 5–11). In Figure 5–12, however, this same section of the frontal lobe is seen before we reach the splenium; on the other hand, in Figure 5–13, it only happens after the callosum has disappeared.

It is important to make clear that modern MR scanners are not limited to these orthogonal planes. Almost any angulation can be obtained, but unless it is especially requested, it will not be attempted routinely. Furthermore, the collaboration of the patient or his physical limitations (neck mobility) may dictate the position of the patient in the scanner.

DYNAMIC NEUROIMAGING STUDIES

Elsewhere in this volume (Chapter 14) the use of dynamic imaging methods in the study of the frontal lobe is discussed (Weinberger et al., this volume). My remarks here are general.

Both SPET and PET are exciting new tools and they have already given us interesting new information on the frontal lobe as can be judged from Weinberger's activation studies in schizophrenics, and our own and Raichle's work with language activation tasks (Damasio et al., 1986; Petersen et al., 1988). It is important to realize, however, that PET studies still face problems in their development. Leaving aside theoretic assumptions behind the activation paradigms, I will highlight two critical areas: (1) The poor resolution of available scanners, and (2) the defective anatomic localization of activation areas. The former will easily be solved by technologic developments. But the latter is more difficult to overcome. PET does not have anatomic landmarks, and current localization methods are largely guesswork. This applies to all available methods including the stereotactic method, which may be reasonably on target when subcortical gray areas are the aim of the studies, but which is not reliable when the focus is on cortical activity.

ACKNOWLEDGMENTS

This study was supported by NINCDS Grant P01 NS19632.

REFERENCES

Beck E. A cytoarchitectural investigation into the boundaries of cortical areas 13 and 14 in the human brain. Journal of Anatomy 83:147–157, 1949.

Braak H. Architectonics of the Human Telencephalic Cortex. New York, Springer-Verlag, 1980.

Brodmann K. Vergleichende Lokalisations Lehre der Grosshirninde. Leipzig, JA Barth, 1909, 1925.

Crosby EC, Humphrey T, Lauer EW. Correlative Anatomy of the Nervous System. New York, Macmillan, 1962.

Damasio H, Damasio AR. Lesion Analysis in Neuropsychology, New York, Oxford University Press, 1989.

Damasio H, Rezai K, Eslinger PJ, Kirchner P, Van Gilder J. SPET patterns of activation in intact and focally damaged components of a language-related network. Neurology 36:316, 1986.

Fuster JM. The Prefrontal Cortex, 2nd Ed. New York, Raven Press, 1989.

Lazorthes G, Gouaze A, Salamon G. Vascularisation et Circulation de l'Encéphale, Paris, Masson, 1976.

Matsui T, Hirano A. An Atlas of the Human Brain for Computerized Tomography. Tokyo, Igaku-Shoin Ltd., 1978.

Mesulam M-M. Patterns in behavioral neuroanatomy: Association areas, the limbic system, and hemispheric specialization. Principles of Behavioral Neurology. Philadelphia, FA Davis, 1987.

Petersen SE, Fox PT, Posner MI, Mintun M, Raichle ME. Positron emission tomographic studies of the cortical anatomy of single-word processing. Nature 331:585–589, 1988.

Roberts M, Hanaway J. Atlas of the Human Brain in Section. Philadelphia, Lea & Febiger, 1970.

Sanides F. The cyto-myeloarchitecture of the human frontal lobe and its relation to phylogenetic differentiation of the cerebral cortex. Journal für Hirnforschung 6:269–282, 1964.

Stuss DT, Benson DF. The Frontal Lobes. New York, Raven Press, 1986.

Truex RC, Carpenter MB. Human Neuroanatomy. Baltimore, Williams & Wilkins Co., 1969.

Waddington MM. Atlas of Cerebral Angiography with Anatomic Correlation. Boston, Little, Brown, 1974.

Weinberger D, Berman KF, Daniel DG. Prefrontal Cortex Dysfunction in Schizophrenia. *In* Frontal Lobe Function and Dysfunction, Levin HS, Eisenberg HM, Benton AL (eds), Oxford University Press, 1991.

III

Cognitive Functioning in Patients with Frontal Lobe Lesions

6

Higher-Order Cognitive Impairments and Frontal Lobe Lesions in Man

TIM SHALLICE
AND PAUL BURGESS

It has long been well known that some patients with lesions to the prefrontal cortex can perform well on some types of demanding cognitive tasks such as WAIS IQ tests, but can have difficulties on some specific problem-solving tasks or in dealing with the types of practical problems that occur in everyday life (Eslinger and Damasio, 1985; Milner, 1964; Stuss and Benson, 1986). The theories that have been put forward to account for this dissociation have tended to be couched in descriptive language and in one case in gestalt terminology. Thus Jouandet and Gazzaniga (1979) characterized the frontal lobes as a system that sequences or guides behavior toward the attainment of some more immediate or distant goal. Damasio (1985) viewed the dorsolateral region of the frontal lobes as critical for "the coherent organization of mental contents on which creative thinking and language depend, and that permit, in general, artistic activities and the planning of future actions" (p. 369).

Fuster (1980) gives a more detailed theoretical account. However, his basic position is that the frontal lobes are critical for the formation and realization of temporal gestalts; he therefore employed a theoretical framework little used in modern studies of normal problem solving. Yet, to develop an adequate theory of the difficulties experienced by patients with frontal lobe lesions it is necessary to relate their problems to cognitive science theorizing on normal problem solving in an analogous way to that through which conceptual correspondences have been obtained between normal and abnormal processing for perceptual, memory, and language functions.

One neuropsychological theory that seems promising in this respect is Luria's (1966) approach to the frontal lobes as a system for the programming, regulation, and verification of activity. A model developed by Norman and Shallice (1986, Shallice, 1982; 1988) can be viewed as one possible realization of Luria's theory in information-processing terms. When we developed our model we were attempting to explain not only neuropsychological findings on frontal lobe patients but also empirical phenomena in the experimental psychology of attention and in the phenomenology of attention to action. It was therefore linked directly with studies of normal subjects.

The most important assumption of our model is also present in artificial intelligence models of problem solving such as those of Fahlman (1974), Sussman (1975), and more especially the best developed and tested general problem-solving model at present available, i.e., SOAR (Laird et al., 1987). This assumption is that the processes involved in the cognitive control of action and thought operations are divisible into two levels or modes. One mode is where potentially demanding but routine action or thought operations when selected by well-learned triggering procedures are sufficient to carry out a task satisfactorily. The second is where such routine operations are insufficient for achieving the goal and some form of explicit modulation or novel activity must be carried out. In addition, these models have in common the assumption that the higher-level processes—for instance those involving the Supervisory System of the Norman and Shallice model or the post-impasse procedures of Laird et al.—come into effective operation only when the routine lower levels of the system cannot solve whatever problem they have been presented.

The way the lower and higher levels of the system operate differs between the models. With respect to the lower level the Norman/Shallice model differs from the others in attempting to incorporate two assumptions compatible with work in the neurosciences. The first is that on-line cognitive operations are carried out by a large set of specific resources (modules?). The second is that a routine mutual inhibitory device exists for selecting which action is to be carried out when there are competing possibilities (Fig. 6–1). The basic control elements in the model have certain similarities to classic S-R bonds but are more directly derived from condition-action pairs of production system models of problem solving (e.g., Newell and Simon, 1972). The position is that a very large but finite set of action and thought schemas—like programs—can each be activated if the respective well-learned triggers (either from the perceptual system or from the output of just recently active schemas) are excited. A selected schema, one for which the activation level has reached threshold, in turn activates its component (child) schemas and can exercise control over any of the special-purpose processing resources it requires. Competition between schemas for control of the cognitive apparatus is effected by means of a lateral inhibitory mechanism—so-called Contention Scheduling—which prevents two competing schemas that require the same resource being selected.[1] Modulating the activation level of schemas and so biasing their probability of being selected in Contention Scheduling is the function of the Supervisory System.

How could one assess on such a model whether damage to the Supervisory System would be an adequate explanation of disorders seen after prefrontal lesions? This question can be addressed on four different levels. The first procedure would be to ask what sort of characteristics the lower level of the system, Contention Scheduling, would have if operating without modulation from a Supervisory System and to consider whether these correspond to characteristics of patients with prefrontal lesions. A second approach is to develop tasks that intuitively appear to require the processes the Supervisory System is held to carry

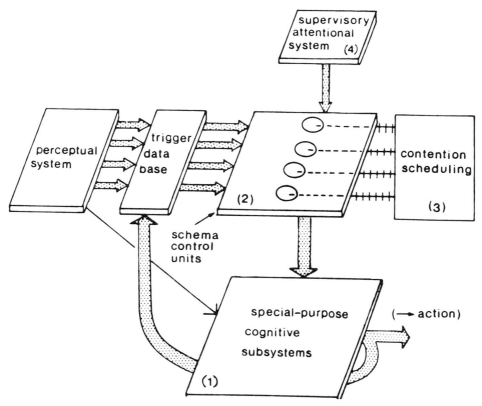

Figure 6–1 The Norman and Shallice model. The thick dotted lines refer to control information, the thin continuous line to the specific information ("encapsulated") required by particular special-purpose cognitive subsystems in their on-line operation, and the hatched lines to the primarily inhibitory interaction between the activation levels of schemas in contention scheduling. (Reprinted from Shallice et al. 1989.)

out and consider whether frontal patients have specific difficulties with such tasks. A third line of attack is to derive tasks from artificial intelligence modeling of such Supervisory processes; again frontal patients should have problems with the tasks. Finally, we can attempt to consider the processes carried out by the Supervisory System in more detail and assess whether selective deficits following frontal lesions exist that correspond to damage to particular subprocesses postulated. In the present paper we will review one line of empirical work using each of these four approaches.

UNMODULATED CONTENTION SCHEDULING

In an earlier paper it was argued that the characteristics of the way that Contention Scheduling would operate if unmodulated by the Supervisory System, will depend upon the overall task situation (Shallice, 1982). In particular, if there are strong trigger-schema contingencies present, when there is a well-learned set of responses in the situation, it will be difficult to switch to a different set of responses, i.e., "stuck-in-set" perseveration (Sandson and Albert, 1984) will occur. By contrast, if all trigger-schema contingencies are weaker, irrelevant aspects of the stimulus situation would be liable to capture control of action or thought, and so, inappropriate behavior would result.

Ample evidence exists that the first type of behavior results from frontal lesions (e.g., Cicerone et al., 1983; Milner, 1964; Nelson, 1976). In the earlier discussion the evidence for distractibility was based on the animal literature and on clinical reports. Solid experimental evidence now exists for a reduction in the ability to concentrate—the complement of distractibility—in frontal patients (e.g., Knight, 1984; Knight et al., 1981; Salmaso and Denes, 1982; Stuss et al., 1981; but see also Wilkins et al., 1987).

One type of behavior that is observed in frontal lobe patients appears to correspond more precisely to what the model would predict should occur when no strong trigger-schema relations exist; actions should be triggered by irrelevant stimuli in the environment. This is utilization behavior (the tendency to pick up and use objects when they are presented), which Lhermitte (1983) has claimed to be a frequent frontal syndrome.

Lhermitte's procedure is, however, subject to alternative interpretations. It involves the patient sitting on the opposite side of the desk to the examiner, who remains silent throughout, and places a common object such as a glass in front of the patient or even stimulates the palm and fingers of the patient's hand with it or holds it and abruptly withdraws it. The patient who exhibits utilization behavior will grasp the glass and begin to use it. If a second object such as a flask of water is introduced in a similar fashion the patient will pour the water into the glass and drink it. Other objects are treated in an analogous fashion. However, another obvious possible interpretation can be made in terms of demand characteristics. The patients confused by the strange behavior of the examiner believe that they are supposed to use the object—and frontal patients make this error more frequently than posterior patients.

In a single-case study (Shallice et al., 1989) carried out with a patient who had bilateral lesions of the inferior and medial aspects of both frontal lobes, this demand characteristic explanation could be excluded. The patient presented with an acute onset behavior pattern of moving furniture, opening cupboards, turning light switches and taps on and off, continually making tea, and so forth. When objects were left lying on the ends of the testing desk while he was being tested he would spontaneously and without prompting begin to use them—picking up pen and paper and writing, picking up a pack of playing cards and dealing a hand to all in the room, picking up matches and lighting a candle, and so on. In one session in which he was carrying out psychometric tasks he produced 23 examples of incidental utilization behavior of which 13 involved a set of actions integrated in a fashion typical of the relevant object, and 10 involved some form of toying with an object or objects. By contrast a second patient who had a comparable IQ as a result of a left parietotemporal lesion and produced utilization behavior when tested in Lhermitte's fashion showed no incidental utilization behavior when our method was used.

In the first patient, utilization behavior occurred when he was supposed to carry out psychometric tasks. Such actions can hardly be attributed to demand characteristics and are therefore the type of behavior that fits with what would be expected from the operation of Contention Scheduling operating unmonitored due to a severe impairment of the Supervisory System.

INTUITIVELY SPECIFIED PROPERTIES OF THE SUPERVISORY SYSTEM—THE COGNITIVE ESTIMATION TASK

In the original specification of the model (Norman and Shallice, 1980; 1986) the Supervisory System was held to be required in five types of situations:

1. Ones that involve planning or decision making.
2. Ones that involve error-correction or troubleshooting.
3. Ones where responses are not well learned or contain novel sequences of actions.
4. Ones judged to be dangerous or technically difficult.
5. Ones that require the overcoming of a strong habitual response or resisting temptation.

A more general characterization can be given that reduces these five types to two. One type is where an incorrect response has been or is liable to be produced by unmodulated contention scheduling, the situations discussed in the last section. The second type of relevant situation is where no routine procedure is available to produce an appropriate response, i.e., the situation is in some essential respect novel. Patients with damage to the Supervisory System should have problems in these situations.

Novelty is difficult to operationalize as to do so would involve the listing of all knowledge and skills available to the subject. In the study of Shallice and Evans (1978) the intuitive procedure was adopted of devising questions about everyday magnitudes where no rote knowledge or routine method seems available for obtaining the answer and yet a strategy fairly easily comes to mind that, when adopted, quickly provides a reasonable answer. Examples would be "How fast does a racehorse gallop?" or "What is the height of the Post Office Tower?" (a well-known building in London). Thus if asked what the average length of the spine is, one can calculate body - head - legs, or imagine a shirt. Moreover if by miscalculation or guessing a normal subject obtained the answer 5 feet, its unreasonableness should be immediately apparent and the answer changed.

Obviously normal subjects answering questions of this sort will show considerable variability. What we were concerned about was the rate at which extremely inaccurate answers occur. These would be more likely to occur if an appropriate strategy was not selected. Three levels of inaccuracy were drawn up for each question, which correspond to the 8th, 16th, and 25th percentile performance as estimated from a control group. With an unselected series of patients with unilateral lesions, patients whose lesions involved the frontal lobes had a significantly higher score than those with posterior lesions for each of the cut-off points. This was still the case when WAIS Arithmetic and Matrices scores were treated as covariates, so the effect is not simply secondary to an inability to calculate or reason.

In an unpublished study Kartsounis and Poynton tested 23 patients with severe intractable nonresponsive depression before a subcaudate tractotomy was carried out, and repeated testing was carried out 2 weeks after the operation and 6 months later. NMR showed widespread bilateral swelling in the frontal lobes at 2 weeks postoperation, but this was not present at the 6-month follow-up. Moreover, whereas traditional frontal lobe tests such as Wisconsin Card Sorting and Word Fluency were impaired at 2 weeks postoperation but not 6 months later, this was not the case for tests like WAIS Digit Span or Ravens Matrices, which remained static. A version of Cognitive Estimation showed a similar pattern to the Wisconsin. Ten questions were used rather than the original 15, and a scoring system adopted of 3, 2, 1 for the three levels of bizarreness of response from the preceding study. The average score of the patients rose significantly from 5.6 to 9.5 (at 2 weeks) and then fell to 7.2. This corroborated the findings of the earlier study.

A different type of estimation procedure has been adopted by Smith and Milner (1984). They showed subjects a series of toy objects and asked them to estimate the cost of the real item the toy represented. Extreme answers were defined more strictly than in the Shallice and Evans study in that only answers more than 2 standard deviations from the normal mean were treated as bizarre. Subjects were patients with left or right unilateral frontal or temporal lobectomies (subdivided into large and small hippocampal excisions) and normal controls, seven groups in all. There was a significant group effect with the right frontal group (23% of all answers being bizarre) performing nearly twice as badly as the worst of the nonfrontal groups. It was argued by Smith and Milner that the effect could not be attributed to inattentiveness or lack of interest, as the right frontal group performed as well as normal controls on free recall of the 16 objects carried out after the estimation procedures had all been carried out.

The most plausible explanation of the deficits found on these two types of estimation task is that the frontal patient is impaired in devising an appropriate strategy to deal with a problem situation where no routine procedure is available. One difference is that in the Shallice and Evans study the effects were significant for the left frontal group but not for the right, but in the Smith and Milner study the complementary pattern was found. However, in neither case was the difference between the two frontal lobe groups significant. Thus, in general, these studies provide support for the Supervisory System position.

A TEST DERIVED FROM ARTIFICIAL INTELLIGENCE—THE TOWER OF LONDON

In a test like Cognitive Estimation the degree of novelty required in answering one of the questions can only be intuitively assessed. One possibility of improving on this means of devising situations that should stress a Supervisory System is to turn to the artificial intelligence literature. If theorists have used a certain task to test a model that has a general supervisory component and there is no

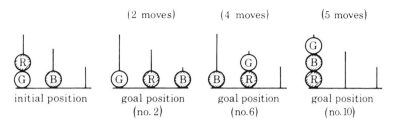

Figure 6–2 Three subproblems of the Tower-of-London test. (Reprinted from Shallice, 1982, p. 204.)

obvious reason to assume that humans have relevant special-purpose knowledge or skills that the program lacks, then such a task would seem an appropriate one to use to assess whether frontal lobe lesions impair the question of a Supervisory System.

In artificial intelligence simulation of problem solving, one type of task that has been frequently used is where stacks of blocks have to be moved into a new configuration in a minimum number of moves. The best known example of this type of task is the Tower-of-Hanoi. Anzai and Simon (1979) simulated the protocol of a subject tackling this task using a model with a supervisory component, which contained a learning mechanism "completely independent of the particular task and fully applicable to other problem solving environments in which heuristic search occurs." However, the Tower-of-Hanoi is not very suitable for psychometric use as a problem-solving task, as the paradigm does not have the potential to have a number of qualitatively different versions of comparable difficulty. For this reason a related task—the Tower of London—was developed, which allows for a variety of qualitatively different problems to be posed with the same basic layout (Fig. 6–2). In the standard version the primary measure is the number of problems solved without error in less than 60 seconds.

In collaboration with Dr. R. McCarthy, the 12 problems of the Tower-of-London were given to 61 patients with unilateral lesions (mainly tumors) and to 20 control subjects (Shallice, 1982). Patients were allocated to the anterior groups if their lesion involved the frontal lobe and its center of gravity was in the anterior half of the cortex. Otherwise they were placed in the posterior group. Considering the scores of the lesion patient groups there was a significant interaction between anterior/posterior location of the lesion and hemisphere with the left anterior group being significantly worse on the task than both the left posterior and right anterior groups. Moreover, the result remained the same when Block Design and Matrices scores were separately covaried, indicating that it could not be reduced to an impairment of control of action or of general reasoning skills.

There have been three other studies using the task with patients having cortical lesions. Their results have not been clear-cut. One unpublished study of Shallice et al. used a patient sample similar to the preceding one, except that patients were excluded whose WAIS score was less than 85 or more than 12 lower than their New Adult Reading Test score (Nelson and O'Connell, 1978)—

a measure of premorbid IQ—12 being the 5% cut-off for the difference measure in the general population. The clinical point behind this procedure is that it is frontal patients with intact IQ who present the greatest diagnostic difficulty. The scientific idea behind the procedure was to eliminate patients with major specific cognitive problems whose results would, it was argued, create noise for a comparison between the effects of anterior and posterior lesions. In fact, a considerable proportion of the anterior as well as the posterior patients were excluded. A set of eight tests were selected because (from the literature) one would expect them to have an important frontal component, but none gave significant anterior/posterior differences. As far as the Tower-of-London was concerned, the anterior groups did not perform significantly worse than the controls.

The Tower-of-London test was also used in the Kartsounis and Poynton study of subcaudate tractotomy operations discussed earlier. No significant difference was found between performance in the preoperative phase and in the immediate postoperative phase. However, in the pre-op phase the subjects were depressed, and Watts et al. (1988) have shown that depressed patients perform significantly less well than controls matched on age and the Mill Hill vocabulary test on the standard measure of the Tower-of-London. In this study there was also a significant correlation between planning time and ratings of whether patients experienced their mind going "blank." It therefore appears that the beneficial effects of change in mood may have masked any negative effect of the acute lesion in Kartsounis and Poynton's investigation.

A third study that used patients with similar etiologies and selected by a procedure similar to the original one gave results that partially confirmed it. Owen et al. (in press) gave a computerized version of the Tower-of-London task to 29 patients who had undergone unilateral or bilateral surgery and had lesions confined to the frontal lobe; 29 control subjects were also tested, matched for age and premorbid IQ as estimated by the New Adult Reading Test score. On a test of posterior function—a spatial short-term memory test that is a computerized version of the Corsi Block Tapping Test (Milner, 1971)—the groups did not differ significantly, indicating that they were well matched. Both groups were on the average able to retain about five block positions, an amount sufficient to retain the whole sequence of the most difficult Tower-of-London problems. However, on the Tower-of-London test, the frontal patients took significantly more moves to solve problems and solved significantly fewer problems without error.

A detailed examination was made of the times to reach solutions. Yoked control trials were used where the subject merely had to copy a sequence of moves on the screen. The frontal group was significantly slower than the control group at carrying this out, which fits with their slower performances on choice reaction time as found by Alivisatos and Milner (1989). When the yoked control times were subtracted, there was no difference between the groups in the planning time—the time spent thinking before making the first move. However, the frontal group was slower to make moves after the first when the yoked control times were subtracted. This finding occurred even when only the minimum number of moves solutions were considered. This suggests that the frontal group had an impairment in planning and had planned what followed their first move less well than the controls even when they made the move correctly, for they then had to think longer on subsequent moves.

The empirical situation is considerably less clear as far as the existence of a frontal deficit on the Tower-of-London is concerned than for the Cognitive Estimation task. Two studies that obtained a positive effect differed in that one—that of Shallice and McCarthy—produced a specifically left frontal problem but that of Owen and colleagues found no difference between the effects of lesions to left and right frontal lobes. The lack of effect in the Kartsounis and Poynton study can perhaps be explained by the contrasting effect of the obtained reduction of depression on performance, whereas that in the Shallice and colleagues study could have arisen because the selection procedure excluded the more severely frontal patients, who are the ones that are most likely to manifest a difficulty on the Tower-of-London.

Overall the task appears not to be clinically very sensitive as a test of frontal lobe dysfunction. However, the clearest evidence that Supervisory functions are impaired in the performance of frontal lobe patients on the task comes from the detailed analyses carried out by Owen and associates. The results of their control task based on the Corsi procedure showed that visuospatial short-term memory load is unlikely to be a critical factor. The way that normal subjects hardly needed to think after their first correct move, but the frontal patients were considerably slower, indicates that even when they made the correct first move frontal patients had planned less well.

FRACTIONATION OF THE SUPERVISORY SYSTEM?

For both empirical and theoretical reasons the attempt to correlate Supervisory Systems impairments with the effect of frontal lobe lesions in group studies is rather limited. Theoretically the processes involved in producing an appropriate solution when routinely selected rote methods do not work or have failed are likely to be complex. Thus an early simulation by Sussman (1975) of a block-stacking program that learned from its mistakes contains a so-called programming component with a variety of computationally distinct subcomponents. Moreover, if, from a more cognitive framework, one considers the subprocesses involved in the supervisory aspects of the problem-solving process they too are complex.

Figure 6–3 illustrates one possible breakdown of the processes involved. It is assumed that given an everyday life problem that cannot be immediately dealt with by routine selection of rote-learned procedures, the Supervisory process proceeds through a series of stages. These we have derived from standard approaches to problem solving (e.g., Ben-Yishay and Diller, 1983; De Groot, 1965) together with Schank's (1982) theory that longer-duration, well-learned multiple stage activities such as going to a restaurant, which do not require temporally continuous control of cognitive processing resources by the activity, are organized by a hierarchy of structures called memory organization packets (or MOPs).[2] It is further assumed that at specific stages of the problem-solving process the Supervisory System can activate schemas in contention scheduling to

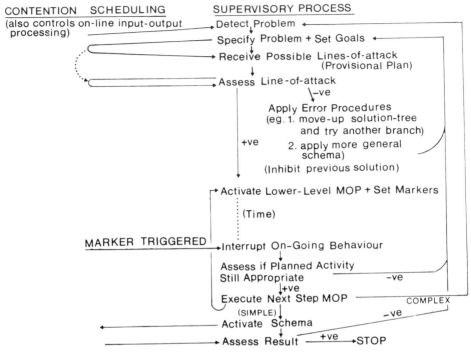

Figure 6–3 Different processes involved in coping with a novel situation from the context of the Norman and Shallice model. The vertical lines indicate the succession in the stages involved. The horizontal lines indicate the flow of information between Supervisory Process and Contention Scheduling at a particular stage.

carry out specific computations or provide particular pieces of information. It seems possible that different stages of Supervisory control would involve materially distinct subsystems.

Empirically, too, it is now becoming apparent that one can isolate particular impairments within the general set of frontal cognitive operations. Suggestions that this is so can be obtained from the clinical literature. A clear example is Eslinger and Damasio's (1985) patient who performed well on a wide variety of neuropsychological tests, including some held to be sensitive to frontal lobe damage, but who had many severe practical difficulties in everyday life that seemed to arise from lack of judgmental and organizational skills.

In a recent study we have, we believe, isolated an analogous impairment quantitatively (Shallice and Burgess, in press). We described three head injury patients in whom there was CT evidence of focal frontal lobe damage. All had WAIS IQs between 120 and 130. On 13 tests that are held to have a frontal component, two of the patients were well within the normal range on all 13 tests, but one patient (C) was below the normal range on three (Personal Orientation, Butters et al., 1972; the Alternation Test, Chorover and Cole, 1966; Stevenson, 1967; and Trail-Making, Reitan, 1958). Thus all three patients scored at around the mean level or better on Bilateral Hand Movements, Cognitive Estimation,

Proverb Interpretation, the Stroop Test (see Perret, 1974), the Tower-of-London, Word Fluency (Milner, 1964), and the Modified Wisconsin Test (Milner, 1964; Nelson, 1975). One patient (A) performed well on a wide range of memory tests; B, however, was impaired on some visual memory tests (e.g., Rey [1964] figure reproduction) but on a variety of verbal memory tests was well within the normal range. C, too, performed well on a variety of memory tests (e.g., Coughlan and Hollows [1985] list learning) but was impaired on certain others that can be held to have a frontal component (e.g., Wechsler Memory Battery Hard Paired Associates).

All three patients showed little spontaneous organization in everyday life, and two at least had made a number of gross oversights with major practical consequences. Two tests were developed of their ability to schedule a number of relatively straightforward activities in a restricted period of time. Thus, in one test they had to carry out six open-ended but not difficult tasks in 15 minutes; two involved dictating routes, two involved writing down the names of pictures of objects, and two involved the carrying out of a series of fairly simple sums. However, to complete all six tasks would take much longer than the limited time available. The patients had to judge how much time to devote to each task so as to optimize their performance given some simple rules, of which the most important was that the scoring system guaranteed diminishing returns on a task as it continued to be carried out; for example, the initial sums scored more than later ones. Normal subjects switched between the tasks tackling on average 5.7 (S.D. 0.5) of them and spent an average of 5 minutes 35 seconds (S.D. 0–53) on the task to which they devoted most time. The three patients were outside the normal range on both measures except for one score (A 3, 7–30; B 5, 10–11; C 3, 7–18). In addition, they performed in a qualitatively inappropriate fashion. Thus A started the test by making notes for 4 minutes, which he never subsequently used, and B spent 10 minutes on one task and did not even tackle a second that was very similar. The three patients performed equally poorly on the second test, which involved scheduling a set of simple shopping activities in real time in a street. They also had analogous problems in practical everyday life situations.

It did not seem possible to explain the poor performance of these patients on these two tests in terms of memory, motivational or posterior cognitive problems. Thus they tackled very satisfactorily complex and demanding tasks such as carrying out Raven's Matrices unsupervised. Their difficulty appeared to lie within the domain of the Supervisory System.

It is possible to subdivide the set of Supervisory processes illustrated in Figure 6–3 into four broad classes: (1) Plan formulation or modification, (2) marker creation or triggering, (3) evaluation and goal articulation, and (4) MOP organization. As the tasks we used did not have subcomponents that are routinely required to operate over a considerable period of time, as, for instance, in the stages involved in going to a restaurant, the fourth of these is not relevant to the present tests. If one contrasts the two scheduling tests with more standard frontal lobe tests, then it is the second of these broad classes on which they are especially loaded. Thus a dissociation between performance on these and other frontal lobe tests, such as that exhibited by patient A and less clearly by patient B, suggests that the marker creation, maintenance, or triggering process can be specifically impaired, where a marker is a tag to treat some future behavior or event as non-routine so that if it occurs, on-going behavior is interrupted and some appropriate nonroutine action initiated. This, we would argue, is a process related to the maintenance of intentions and more critically to their later realization at an appropriate time. In patients like A and B these processes seem to be more impaired than the Supervisory ones.

More fundamentally, though, this study provides quantitative support for the types of dissociation within executive processes described, for instance, by Eslinger and Damasio. Whether there is any correspondence between the present dissociation and that observed in animals between the effects of lesions to orbital and dorsolateral parts of the frontal cortex (e.g., Fuster, 1980) remains to be investigated. The results do, however, suggest that a fractionation of Supervisory System functions will prove possible.

NOTES

1. In a later article Norman (1986) has suggested that the contention scheduling/schema mechanism could be replaced by a large connectionist network. For the present purposes the two approaches are essentially interchangeable.

2. The MOP/schema distinction is discussed in Shallice (1988). Grafman (1985, unpublished) has argued that MOPs are frontally stored.

REFERENCES

Alivisatos B, Milner B. Effects of frontal or temporal lobectomy on the use of advanced information in a choice reaction time task. Neuropsychologia 27:495–504, 1989.

Anzai Y, Simon H. The theory of learning by doing. Psychol Rev 86:124–140, 1979.

Ben-Yishay Y, Diller L. Cognitive remediation. *In* Griffith ER, Bond MR, Miller JD (eds), Rehabilitation of the Head Injured Adult. Philadelphia, FA Davis Company, 1983.

Butters N, Soeldner C, Fedio P. Comparison of parietal and frontal lobe spatial deficits in man: Extrapersonal vs personal (egocentric) space. Percept Mot Skills 34:27–34, 1972.

Chorover SL, Cole M. Delayed alternation performance in patients with cerebral lesions. Neuropsychologia 4:1–7, 1966.

Cicerone KD, Lazar RM, Shapiro WR. Effects of frontal lobe lesions on hypothesis sampling during concept formation. Neuropsychologia 21:513–524, 1983.

Coughlan AK, Hollows SE. The Adult Memory and Information Processing Battery. Leeds, St. James's University Hospital, 1985.

Damasio AR. The frontal lobes. *In* Heilman KM, Valenstein E (eds), Clinical Neuropsychology, 2nd Edition. New York, Oxford University Press, 1985.

De Groot AD. Thought and choice in chess. The Hague, Mouton, 1965.

Eslinger PJ, Damasio AR. Severe disturbance of higher cognition after frontal lobe ablation: Patient EVR. Neurology 35:1731–1741, 1985.

Fahlman SE. A planning system for robot construction tasks. Artif Intell 5:1–49, 1974.

Fuster JM. The prefrontal cortex. New York, Raven Press, 1980.

Jouandet M, Gazzaniga MS. The frontal lobes. *In* Gazzaniga MS (ed), Handbook of Behavioural Neurobiology, Vol 2. New York, Plenum Press, 1979.

Knight RT. Decreased response to novel stimuli after prefrontal lesions in man. EEG Clin Neurophys 52:571–582, 1984.

Knight RT, Hillyard SA, Woods DL, Neville HJ. The effects of frontal cortical lesions on event-related potentials during auditory selective attention. EEG Clin Neurophysiol 59:571–582, 1981.

Laird J, Newell A, Rosenbloom P. SOAR: An architecture for general intelligence. Artif Intell 33:1–64, 1987.

Lhermitte F. "Utilization behaviour" and its relation to lesions of the frontal lobes. Brain 106:237–255, 1983.

Luria AR. Higher Cortical Functions in Man. English translation of 1st edition by Haigh B. New York, Basic Books and Plenum Press, 1966.

Milner B. Some effects of frontal lobectomy in man. *In* Warren JM, Akert K (eds), The Frontal Granular Cortex and Behaviour. New York, McGraw-Hill, 1964.

Milner B. Interhemispheric differences in the localisation of psychological processes in man. Brit Med Bull 27:272–277, 1971.

Nelson HE. A modified card sorting task sensitive to frontal lobe defects. Cortex 12:313–324, 1976.

Nelson HE, O'Connell A. Dementia: The estimation of premorbid intelligence levels using the new adult reading test. Cortex 14:234–244, 1978.

Newell A, Simon H. Human Problem Solving. Englewood Cliffs, N.J., Prentice-Hall, 1972.

Norman DA. Reflections on cognition and parallel distributed processing. *In* McClelland J, Rumelhart DE (eds), Parallel Distributed Processing: Exploration in the Microstructure of Cognition, Vol 2. Cambridge, Mass, MIT Press, 1986.

Norman D, Shallice T. Attention to action: Willed and automatic control of behaviour. Center for human information processing (Technical Report No. 99). (Reprinted in revised form in Davidson RJ, Schwartz GE, Shapiro D (eds), Consciousness and Self-Regulation, Vol 4. New York, Plenum Press, 1986.)

Owen A, Downes JJ, Sahakian BJ, Polkey CE, Robbins TW. Planning and spatial working memory following frontal lobe lesions in man. Neuropsychologia (in press).

Perret E. The left frontal lobe in man and suppression of habitual responses in verbal categorical behaviour. Neuropsychologia 12:323–330, 1974.

Reitan RM. Validity of the trail-making test as an indication of organic brain damage. Percept Mot Skills 8:271–276, 1958.

Rey A. L'Examen Clinique en Psychologie. Paris, Presses Universitares de France, 1964.

Salmaso D, Denes G. Role of the frontal lobes on an attention task: A signal detection analysis. Percept Mot Skills 54:1147–1150, 1982.

Sandson J, Albert ML. Varieties of perseveration. Neuropsychologia 22:715–732, 1984.

Schank RC. Dynamic memory. Cambridge, Cambridge University Press, 1982.

Shallice T. Specific impairments of planning. Philos Trans R Soc Lond (Biol) 298:199–209, 1982.

Shallice T. From Neuropsychology to Mental Structure. Cambridge, Cambridge University Press, 1988.

Shallice T, Burgess PW. Deficits in strategy application following frontal lobe lesions in man. Brain (in press).

Shallice T, Burgess PW, Baxter DM, Schon F. The origins of utilisation behaviour. Brain 112:1587–1598, 1989.

Shallice T, Evans ME. The involvement of the frontal lobes in cognitive estimation. Cortex 4:294–303, 1978.

Smith ML, Milner B. Differential effects of frontal-lobe lesions on cognitive estimation and spatial memory. Neuropsychologia 22:697–705, 1984.

Stevenson J. Some psychological effects of frontal lobe lesions in man. MSc Thesis. Cambridge University, 1967.

Stuss DT, Benson DF. The frontal lobes. New York, Raven Press, 1986.

Stuss DT, Kaplan EF, Benson DF, Wier WS, Naeser MA, Levine HL. Long-term effects of prefrontal leucotomy: An overview of neuropsychologic residuals. J Clin Neuropsychol 3:13–32, 1981.

Sussman GJ. A computational model of skill acquisition. New York, American Elsevier, 1975.

Watts FN, MacLeod AK, Morris L. Associations between phenomenal and objective aspects of concentration problems in depressed patients. Br J Psychol 79:241–250, 1988.

Wilkins AJ, Shallice T, McCarthy R. Frontal lesions and sustained attention. Neuropsychologia 25:259–365, 1987.

7

Evoked Potential Studies of Attention Capacity in Human Frontal Lobe Lesions

ROBERT T. KNIGHT

Ensembles of neurons active during sensory and cognitive processing generate field potentials that can be recorded from the scalp of humans. Evoked potentials (EPs) generated 0 to 50 msec poststimulation reliably assess stimulus-dependent neural activity in sensory pathways and primary sensory cortex.

In the last 15–20 years, cognitive event-related potentials (ERPs) have been discovered that index mental processes independent of sensory parameters. ERPs have been employed to study motor preparation, orientation, attention, memory, and semantic analysis (for review: Hillyard and Picton, 1987). Cognitive potentials are generated from 50 to 1000 msec poststimulation and have been widely applied to neurophysiologic analysis of both normal and abnormal populations. For instance, ERPs have been used to assess development (Courchesne, 1977), psychiatric disease (Baribau-Braun et al., 1983; Pritchard, 1986), dementia (Goodin et al., 1978), and neuropsychologic populations (Knight, 1985). The current review will focus on EP and ERP studies of patients with frontal lobe damage.

FRONTAL LOBE SYNDROMES

Human prefrontal cortex syndromes can be subdivided into at least three subtypes. Orbitofrontal damage (Brodmann areas, 11, 12) results in prominent affective disturbances. Emotional lability and decreased impulse control contribute to poor social integration. Problems such as loss of control of anger and inappropriate laughing, crying, or sexuality are often observed. Attention capacity is usually preserved, frontal release signs are absent, and the patient is typically aware of the problem but is unable to control his or her behavior.

Bilateral mesial prefrontal damage involving supplementary motor and cingulate cortex (Brodmann areas 24, 25, 32, 33, and mesial 6, 8, 9) produces an amotivational, akinetic state with motor programming deficits manifesting clinically as apractic disturbances. Unilateral mesial or mild bilateral disease yields lesser degrees of difficulty in the initiation and sustaining of motor and mental activity.

Damage in dorsolateral prefrontal cortex (Brodman areas 6, 8, 9, 10, 44, 45, 46) leads to a complex range of behavioral disturbances. In early disease due either to tumors (i.e., glioma) or to degenerative disease (i.e., Picks) sparing language cortex, subtle deficits in creativity and mental flexibility are often noted by the patient or family. As unilateral disease progresses or becomes bilateral, pronounced behavioral problems become apparent. Abnormalities emerge in planning, goal-directed behavior, temporal coding of external and internal events, metamemory, judgment, and insight. Attention capacity is invariably impaired in advanced disease.

A common cause of acute unilateral dorsolateral prefrontal damage is infarction of the precentral branch of the middle cerebral artery. This occlusion results in variable amounts of damage to areas 6, 8, 9, 10, 44, 45, 46. Damage typically centers in area 46, which is likely equivalent to the sulcus principalis region in monkeys critical for delayed-response performance (Jacobsen 1935, Fuster this volume, Chapter 3, and Goldman-Rakic and Friedman this volume, Chapter 4).

Acute unilateral infarcts involving area 46 and the frontal eye field (area 8) are often associated with a transient syndrome of mild global confusion and attention dysfunction. Right-sided prefrontal infarcts are more likely to result in contralateral hemispatial neglect than comparable volume left-sided infarcts (Mesulam, 1981). When motor and language cortex is spared, patients may not seek acute medical treatment. However, when seen at a later date they may complain of continued problems with attention, memory, and mental quickness. In advanced bilateral dorsolateral disease due to tumor, degeneration, or vascular disease, perseveration and frontal release signs (snout, grasp, palmomental) are often present. The following physiologic sections will focus on studies of patients with unilateral dorsolateral infarcts, since these lesions are nonprogressive and can be well defined anatomically by computerized tomography (CT) and magnetic resonance imaging (MRI) techniques.

GATING DEFICITS

Distractibility is a prominent feature of prefrontal lesioned animals (Bartus and Levere, 1977; Brutkowski, 1965) and humans (Fuster, 1980; Milner, 1982; Woods and Knight, 1986) and is due to inability to inhibit attending and responding to irrelevant events in the internal and external environment. Neurophysiologic studies have documented a net inhibitory prefrontal modulation of remote subcortical and cortical structures (Alexander et al., 1976; Edinger et al., 1975). An elegant series of studies by Skinner and Yingling (Skinner and Yingling, 1977; Yingling and Skinner, 1977) has revealed that prefrontal cortex exerts modality-specific suppression of sensory transmission through thalamic relay nuclei. Prefrontal cortex excites the nucleus reticularis thalami, which in turn sends gaba-ergic inhibitory fibers to thalamic relay nuclei. Through this net inhibitory pathway to thalamic relay nuclei prefrontal cortex is able to gate transmission to primary sensory regions.

Cryogenic suppression of prefrontal cortex decreases nucleus reticularis thalami suppression of thalamic relay nuclei resulting in disinhibition of sensory input measured by enhancement of the amplitude of primary sensory cortex evoked potentials. This prefrontal-thalamic gating mechanism provides a powerful neurophysiologic system for early filtering of sensory inputs capable of intra- and intermodality suppression of irrelevant stimuli.

Evidence supporting an early prefrontal sensory gating mechanism in humans has been provided by evoked potentials studies in patients with focal damage in dorsolateral prefrontal cortex. The P30 component of the auditory evoked response (AEP) occurs at 25–30 msec poststimulation and is generated predominantly in primary auditory cortex (Kraus et al., 1982; Pelizzone et al., 1987). Discrete prefrontal damage results in amplitude disinhibition of the P30 component of the AEP (Knight et al., 1989a) (Fig. 7–1).

Figure 7–1 On the left are auditory evoked potentials from controls (solid; n = 13, mean age 62 yr) and unilateral prefrontal lesioned subjects (dashed; n = 13, mean age 59 yr). The average lateral lesion extension for the group is shown on the bottom. Lesion volume averaged 42.1 cc. Wave V from the inferior colliculus is unaffected, whereas the P30 generated in auditory cortex (AudCx) shows amplitude disinhibition after prefrontal damage. On the right are somatosensory evoked potentials recorded from a similar patient group. There is amplitude disinhibition of the P27 generated in areas 1, 2 of the postcentral gyrus.

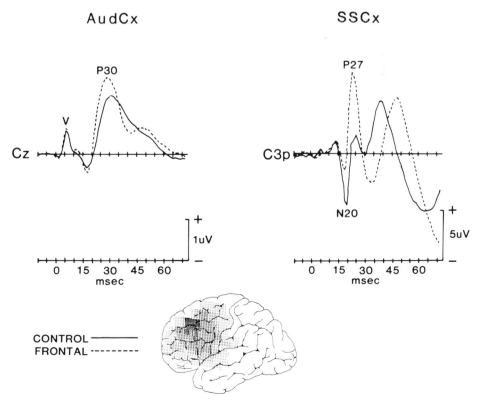

Parallel findings have been obtained in the somatosensory modality. Unilateral focal dorsolateral prefrontal damage results in amplitude disinhibition of the P27 component of the primary somatosensory evoked response generated in areas 1, 2 of the postcentral gyrus (Yamaguchi and Knight, 1990; see Fig. 7–1). Thus, human prefrontal damage results in disinhibition of sensory input to both primary auditory and somatosensory cortex, a finding similar to that observed in frontal lesioned animals.

In normals, focused sustained attention increases the amplitude of auditory and somatosensory evoked potentials as early as 25 msec poststimulation (Desmedt et al., 1983; McCallum et al., 1983; Woldorff et al., 1987). The finding that primary cortical sensory input is modulated by prefrontal cortex suggests that early attention effects (25–50 msec) in normals may be controlled by dorsolateral prefrontal regions.

Input modulation of attended spatial locations and modalities would provide a beneficial mechanism for normal focused attention ability. An early selection mechanism would permit the organism to rapidly focus energy on analyzing events in the attended channel. This would obviate the need to take in multiple parallel channels of irrelevant information, sort these inputs, and then select the desired one for further processing.

Conversely, chronic disinhibition of sensory input would be detrimental to attention capacity in both prefrontal lesioned animals and humans, since all environmental events would initially assume equal biologic valence. This would require that both relevant and irrelevant stimuli be processed before making a response decision. It is likely that these sensory gating deficits contribute to the distractibility and attention dysfunction found in frontal lesioned animals and humans. Chronic leakage of irrelevant sensory stimuli would also be expected to habituate the novelty detection system, a finding frequently observed in prefrontal patients (Knight, 1984; Sokoloff, 1963).

FOCUSED SUSTAINED ATTENTION DEFICITS

Sustained attention to one ear, one limb, or one visual field results in systematic increased amplitudes of evoked potentials to stimuli in the attended channel. This phenomenon appears to be due to a combination of enhancement of neural activity to the attended channel (i.e., an ear, a hand, a field) and active suppression of neural processing in the nonattended channel (for review: Woods, 1990). Selective, sustained attention to stimuli in an attended channel has been most widely studied in the auditory modality (Hillyard et al., 1973).

In dichotic auditory experiments, attended stimuli generate a negative ERP onsetting at about 50 msec poststimulation and lasting at least 500 msec. This electrophysiologic marker of focused attention has been labeled the processing negativity (Nd) and is the purest neurophysiologic measure of focused sustained auditory attention recordable in humans.

Generation of an Nd to a stimulus also predicts enhanced performance in the attended channel. For instance, rare events that the subject must discriminate are better detected in the channel wherein stimuli have Nd enhancement.

These rare detected targets generate P300 ERP components that index phasic attention capacity. The P300 ERP will be discussed in later sections.

The auditory Nd has been studied in patients with focal damage in left or right dorsolateral prefrontal cortex. A pattern of results emerged converging with the extensive literature on prefrontal attention asymmetries in humans (Mesulam, 1981; Heilman et al., 1983). In controls, comparable Nd effects were generated for focused attention to the left or right ear. Patients with left prefrontal damage were also able to generate comparable attention negativity to left and right ear stimuli. There was a slight reduction in the Nd relative to controls but these differences were nonsignificant. A different pattern was found in right prefrontal damaged patients. There was a complete absence of the Nd component to left ear stimuli with concomitant decrease in the selective attention detection capacity in that ear (Knight et al., 1981) (Fig. 7–2).

A detailed analysis of the temporal microstructure of the attention deficit in the right prefrontal patients revealed further interesting effects. First, when attended stimuli were presented at interstimulus intervals less than 200 msec, both right and left lesioned subjects had normal attention capacity in both ears. Abnormalities emerged only at interstimulus intervals greater than 200 msec. This indicated that attention deficits in the right lesioned subjects were not due simply to slowed processing capacity, since the patients could generate an Nd to rapidly presented stimuli. The finding that attention deficits were apparent only at long interstimulus intervals provides support for Fuster's hypothesis that frontal lesions impair the "synthetic temporal function" necessary for bridging temporal discontinuities in the environment (Fuster, 1980).

Stimulus by stimulus evaluation of the data provided additional insights into the prefrontal abnormalities. In normals if a subject attends to an ear an irrelevant stimulus delivered to the nonattended ear has no effect on the capacity to generate a processing negativity to a subsequent stimulus in the attended ear. Normals are capable of suppressing the distracting effect of irrelevant stimuli on focused attention capacity. In the right frontal patients irrelevant stimuli eliminated the processing negativity to the next attended stimuli in both the left ear contralateral to the lesion and in the "normal" ipsilateral right ear. This effect was particularly evident at long interstimulus intervals. A tendency for inappropriate distractibility by irrelevant stimuli was also observed in the contralateral right ear of left prefrontal lesioned patients (Woods and Knight, 1986). These data support the notion that distractibility is a key component of the attention deficits seen after prefrontal damage. The inability to inhibit irrelevant signals may be linked to the previously described early gating deficits found in these patients.

These results also provide neurophysiologic support for asymmetric organization of attention capacity in human prefrontal cortex. Other data from clinical observation of neglect behavior (Hier et al., 1983; Kertesz and Dobrowolski, 1981; Stein and Volpe, 1983) support right prefrontal predominance in attention capacity. Human postmortem (Wada et al., 1975; Weinberger et al., 1982) and CT evidence (Lemay and Kido, 1978) have documented that the right frontal lobe is larger than the left. This asymmetry has been suggested to provide the anatomic substrate for the attention asymmetries observed between left and right prefrontal cortex lesioned patients (Knight, 1990).

Selective Attention

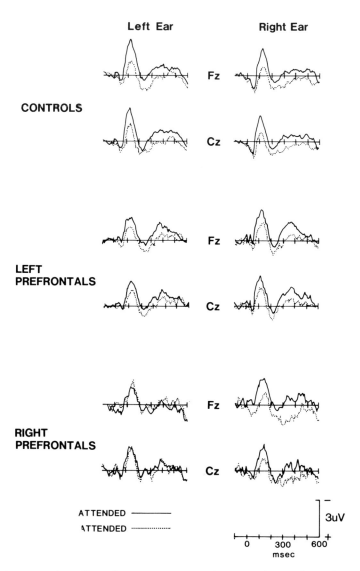

Figure 7–2 Attention effects for controls (n = 12) and patients with unilateral prefrontal lesions. Normal subjects generate enhanced amplitude of attended stimuli (processing negativity; Nd), which is comparable for left and right ear attention. Left prefrontal lesioned patients generate a slightly diminished processing negativity equal in amplitude for left and right ear attention. Right prefrontal patients show a hemi-inattention to left ear stimuli. Note that the amplitude of the response to the unattended tones are larger in the ear contralateral to the lesion for both left and right lesioned patients.

PHASIC ATTENTION DEFICITS

Evoked potential methods can also be used to study phasic attention shifts. The P300 component of the ERP is generated upon detection of discrete sensory stimuli. There is controversy regarding the psychologic underpinning of the P300 with constructs including stimulus evaluation, attention, orientation, and memory proposed as the psychobiologic basis of the P300 (Fabiani et al., 1986; Hillyard and Picton, 1987; Karis et al., 1986; Paller et al., 1987). Irrespective of whether the P300 indexes neural activity from attention, memory, or other neural systems, it cannot be generated without initial phasic attention to a discrete stimulus. Thus, the P300 can be used as a neurophysiologic index of phasic attention capacity in humans.

The neural origin of the P300 has also been a subject of debate. Data from scalp topographic analysis, intracranial recording, and neuromagnetic studies have proposed neural sources in cortical (Knight et al., 1989b; Scabini et al., 1989; Knight, 1990), limbic (Halgren et al., 1980; Okada et al., 1983; McCarthy et al., 1989), and subcortical regions (Yingling and Hosobuchi, 1984; Katayama et al., 1985; Velasco et al., 1986). Resection of the anterior temporal lobe in chronic epileptics does not alter the scalp P300 at central scalp sites, indicating that anterior limbic regions are not crucial for the P300 recorded midline scalp sites (Johnson, 1988).

Some of the controversy regarding the neural origin of the P300 may be due to the fact that multiple brain regions contribute to the scalp recorded P300. For instance, at least two types of P300 responses are recorded in normal subjects in the visual (Beck et al., 1980; Courchesne et al., 1975), auditory (Knight, 1984; Squires et al., 1975), and somatosensory modalities (Barrett et al., 1987; Yamaguchi and Knight, 1991). During sustained attention tasks, correct detection of an infrequent target stimulus in the attended channel generates a P300 (P3b) maximal at centroparietal scalp sites. Delivery of an unexpected deviant stimulus with no particular task significance but which is novel enough to attract attention also generates a P300 (P3a). The P3a is maximal at frontocentral scalp sites and is generated from 20 to 50 msec earlier than the P3b. The P3b indexes voluntary phasic attention, whereas the P3a indexes involuntary automatic attention to potentially significant environmental events.

Cortex in dorsolateral prefrontal and temporal-parietal junction has been implicated in sustained and phasic attention capacity in animals and humans (Andersen 1987; Fuster, 1980; Hikosaka et al., 1988; Lynch, 1980; Mesulam, 1981). To assess voluntary and automatic phasic attention capacity, P3a and P3b ERPs were recorded in patients with focal lesions in either dorsolateral prefrontal cortex or temporal-parietal junction. Auditory, visual, and somatosensory experiments were conducted to assess whether these regions are involved in modality specific or nonspecific attention allocation.

The typical experimental paradigm employed is shown in Figure 7–3. Briefly, the subject is asked to attend to repetitive, identical sensory stimuli occurring every 1 to 2 seconds. Interspersed among these repetitive stimuli are target stimuli occurring randomly on about 10% of the trials. The subject is instructed to press a button upon detection of these target events. A parietal

P300 EXPERIMENT

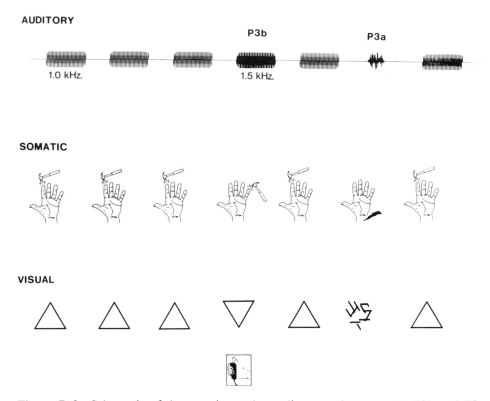

Figure 7–3 Schematic of the experimental paradigms used to generate P3b and P3a potentials in the auditory, somatosensory, and visual modalities. Repetitive background stimuli are delivered on 80% of the trials at 1-second interstimulus intervals. On 10% of the trials a randomly occurring target stimulus is presented (auditory: 1.5 KHz toneshift; somatosensory: tap to a designated finger; visual: inversion of a triangle). The subject is instructed to press a button upon detection of a target stimulus. Correctly detected targets generate a P3b. On the remaining 10% of the trials deviant stimuli requiring no behavioral response are randomly presented (auditory: complex tones; somatosensory: wrist shocks; visual: complex visual shapes). These deviant, novel stimuli generate a P3a.

maximal P3b is generated to correctly detected target stimuli in the auditory, visual, and somatosensory modalities.

Deviant novel stimuli are randomly interspered in the trains of background and target stimuli on about 5–10% of the trials. These deviant stimuli require no overt behavioral response but still generate large P3a potentials maximal over frontocentral scalp sites.

P3b responses are minimally affected by prefrontal lesions (Knight, 1984). The relatively preserved target P3b in prefrontal subjects is in accord with studies

NOVEL P3a

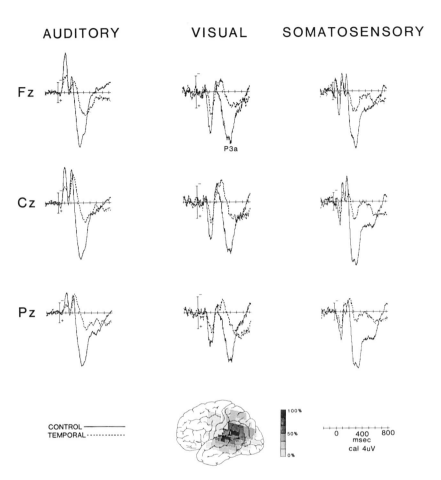

Figure 7-4   P3a potentials from controls (solid) and patients with unilateral lesions in the temporal-parietal junction. The averaged lateral lesion extent for the patients participating in the auditory study is shown at the bottom (lesions averaged about 40 cc in volume for the groups in each experiment: n = 13 auditory, n = 11 visual, n = 8 somatosensory). Recordings are shown from midline scalp sites (Fz, Cz, Pz). The P3a is markedly attenuated in all three modalities.

reporting that prefrontal subjects perform normally on simple sensorimotor tasks such as the button press to an easily discriminable target typically employed in P3b studies (Stuss and Benson, 1984). Conversely, temporal-parietal junction lesions abolish the P3b at posterior scalp sites in both the auditory and somatosensory modality (Knight et al., 1989b; Yamaguchi and Knight, in press) (Fig. 7-4). The visual P3b is also reduced by temporal-parietal junction lesions, although not to the degree found in the auditory and somatosensory modalities (Knight, 1990). The relative visual P3b preservation in patients with

AUDITORY

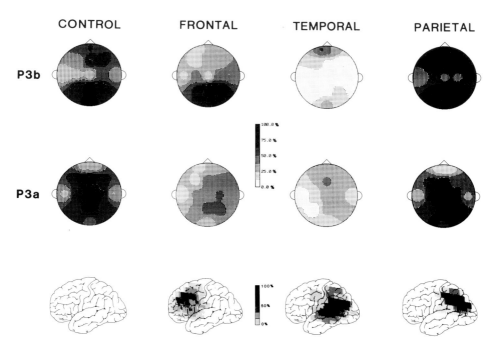

Figure 7–5   Scalp voltage topographies for the auditory P3b and P3a in dorsolateral prefrontal, temporal-parietal junction, and lateral parietal cortex lesioned groups. In controls the P3b is maximal at parietal scalp sites and the P3a has comparable amplitude at Fz, Cz, and Pz electrodes. On the far right of the figure, lateral parietal lesioned subjects (parietal) show topographies comparable with controls. Temporal-parietal lesioned subjects (temporal) have a marked reduction of both the P3b and P3a particularly evident over the lesioned hemisphere (left side of voltage maps). Prefrontal subjects (frontal) have mild P3b reductions and pronounced reduction of the P3a particularly evident over the lesioned hemisphere (left side of voltage map).

temporal-parietal junction lesions implies that modality specific circuits contribute to the P3b.

A different pattern of results was observed for the P3a generated to unexpected, novel stimuli. Lesions in the temporal-parietal junction markedly reduced the P3a in the auditory, visual, and somatosensory modalities (Knight et al., 1989a; Knight, 1990; Yamaguchi and Knight, 1990) (see Figs. 7–4 and 7–5). This P3a reduction was particulary prominent over lesioned temporal-parietal junction. These results converge with single unit studies reporting multimodal cells in the caudal superior temporal sulcus polysensory region (cSTP) of the primate temporal-parietal junction (Hikosaka et al., 1988) which respond selectively to novel stimuli (Chitty et al., 1985). Prefrontal lesions also reduced the P3a in the auditory, visual, and somatosensory modalities. P3a reductions were more prominent over the lesioned hemisphere (Figs. 7–5 and 7–6).

Behavioral findings in these subjects provide some insight into the biologic

NOVEL P3a

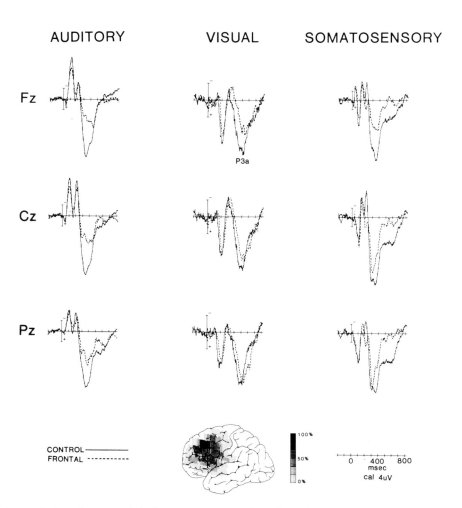

Figure 7–6 P3a potentials from controls and prefrontal damaged subjects (n = 13, mean volume about 40 cc in volume for the groups studied in each experiment). The P3a is reduced in all three sensory modalities with reductions more evident over frontal electrode sites.

significance of the ERP results. Subjects with P3a reductions have evidence of deficits in both automatic attention (Woods et al., 1987) and identity priming at rapid 1–10 sec interstimulus intervals (Kersteen-Tucker and Knight, 1989). Thus, both attention and memory capacity are impaired in subjects with reduced P300 components. This suggests that cortex in dorsolateral prefrontal, and temporal-parietal junction are components of a multimodal network involved in the detection and rapid encoding of significant environmental events. Prefrontal cortex appears critical for involuntary access to this system, whereas temporal-parietal cortex is crucial for both involuntary and voluntary processing.

The neural activity of this network manifested as the scalp P300 may index the recently proposed perceptual priming system thought to underlie rapid presemantic memory capacity in humans (Tulving and Schacter, 1990). Activity from these multimodal association regions is then read out to mesial temporal regions (Amaral et al., 1983) for further memory processing, indexed perhaps by intracerebral ERP activity (McCarthy et al., 1989).

ACKNOWLEDGMENTS

Special thanks to Clay Clayworth for technical assistance in all phases of the work. The work was supported by NINDS Javits Award NS21135 and the Veterans Administration Medical Research Service.

REFERENCES

Alexander GE, Newman JD, Symmes D. Convergence of prefrontal and acoustic inputs upon neurons in the superior temporal gyrus of the awake squirrel monkey. Brain Research 116:334–338, 1976.

Amaral DG, Insausti R, Cowan WM. Evidence for a direct projection from the superior temporal gyrus to the entorhinal cortex in the monkey. Brain Research 275:263–277, 1983.

Andersen RA. Inferior parietal lobule function in spatial perception and visuomotor integration. In Handbook of Physiology. F Plum (ed), American Physiological Society, Baltimore, MD, 1987, pp. 483–518.

Baribeau-Braun J, Picton TW, Gosselin J. Schizophrenia: A neurophysiological evaluation of abnormal information processing. Science 219:874–876, 1983.

Barrett G, Neshige R, Shibasaki H. Human auditory and somatosensory event-related potentials: effects of response condition and age. Electroencephalography Clinical Neurophysiology 66:409–419, 1987.

Bartus RT, Levere TE. Frontal decortication in rhesus monkeys. A test of the interference hypothesis. Brain Research 119:233–248, 1977.

Beck EC, Swan C, Dustman RE. Long latency components of the visually evoked potential in man: effects of aging. Experimental Aging Research 6:523–545, 1980.

Brutkowski S. Functions of prefrontal cortex in animals. Physiological Review 45:721–746, 1965.

Chitty AJ, Mistlin AJ, Perrett DI. Somatosensory and associated visual properties of neurones in a polysensory region of macaque temporal cortex. J Physiology (Abs) 367:301, 1985.

Courchesne E. From infancy to adulthood: the neurophysiological correlates of cognition. In Cognitive Components in Cerebral Event-Related Potentials and Selective Attention. JE Desmedt (ed). S Karger, Basel, 1977, pp. 224–242.

Courchesne E, Hillyard SA, Galambos R. Stimulus novelty, task relevance, and the visual evoked potential in man. Electroencephalography Clinical Neurophysiology 39:131–143, 1975.

Desmedt JE, Hut NT, Bourguet M. The cognitive P40, N60 and P100 components of somatosensory evoked potentials and the earliest electrical signs of sensory processing in man. Electroencephalography Clinical Neurophysiology 56:272–282, 1983.

Edinger HM, Siegel A, Troiano R. Effect of stimulation of prefrontal cortex and amygdala on diencephalic neurons. Brain Research 97:17–31, 1975.

Fabiani M, Karis D, Donchin E. P300 and recall in an incidental memory paradigm. Psychophysiology 23:298–308, 1986.

Fuster JM. The Prefrontal Cortex. Raven Press, New York, 1980.

Goodin DS, Squires KC, Starr A. Long latency event-related components of the auditory evoked potential in dementia. Brain 101:635–648, 1978.

Halgren E, Squires NK, Wilson CL. Rohrbaugh JW, Crandall PH. Endogenous potentials generated in the human hippocampal formation and amygdala by infrequent events. Science 210:803–805, 1980.

Heilman KM, Watson RT, Valenstein E, Damasio AR. Localization of lesions in neglect. In Localization in Neuropsychology. A Kertesz, (ed). Academic Press, New York, 1983, pp. 471–492.

Hier DB, Mondlock J, Caplan LR. Recovery of behavioral abnormalities after right hemisphere stroke. Neurology 33:345–350, 1983.

Hikosaka K, Iwai E, Saito H, Tanaka K. Polyresponse properties of neurons in the anterior bank of the caudal superior temporal sulcus of the Macaque monkey. Journal of Neurophysiology 60:1615–1637, 1988.

Hillyard SA, Hink RF, Schwent VL, Picton TW. Electrical signs of selective attention in the human brain. Science 182:177–180, 1973.

Hillyard SA, Picton T. Electrophysiology of cognition. In Handbook of Physiology. F Plum (ed). American Physiological Society, Baltimore, 1987, pp. 519–584.

Jacobsen CF. Functions of frontal association area in primates. Archives Neurology Psychiatry 33:558–569, 1935.

Johnson Jr, RJ. Scalp-recorded P300 activity in patients following unilateral temporal lobectomy. Brain 111:1517–1529, 1988.

Karis D, Fabiani M, Donchin E. "P300" and memory: Individual differences in the Von Restorff effect. Cognitive Psychology 16:177–216, 1986.

Katayama Y, Tsukiyama T, Tsubokawa T. Thalamic negativity associated with the endogenous late positivity component of cerebral evoked potentials (P300): recording using discriminative aversive conditioning in humans and cats. Brain Research Bulletin 14:223–226, 1985.

Kersteen-Tucker ZA, Knight RT. Cortical lesions dissociate short and long term components of repetition priming. Society Neuroscience (Abs) 15:245, 1989.

Kertesz A, Dobrowolski S. Right-hemisphere deficits, lesion size and location. Journal Clinical Neurophysiology 3:283–299, 1981.

Knight RT, Hillyard SA, Woods DL, Neville SJ. The effects of frontal cortex lesions on event-related potentials during auditory selective attention. Electroencephalography and Clinical Neurophysiology 52:571–582, 1981.

Knight RT. Decreased response to novel stimuli after prefrontal lesions in humans. Electroencephalography and Clinical Neurophysiology 59:9–20, 1984.

Knight RT. Electrophysiology in behavioral neurology. In Principals of Behavioral Neurology. MM Mesulam (ed). Contemporary Neurology Series. FA Davis, Philadelphia, 1985, pp. 327–346.

Knight RT. ERPs in patients with focal brain lesions. Electroencephalography and Clinical Neurophysiology (Abs) 75:72, 1990.

Knight RT. Neural mechanisms of event-related potentials: evidence from human lesion studies. *In* J Rohrbaugh, R Parasuman, and R Johnson, Jr (eds). Oxford University Press, New York, 1990, pp. 3–18.

Knight RT, Scabini D, Woods DL. Prefrontal cortex gating of auditory transmission in humans. Brain Research 504:338–342, 1989a.

Knight RT, Scabini D, Woods DL, Clayworth CC. Contribution of temporal-parietal junction to the human auditory P3. Brain Research 502:109–116, 1989b.

Kraus N, Ozdamar O, Stein L. Auditory middle latency responses (MRLs) in patients with cortical lesions. Electroencephalography and Clinical Neurophysiology 54:275–287, 1982.

Lemay M, Kido DK. Asymmetries of the cerebral hemisphere on computed tomograms. Journal Computed Assisted Tomography 2:471–476, 1978.

Lynch JC. The functional organization of posterior parietal association cortex. Behavioral Brain Science 3:485–534, 1980.

McCallum WC, Curry SH, Cooper R, Pocock PV, Papakostopoulos D. Brain event-related potentials as indicators of early selective processes in auditory target localization. Psychophysiology 20:1–17, 1983.

McCarthy G, Wood CC, Williamson PD, Spencer DD. Task-dependent field potentials in human hippocampal formation. Journal of Neuroscience 9:4253–4260, 1989.

Mesulam MM. A cortical network for directed attention and unilateral neglect. Annals of Neurology 10:309–325, 1981.

Milner B. Some cognitive effects of frontal lesions in man. Philosophical Transactions Royal Society London 298:211–226, 1982.

Okada YC, Kaufman L, Williamson SJ. The hippocampal formation as a source of the slow endogenous potentials. Electroencephalography and Clinical Neurophysiology 55:417–426, 1983.

Paller KA, Kutas M, Mayes AR. Neural correlates of encoding in an incidental learning paradigm. Electroencephalography and Clinical Neurophysiology 67:360–371, 1987.

Pelizzone M, Hari R, Makela JP, Huttunen J, Hamalainen M. Cortical origin of middle-latency auditory evoked responses in man. Neuroscience Letters 82:303–307, 1987.

Pritchard WS. Cognitive event related potential correlates in schizophrenia. Psychologic Bulletin 100:43–66, 1986.

Scabini D, Knight RT, Woods DL. Frontal lobe contributions to the human P3a. Society Neuroscience (Abs) 15:477, 1989.

Skinner JE, Yingling CD. Central gating mechanisms that regulate event-related potentials and behavior. Progress Clinical Neurophysiology 1:30–69, 1977.

Sokolov EN. Higher nervous functions: the orienting reflex. Annual Review Physiology 25:545–580, 1963.

Squires N, Squires K, Hillyard SA. Two varieties of long-latency positive waves evoked by unpredictable auditory stimuli in man. Electroencephalography and Clinical Neurophysiology 38:387–401, 1975.

Stein S, Volpe BT. Classic "parietal" neglect syndrome after subcortical right frontal lobe infarction. Neurology 33:797–799, 1983.

Stuss DT, Benson DF. Neurophysiolgical studies of the frontal lobe. Psychological Bulletin 95:3–28, 1984.

Tulving E, Schacter DL. Priming and human memory systems. Science 247:301–306, 1990.

Velasco M, Velasco F, Velasco AL, Almanza X, Olivera A. Subcortical correlates of the P300 potential complex in man to auditory stimuli. Electroencephalography and Clinical Neurophysiology 64:199–210, 1986.

Wada JA, Clarke R, Hamm A. Cerebral hemispheric asymmetry in humans. Archives Neurology 32:239–246, 1975.

Weinberger DR, Luchins DJ, Morisha J, Wyatt RJ. Asymmetric volumes of the right and left frontal and occipital regions of the human brain. Annals of Neurology 11:97–100, 1982.

Woldorff M, Hansen JC, Hillyard SA. Evidence for effects of selective attention in the mid-latency range of the human auditory event-related potential. *In* Current Trends in Event-Related Potential Research (EEG Suppl 40). R Johnson Jr, JW Rohrbaugh, and R Parasuraman (eds). Elsevier Science Publisher BV, Ireland, 1987, pp. 146–154.

Woods DL. The physiological basis of selective attention: implications of event-related potential studies. Event-Related Brain Potentials, J Rohrbaugh, R Johnson, Jr, and R Parasuraman (eds). Oxford University Press, New York, 1990, pp. 178–210.

Woods DL, Knight RT. Electrophysiological evidence of increased distractibility after dorsolateral prefrontal lesions. Neurology 36:212–216, 1986.

Woods DL, Knight RT, Scabini D, Clayworth CC. Automatic shifts of auditory attention are impaired by parietal-temporal lesions. Society Neuroscience (Abs) 13:852, 1987.

Yamaguchi S, Knight RT. Gating of somatosensory inputs by human prefrontal cortex. Brain Research 521:281, 1990.

Yamaguchi S, Knight RT. P300 generation by novel somatosensory stimuli. Electroencephalography and Clinical Neurophysiology 78:50–55, 1991.

Yamaguchi S, Knight RT. Anterior and posterior association cortex contributions to the somatosensory P300. Journal of Neuroscience (in press).

Yingling CD, Hosobuchi Y. A subcortical correlate of P300 in man. Electroencephalography and Clinical Neurophysiology 59:72–76, 1984.

Yingling CD, Skinner JE. Gating of thalamic input to cerebral cortex by nucleus reticularis thalami. *In* Progress Clinical Neurophysiology (Vol 1). JE Desmedt (ed). S Karger, Basel, 1977, pp. 70–96.

IV
The Role of the Frontal Lobes in Memory

8

Interference Effects on Memory Functions in Postleukotomy Patients: An Attentional Perspective

DONALD T. STUSS

The role of interference on memory functions in patients who have suffered focal frontal lobe damage has been frequently inferred from the results of clinical observations and experimental research. What type of interference and how this phenomenon relates to theoretic constructs has been less frequently presented. This chapter begins with a brief historical review of the detrimental effects of interference on behavior in patients who have frontal lobe damage. This history includes a more detailed presentation of interference effects in postleukotomy patients. The final section addresses theoretic issues possibly related to these basic data.

INTERFERENCE AND FRONTAL LOBE FUNCTION: A HISTORICAL REVIEW

The ability of frontal lobe damaged monkeys to perform immediate discrimination tasks stands in marked contrast to their striking deficit on tasks of apparent similar difficulty where a delayed response is required. To early researchers, this suggested that these animals suffered a "loss of recent memory" (Jacobsen, 1935; 1936). With experimental refinement, it was concluded that other factors were more relevant. These variables included drive (Pribram, 1950), distractibility (Finan, 1942; Malmo, 1942), and stimulus and task specificity (Jacobsen and Nissen, 1937; Pribram, 1961). When there were no distracting factors during the delay, the frontal lobe damaged monkeys were not impaired. It appeared that the deficit was an "inability to inhibit its orienting reflexes to irrelevant stimuli, inhibiting the retention of the necessary selective traces" (Luria, 1967, p. 737).

Fuster (1985), reviewing many delayed response studies, postulated that at least two factors influence results on the delayed response tasks. One of the deficient functions did indeed appear to be short-term memory, since the severity of the deficit was related to the length of the delay. The second, apparently more relevant, factor was termed attention/interference control. Regardless of the duration of delay, no deficit would be revealed on delayed-response tasks by frontal lobe damaged monkeys if there were no competing alternatives creating interference. An inability to maintain consistent, directed attention over time because of vulnerability to interference appeared to be a basic deficit in monkeys with frontal lobe damage (Fuster, 1985). This was also called a defect in the normal capacity to suppress (Fuster, 1981).

The history of the effects of interference in humans with frontal lobe damage has been less consistent. This has perhaps been due to the fact that the impairment has been described in different ways. Some authors expressed the disorder as an inability to persist in working on a problem; other authors stressed the impairment in the control of reactions to distracting stimuli. "On the one hand, the patient does not maintain the facilitative set for staying at work; on the other, he does not sustain the inhibitive set against reacting to distracting stimuli" (Arnot, 1952, pp. 490–491). The deficit in this view is a double-edged sword. Regardless of the cause, the end result in behavioral terms appeared to be similar (Denny-Brown, 1951).

An excellent clinical description of the type of change that occurred after frontal lobe damage was articulated by Harlow (1868). Phineas Gage prior to the accident that caused significant medial frontal pathology was, to all accounts, "persistent in executing all his plans of operation." Subsequently, however, he was "capricious and vacillating." Many other authors emphasized the impairment in persistence, maintenance or sustaining of a function (Arnot, 1952; Malmo, 1948). The operational definitions, however, were quite broad. Robinson (1946) suggested that prefrontal lobotomy resulted in decreased "deliberative" behavior and impaired ability to maintain and prolong attention. This was revealed in three ways: Resistance to distraction; capacity for deliberation; motor capacity to behave deliberately. Arnold (1960) labeled the problem an "interference with the appraisal of action," the frontal lobe patient giving in to every impulse as it arose. Incongruously, the patient may persist in some inappropriate action.

Malmo (1948; Malmo and Amsel, 1948) stressed the effects of interference during learning tasks. Assessing serial position in learning, he demonstrated that frontal gyrectomy patients had increased susceptibility to intraserial interference, a result he labeled "associative interference." Patients with frontal lobe damage had increased "oscillations," defined as the alternation between successful and unsuccessful responses.

The detrimental influence of interference has perhaps been most frequently noted during more recent studies of the effects of frontal lobe damage on memory functions, although there have been exceptions (Eslinger and Damasio, 1985). Prisko, in Milner's laboratory (1964; Milner et al., 1985), used a delayed comparison technique in which two easily discernible stimuli in the same sensory modality (pairs of colors, clicks, tones, and nonsense stimuli) were presented with intertrial delays of 60 seconds. A frontal lobe deficit was revealed whenever the same stimuli recurred in different pairings. This occurred for all but the novel nonsense stimuli, in which each stimulus pair was unique. "This contrast appears to indicate that the patients with frontal-lobe lesions had a heightened susceptibility to interference from the effects of preceding trials, rather than an inability to retain new information over a short time interval" (Milner et al., 1985, p. 137). A similar general pattern of results was observed on tests of recurring figures, or continuous recognition, which maximize interference effects. In this procedure, a series of single stimuli is presented consecutively, with a defined number of the stimuli repeated in the series (Kimura, 1963). For each stimulus the subject indicates whether it is old (repeated) or new. Frontal lobe patients were impaired on certain subtests but not others (Milner, 1964; Milner and Teuber, 1968). It appeared that frontal patients did have a heightened susceptibility to proactive interference, but that this could not explain the disorder nor the variability in results. The importance of the specific method of testing was emphasized. Lewinsohn and associates (1972) noted that frontal patients were impaired on memory tasks. Each task, however, used interference procedures to control for rehearsal, so that an attribution to an amnesic deficit could not be made. Butters and colleagues (1970), using the Brown-Peterson Test, which has an interference component, reported that left frontal patients had impaired registration of verbal material, but no memory deficit as measured by delayed recall. Right frontal patients, on the other hand, had the opposite pattern. Lesion extent, however, was not controlled.

The strength of the interference effects in patients with frontal lobe damage, as well as the controversy concerning the reliability of such effects, is revealed in the studies on release from proactive interference (PI). In this paradigm, different lists (e.g., five) of words are read to the subject. The first four lists are composed of words derived from the same category, resulting in a buildup of PI, with increasingly poorer performance on each subsequent list. The last list is from a different category, allowing release from PI, as indicated by improved recall of the last list. Moscovitch (1981), comparing patients with different focal lesions, demonstrated that patients with left frontal lobe damage had the least amount of release. It was concluded that failure to release from PI is associated with frontal impairment rather than memory loss. Other research seemed to corroborate this conclusion. The deficit of Korsakoff patients on release from PI tasks is correlated with their degree of frontal impairment (Squire, 1982). Parkin and colleagues (1988) reported impaired release from PI in a patient with an anterior communicating artery aneurysm.

Other studies, however, presented conflicting data. Comparing frontal patients with and without memory deficit, it was concluded that impaired release from PI was present in patients with frontal pathology only if there was a concomitant memory impairment (Freedman and Cermak, 1986). Janowsky and colleagues (1989) went so far as to state failure to release from PI is specifically not a frontal lobe deficit.

In summary, both observational and research evidence suggest that a sensitivity to interference is a prominent deficit after frontal lobe damage. Milner and Teuber (1968) emphasized the importance of the concept of interference in differentiating in frontal lobe patients actual memory loss and difficulty with initial registration. Fuster stated, "Protection against interference from both inside and outside the organism . . . is one of the important functions of prefrontal cortex in the organization of behavior" (Fuster, 1981, p. 1167). This review also outlined important variables influencing the effect of interference: The possibility of different kinds of interference effects; the descriptive nature of the term interference; and the importance of methodologic issues such as test design and administration, and lesion location and extent.

THE NORTHAMPTON LEUKOTOMY STUDY

The data presented here are derived from a series of articles summarizing the Northampton Veterans Administration study of the long-term (approximately 25 years) effects of prefrontal leukotomy (Benson et al., 1981; Naeser et al., 1981; Stuss et al., 1981a,b; 1982).

Twenty-six males were tested and divided into five groups (n = 5, except group 3 where n = 6) equated for experience of military service, age, socioeconomic status, and years of education. Group 5 was a normal control group without central nervous system or psychiatric dysfunction. All four patient groups (1 to 4) were schizophrenics from the same institution. The first three groups, all institutionalized within a similar time period (early 1940s) and diagnosed by the same core of physicians, had been treated by bilateral prefrontal psychosurgery (Fig. 8–1). These groups differed primarily in the degree of recovery after surgery: group 1 = good recovery; group 2 = moderate recovery; group 3 = poor recovery. Group 4 (nonleukotomized psychiatric control group) consisted of schizophrenic patients equated with groups 1, 2, and 3 for diagnosis, age, education, and nonsurgical psychiatric treatment, who had not undergone psychosurgery. They were comparable with group 3 in years of hospitalization and treatment. There was no statistical IQ difference between the good recovery and normal control groups. Because of the possible influence of factors such as the level of recovery, emphasis herein is placed on the comparison between these latter two groups (1 and 5).

The tests relevant to the issue of interference can be grouped into three very general categories. The first is the baseline measures of clinical attention, which have no apparent external interference factor. The second category consists of tests of "attention," which do have an interference component. The third is measures of memory, contrasting those tests with and without overt influence of interference factors. These divisions are established on face validity and do not imply a theoretic basis for differentiation.

General Clinical Measures of Attention

1. Mental control tests of the Wechsler Memory Scale, form 1 (Wechsler, 1945); Serial Seven subtraction (Smith, 1967): The group 1 good recovery leukotomized patients did not differ significantly from the control subjects on time or error measures for either test, all results falling within the normal range. For example, time to complete the count by threes task (1–4–7 . . . 40) was as follows: group 1, $M = 17.6$, $SD = 8.6$; group 5, $M = 13.6$, $SD = 15$. The subjects

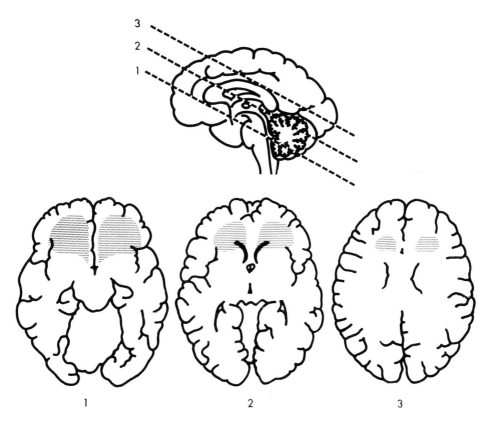

Figure 8-1 This schematic representation depicts the approximate location of frontal leukotomy lesions in the Northampton VA Medical Center series. Lesions were bilateral in the anterior medial-frontal white matter. (From Stuss and Benson, 1983, with permission.)

in group 1, who had large bilateral orbitofrontal lesions, were actually superior on the Serial Seven test (100–93–86 . . . 58) in time (53.6 seconds) and errors (2.2) to the control group 5 (time = 74.8; errors = 3.4).

2. Span Tests: Digit span forward and backward (Wechsler, 1955); Knox Cube Imitation Test (Arthur, 1947). The digit span measurement is a well-known test, incorporated in bedside neurobehavioral examinations and formal clinical investigations. The Knox Cube is a "nonverbal" counterpart of digits forward. Results of these two tests are presented in Figure 8-2. There were no significant differences between the two defined groups.

In summary, on basic clinical tests that did not appear to have any interference component, good recovery leukotomized patients with large bilateral orbitofrontal lesions were not significantly impaired, and indeed performed as well or better than the normal control subjects on certain tests.

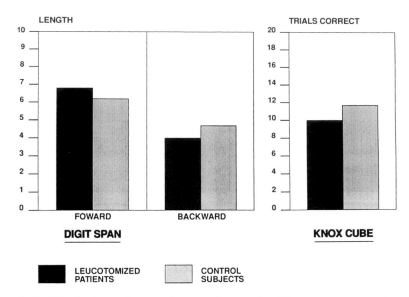

Figure 8-2 The leukotomized patients and control subjects are compared on verbal (Digit Span) and nonverbal (Knox Cube) span tests.

Attentional Tasks with an Interference Component

Two tests were administered that appeared to fit this descriptive category.

1. The Trail-Making Test (Army Individual Test Battery, 1944) consists of two parts. In part A, the subject draws a line joining consecutively numbered circles randomly arranged on a page. In part B, the subject connects letters and numbers in an alternating sequential manner (1–A–2–B . . . 13). The rapid alternation between numbers and letters creates some interference. Reitan (1958) suggested that part B may be particularly sensitive to damage in the frontal lobes. Frontal lobe patients, when impaired on this test, can reveal striking qualitative deficits (Picton et al., 1986) (Fig. 8–3). When the subjects in the two groups defined in this study were assessed, the group 1 patients were somewhat slower on both tasks, but there was no significant difference between the groups (Fig. 8–4). There was a large standard deviation.

2. The Stroop (1935) test more directly assesses the issue of interference. In the version used for the studies described herein, three separate pages contained either (1) three color names, (red, blue, green) typed in black on white (word reading); (2) randomized red, blue, and green rectangles, which the subject named (color naming); and (3) color names printed in a color different from the word itself (interference). For example, the word blue would be printed in red or green, and so on. The subject stated the color of the word, but did not read the word itself. In the past, the Stroop test was reported as sensitive to the effects of focal frontal lobe damage (Perret, 1974). In the study described in this chapter there were no significant differences between the two defined groups (Figure 8–

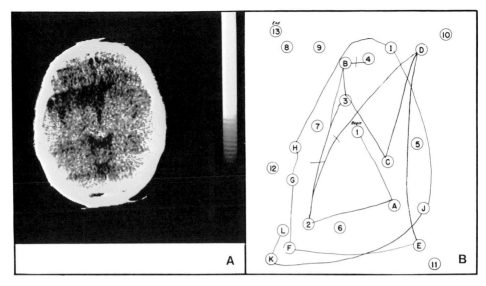

Figure 8–3 The left side of the figure is a computerized tomography scan showing a deep infarct (dark area) in the left frontal lobe. In this figure, left is left. On the right side is the patient's attempt to alternately connect numbers and letters as required on Part B of the Trail-Making Test. (From Picton, et al., 1986, with permission.)

Figure 8–4 Leukotomized subjects are slower, but not significantly so, on both Part A (1–2–3 . . .) and Part B (1–A–2–B . . .) of the Trail-Making Test.

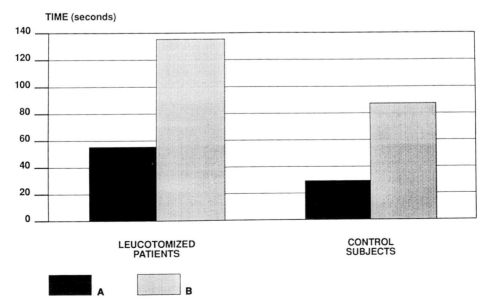

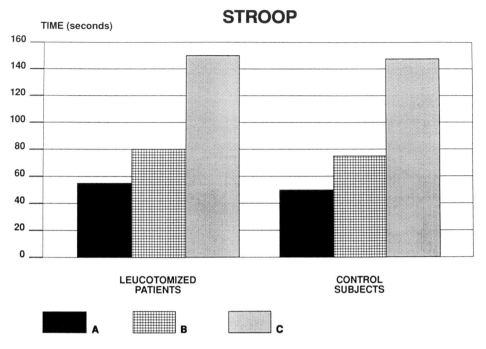

Figure 8-5 There is no significant difference between the leukotomized patients and control subjects on any measures of the Stroop test: A = word reading; B = color naming; C = interference subtest.

5). Again, while the leukotomized subjects were somewhat slower, this was not a statistical difference.

In summary, leukotomized patients did not reveal a striking deficit on attentional tasks that included factors of interference. Possible factors explaining this apparent contradiction with previous results will be presented in the discussion.

Memory Tasks

The Wechsler Memory Scale Form 1 (WMS; Wechsler, 1945) was used as a baseline measure for comparison to memory tasks that have an interference component. There was no significant difference between the leukotomized and normal control groups for the overall memory quotient. For certain subtest measures, such as the difficult Paired Associates, the patient group was actually superior (group 1 = 7.8, SD = 2.9; group 5 = 7.0, SD = 2.6).

Two memory tests with interference were administered.

1. Verbal and Nonverbal Recurring Figures (Kimura, 1963; Milner and Teuber, 1968). In this test, a series of cards (verbal—144; nonverbal—160) were individually presented one every 3–5 seconds. Within each series, a defined

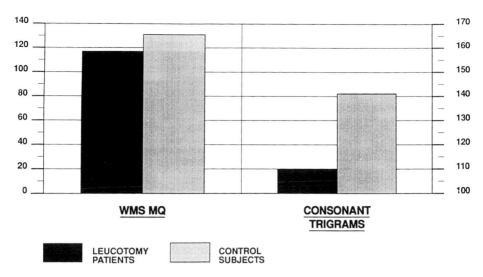

Figure 8–6 Comparison of leukotomy patients with orbital frontal lesions with the control subjects on the Wechsler Memory Scale—Memory Quotient **(left)** and the Brown-Peterson test of short-term memory under interference. The Brown-Peterson score is the sum of three separate versions. (From Stuss, 1987, with permission.)

number of stimuli were repeated. The subject was required to indicate for each stimulus whether it had been presented previously or not. As noted above, frontal lobe patients had previously been shown to be impaired on this test. For the present comparisons, the group 1 leukotomized subjects were not significantly different from the normal control group for all classifications of dependent measures (e.g., words, numbers, nonsense words) in either series. On some measures (e.g., number of false-positive responses for the verbal series) the orbitofrontal damaged patients ($M = 5.6$, $SD = 1.1$) actually performed better than the control group ($M = 6.6$, $SD = 4.3$).

2. Brown-Peterson Test of Short-Term Memory under Interference (Brown, 1958; Cermak and Butters, 1972; Peterson and Peterson, 1959). Sets of three consonants ($Q-L-X$) were presented to the subject in three different modality/order combinations: Oral sequential; visual sequential; visual simultaneous. Each triad was followed by delay of 0, 3, 9, or 18 seconds, after which the subject had to recall the three letters. Interference was caused during the delay by having the subject count backward out loud by threes, starting with a random number.

In other studies of frontal lobe patients, the results on the Brown-Peterson have been equivocal (Butters et al., 1970; Eslinger and Damasio, 1985). The results of the two groups observed in this test are summarized in Figure 8–6, which compares the total of all three versions of the Brown-Peterson to the WMS memory quotient. While groups 1 and 5 were both equivalent on the WMS, the leukotomized subjects were significantly impaired on the Brown-Peterson.

In summary, patients with bilateral orbitofrontal leukotomy did show a striking deficit in memory when interference was presented, at least in certain tasks. As suggested by the historical observations, interference does appear to be a prominent factor affecting the performance of patients with frontal system damage. Both the leukotomy results as well as the history, however, indicate some variability in results. The following section discusses the possible factors influencing the results.

METHODOLOGIC AND THEORETIC ISSUES

The general clinical tests of attention provide an important fulcrum for comparison. While behaviorally the leukotomized patients were apathetic and easily distracted by extraneous stimulation, the good recovery patients (group 1) in particular performed normally on many of the attentional tasks, such as Serial Seven Subtraction, the WMS Mental Control subtests, and the Knox Cube Imitation test. A more detailed evaluation of Digit Span serves as an example. This test has been presented as a general measure of attention, immediate memory, and mental flexibility (Lezak, 1976). One or more of its measures has been shown to be sensitive to brain damage (e.g., Black and Strub, 1978; Costa, 1975; De Renzi and Nichelli, 1975; Russell, 1972; Smith and Kinder, 1959; Spreen and Benton, 1965). However, if the pathology is localized within the frontal cortex, digit span has been most consistently reported as unimpaired (Mettler, 1949; Partridge, 1950; Stuss et al., 1978; Teuber, 1964), with only few exceptions (e.g., Hamlin, 1970). Frontal lobe damage of any etiology does not appear to cause chronic impairment on basic attentional tasks. These negative findings also confirm that, as a group, the leukotomy patients were testable, cooperative, and task oriented.

Two classifications of tests were employed to assess if the focal orbitofrontal damage caused by the leukotomy would reveal the effects of interference on functioning. On the Stroop and Trail-Making tests, the leukotomized patients were not significantly impaired. In striking contrast, the leukotomized patients revealed a significant impairment on the Brown-Peterson test, indicating a susceptibility to the effects of interference. The comparison of the same patients' performance on the WMS and the Brown-Peterson isolated the dramatic effects caused by the interference when trying to recall the three letters.

Why is this deficit not consistent? That is, why is there not a significant impairment on all of the tasks that had an interference component such as the Stroop and the Recurring Figures, particularly when significant impairment in frontal lobe patients had been previously reported on the measures? This problem will be addressed by examining methodologic factors and theoretic issues.

One possibility is the test situation. This was an important factor in the delayed-response paradigms, where performance dramatically improved when distractions were minimized or attention captured (Isaac and De Vito, 1958; Malmo, 1942; Orbach and Fischer, 1959). Perhaps, as previously suggested, "with elimination of distractions and rigid demand for compliance, the examiner may act as the frontal lobes for these patients" (Stuss et al., 1981a, p. 1096). One would have to postulate that the examiner's ability to serve as an external control would be limited, since the Brown-Peterson deficit was not eliminated.

A second factor may be the length of time since the psychosurgery, allowing for recovery and adaptation (Finger and Stein, 1982). This hypothesis alone, however, is also insufficient to explain the variability in results.

Localization of lesion might be an important variable. Localization of function within the frontal cortex is an accepted fact (Milner, 1964; Pandya, 1987; Petrides, 1987; Stuss and Benson, 1983). Luria (1973) had suggested that attentional deficits were prominent with medial basal lesions. The leukotomized patients had pathology maximal in the lower orbitofrontal white matter regions. Fuster (1988) had suggested that in nonhuman animals, suppression of interfering memories could be related particularly to ventral and medial frontal cortex. However, patients with dorsolateral frontal pathology also appear to have a susceptibility to interference (Milner, 1964; Milner et al., 1985). With the evidence available, localization within the frontal cortex cannot yet be considered a deciding variable in relation to interference effects.

Another possible factor may be the structure of the tests themselves. Milner and Teuber (1968) had emphasized the importance of test structure and procedure. The data are not clear in this regard. For example, the Brown-Peterson has been interpreted as creating proactive interference, in the sense that the preceding trials interfere with subsequent trials (Squire, 1987; Stuss et al., 1982). If so, then, the leukotomized patients should also have revealed impairment in the Recurring Figures subtest, which appears to have proactive interference as an inherent quality. There was no such evidence, even in a first-half–second-half comparison. It may be, however, that the Brown-Peterson creates not only proactive but also retroactive interference, the latter reflected in the interference caused by counting before recall. The conjunction of the two types of interference may make it particularly sensitive.

In the leukotomy studies, one must also consider factors such as sample size. On certain tests such as the Trail-Making part B, there was a tendency for the leukotomized subjects to perform more poorly. Decreased power due to small sample size is again an insufficient explanation of the variable effects of interference, since on many tasks such as the Recurring Figures there was minimal difference between the two groups.

It appears that methodologic factors cannot adequately explain the variability in the results. A more profitable approach to the question of interference effects may be from a theoretic perspective. Prisko's results, for example, evolved into the proposal that the frontal lobes are important to the ability to structure and segregate events in memory (Milner and Teuber, 1968; Milner et al., 1985). Another proposed possibility is to examine the detrimental effects of interference from the viewpoint of an attentional disorder. With few exceptions research on the effects of frontal lobe damage in humans has not utilized attentional concepts.

The psychologic process of attention can be viewed in several ways (see Moscovitch, 1981). An arbitrary decision is made in this presentation to define attention as divided, focused, and sustained capabilities. *Divided attention* refers to the ability to handle multiple sources of information simultaneously. The deficit suggests a capacity limitation. *Focused attention* is defined as the ability to inhibit pull to irrelevant information. Automatic response tendencies conflict with the present task demands. *Sustained attention* indicates the ability to maintain attention over time. It is proposed that the term "interference" has been used generically, even though in reality different tests or situations using interference evoked different attentional problems. Historically, Arnot's (1952) concept of facilitative set appears to reflect sustained attention, while inhibitive set is consistent with the notion of focused attention. Perhaps, the Brown-Peterson test should be interpreted as a divided attention deficit (handling multiple sources of information simultaneously), as well as a sustained attention problem due to the extended nature of the test. Fuster and Bauer (1974) described a similar deficit in monkeys as the inability to maintain consistent, directed attention over time because of vulnerability to interfering stimuli.

An interaction between a methodologic issue and the type of attentional disorder might be postulated to explain the variable effects of interference. For example, the interference effects of the Stroop might not be present in the leukotomized subjects because of lesion location and the specificity of the interference effect, i.e., a focused attention rather than divided attention problem.

Another interpretation, borrowed from our work in patients with traumatic brain injury (TBI) (Stuss et al., 1989), is based on an extended definition of attention. A reaction time paradigm was constructed to assess the presence and severity of a focused attention deficit in TBI patients. Two groups of TBI patients were assessed, each compared with age-, sex-, and education-matched control subjects. The first study evaluated patients with varying severity of TBI who had been hospitalized. In the second study, mildly concussed patients were followed during recovery. Patients were tested repetitively, depending on the specific study (study 1 = 2 consecutive weeks; study 2 = 5 times over a 3-month period). As expected, the patients had a divided attention problem. In addition, however, a focused attention deficit was revealed. An unexpected observation was that this deficit was variable and would be revealed inconsistently over repeated assessments (Fig. 8–7). We proposed that the attentional deficit in head-injured patients was not a simple impairment. In addition to a divided attention deficit, there were two superimposed and interactive attentional problems in focused attention and consistency of performance. While head-injured patients as a group could muster resources to meet the demands of a focused attention task, they were inconsistent in maintaining that optimal level of performance. The "top-down" focused attention is apparently reached at a cost that cannot be maintained.

Inconsistency of performance may be an important aspect of attention. It is different from sustained attention, which normally refers to time on task over a limited time period. It does, however, have considerable similarity to the concepts of "persistence" and "maintenance" proposed in the frontal lobe research. The focused attention deficit was variably revealed because of inconsistency of performance. Patients may be able to do a task, but not sustain it over a defined single period of time (sustained attention), or maintain consistent performance over repetitive evaluations (consistent attention). The possibility that inconsistency may be more directly related for frontal executive functions derives as well from the head injury literature. TBI patients, although suffering from diffuse brain damage, may predominantly have frontotemporal pathology (Courville,

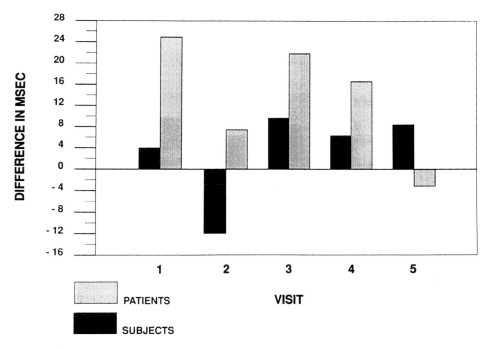

Figure 8-7   The concussed subjects are compared with matched control subjects on the focused attention task over five visits. The higher the score, the greater the vulnerability to distracting stimuli. The figure illustrates the relatively greater focused attention deficit of the concussed subjects, as well as their greater variability in maintaining consistent performance. (From Stuss and Gow, in press, with permission.)

1937; Stuss, 1987; Stuss and Gow, in press). This hypothesis, including the specificity of lesion localization to and within the frontal systems for the concept of inconsistency of attention, requires verification.

In summary, frontal lobe damage results in a susceptibility to interference. This concept, however, is too broad and, consequently, misleading. Interpretation in terms of attentional constructs provides a more logical postulate for understanding the deficit in frontal lobe patients, and for advancing knowledge.

ACKNOWLEDGMENTS

Research funding was provided by the Ontario Mental Health Foundation. P. Mathews is thanked for typing the manuscript. J. Pogue and T. Halpen are thanked for preparation of the figures.

REFERENCES

Army Individual Test Battery. Manual of Directions and Scoring, U.S. Army. Washington, D.C.: War Department, Adjutant General's office, 1944.

Arnold MB. Emotion and Personality, Vol II, Neurological and Physiological Aspects. New York: Columbia University Press, 1960.

Arnot R. A theory of frontal lobe function. Arch Neurol Psychiat 67:487–495, 1952.

Arthur G. A Point Scale of Performance Tests. Revised form II. New York: Psychological Corporation, 1947.

Benson DF, Stuss DT, Naeser MA, Weir WS, Kaplan EF, Levine HL. The long-term effects of pre-frontal leucotomy. Arch Neurol 38:165–169, 1981.

Black FW, Strub RL. Digit repetition performance in patients with focal brain damage. Cortex 14:12–21, 1978.

Brown J. Some tests of the decay theory of immediate memory. Q J Exp Psychol 10:12–21, 1958.

Butters N, Samuels I, Goodglass H, Brody B. Short-term visual and auditory memory disorders after parietal and frontal lobe damage. Cortex 6:440–459, 1970.

Cermak LS, Butters N. The role of interference and encoding in the short-term memory of Korsakoff patients. Neuropsychologia 10:89–95, 1972.

Costa LD. The relation of visuospatial dysfunction to digit span performance in patients with cerebral lesions. Cortex 11:31–36, 1975.

Courville CB. Pathology of the Central Nervous System, part 4. Mountain View, CA: Pacific Publishers, 1937.

Denny-Brown D. The frontal lobes and their functions. *In* Feiling A (ed), Modern Trends in Neurology. London: Butterworth, 1951, pp. 13–89.

De Renzi E, Nichelli P. Verbal and non-verbal short-term memory impairment following hemispheric damage. Cortex 11:341–354, 1975.

Eslinger PJ, Damasio AR. Severe disturbance of higher cognition following bilateral frontal lobe ablation: patient EVR. Neurology 35:1731–1741, 1985.

Finan JL. Delayed response with pre-delay reinforcement in monkeys after the removal of the frontal lobes. Am J Psychiatry 55:202–214, 1942.

Finger S, Stein DG. Brain Damage and Recovery. Research and Clinical Perspectives. New York: Academic Press, 1982.

Freedman M, Cermak LS. Semantic encoding deficits in frontal lobe disease. Brain Cog 5:108–114, 1986.

Fuster JM. Prefrontal cortex in motor control. *In* Brooks VB (ed), Handbook of Physiology—The Nervous System, Vol. II: Motor Control. Bethesda: AM Physiol Soc, 1981, pp. 1149–1178.

Fuster JM. The prefrontal cortex, mediator of cross-temporal contingencies. Human Neurobiol 4:169–179, 1985.

Fuster JM. The Prefrontal Cortex. Anatomy, Physiology, and Neuropsychology of the Frontal Lobe. New York: Raven Press, 1988.

Fuster, JM, Bauer RH. Visual short-term memory deficit from hypothermia of frontal cortex. Br Res 81:393–400, 1974.

Hamlin RM. Intellectual function 14 years after frontal lobe surgery. Cortex 6:299–307, 1970.

Harlow JM. Recovery after severe injury to the head. Publ Mass Med Soc 2:327–346, 1868.

Isaac W, De Vito JL. Effect of sensory stimulation on the activity of normal and prefrontal-lobectomized monkeys. J Comp Physiol Psychiat 51:172–174, 1958.

Jacobsen CF. Functions of the frontal association area in primates. Arch Neurol Psychiat 33:558–569, 1935.

Jacobsen CF. Studies of cerebral functions in primates: I. The functions of the frontal association areas in monkeys. Comp Psychol Monographs 13:3–60, 1936.

Jacobsen CF, Nissen HW. Studies of cerebral functions in primates. IV. The effects of frontal lobe lesions on the delayed alternation habit in monkeys. J Comp Psychol 23:101–112, 1937.

Janowsky JS, Shimamura AP, Kritchevsky M, Squire LR. Cognitive impairment following frontal lobe damage and its relevance to human amnesia. Behav Neurosci 103:548–560, 1989.

Kimura D. Right temporal lobe damage. Arch Neurol 8:264–271, 1963.

Lewinsohn PM, Zieler RE, Libet J, Eyeberg S, Nielson G. Short-term memory: A comparison between frontal and nonfrontal right and left-hemisphere brain-damaged patients. J Comp Physiol Psychol 81:248–255, 1972.

Lezak MD. Neuropsychological Assessment. New York: Oxford University Press, 1976.

Luria AR. The working brain. (B. Haigh, trans.). New York: Basic, 1973.

Luria AR. Frontal lobe syndromes. *In* Vinken PJ, Bruyn GW (eds), Handbook of Clinical Neurology, Vol 2. Amsterdam: North Holland, 1967, pp. 725–757.

Malmo RB. Interference factors in delayed response in monkeys after removal of frontal lobes. J Neurophysiol 5:295–308, 1942.

Malmo RB. Psychological aspects of frontal gyrectomy and frontal lobotomy in mental patients. Res Publ Assoc Res Nerv Men Dis 27:537–564, 1948.

Malmo RB, Amsel A. Anxiety-produced interference in serial rote learning with observations on rote learning after partial frontal lobectomy. J Exp Psychol 38:440–454, 1948.

Mettler FA (ed). Columbia-Greystone Associates. Selective Partial Ablation of the Frontal Cortex: A Correlative Study of its Effects on Human Psychotic Subjects. New York: Hoeber, 1949.

Milner B. Some effects of frontal lobectomy in man. *In* Warren JM, Akert K (eds), The Frontal Granular Cortex and Behavior. New York: McGraw-Hill, 1964, pp. 313–334.

Milner B, Petrides M, Smith ML. Frontal lobes and the temporal organization of memory. Human Neurobiol 4:137–142, 1985.

Milner B, Teuber HL. Alteration of perception and memory in man. *In* Weiskrantz L (ed), Analysis of Behavioral Change. New York: Harper & Row, 1968, pp. 268–375.

Moscovitch M. Multiple dissociations of function in the amnesic syndrome. *In* Cermak LS (ed), Human Memory and Amnesia. Hillsdale NJ: Erlbaum, 1981, pp. 337–370.

Naeser MA, Levine HL, Benson DF, Stuss DT, Weir WS. Frontal leucotomy size and hemispheric asymmetries on CT scans of schizophrenics with variable recovery. Arch Neurol 38:30–37, 1981.

Orbach J, Fischer GJ. Bilateral resections of frontal granular cortex. Factors influencing delayed response and discrimination performance in monkeys. A.M.A. Arch Neurol 1:78–86, 1959.

Parkin AJ, Leng NRC, Stanhope N, Smith AP. Memory impairment following ruptured aneurysm of the anterior communicating artery. Brain Cog 7:231–243, 1988.

Partridge M. Pre-frontal Leucotomy. Oxford: Blackwell, 1950.

Perret E. The left frontal lobe of man and the suppression of habitual responses in verbal categorical behaviour. Neuropsychologia 12:323–330, 1974.

Peterson LR, Peterson MJ. Short-term retention of individual verbal items. J Exp Psychol 58:193–198, 1959.

Petrides M. Conditional learning and the primate frontal cortex. *In* Perecman E (ed), The Frontal Lobes Revisited. New York: IRBN Press, 1987, pp. 91–108.

Picton TW, Stuss DT, Marshall KC. Attention and the brain. *In* Friedman SL. Klivington KA, Peterson RW (eds), The Brain, Cognition, and Education. New York: Academic Press, 1986, pp. 19–79.

Pribram KH. Some physical and pharmacological factors affecting delayed response performance of baboons following frontal lobotomy. J Neurophysiol 13:373–382, 1950.

Pribram KH. A further experimental analysis of the behavioral deficit that follows injury to the primate frontal cortex. Exp Neurol 3:432–466, 1961.

Reitan RM. Validity of the Trail-making test as an indicator of organic brain damage. Percept Mot Skills 8:271–276, 1958.

Robinson MF. What price lobotomy? J Abnorm Soc Psychol 41:421–436, 1946.

Russell EW. WAIS factor analysis with brain-damaged subjects using criterion measures. J Consult Clin Psychol 39:133–139, 1972.

Smith A. The serial sevens subtraction test. Arch Neurol 17:78–80, 1967.

Smith A, Kinder EF. Changes in psychological test performances of brain-operated schizophrenics after eight years. Science 129:149–150, 1959.

Spreen O, Benton AL. Comparative studies of some psychological tests for cerebral damage. J Nerv Ment Dis 140:323–333, 1965.

Squire LR. Comparisons between forms of amnesia: Some deficits are unique to Korsakoff's syndrome. J Exp Psychol: Learning, Memory, and Cognition 8:560–571, 1982.

Squire LR. Memory and Brain. New York: Oxford University Press, 1987.

Stroop JR. Studies of interference in serial verbal reactions. J Exp Psychol 18:643–662, 1935.

Stuss DT. Contribution of frontal lobe injury to cognitive impairment after closed head injury: methods of assessment and recent findings. In Levin HS, Grafman J, Eisenberg HM (eds), Neurobehavioral Recovery from Head Injury. New York: Oxford University Press, 1987, pp. 166–177.

Stuss DT, Alexander MP, Lieberman A, Levine H. An extraordinary form of confabulation. Neurology 28:1166–1172, 1978.

Stuss DT, Benson DF. Frontal lobe lesions and behavior. In Kertesz A (ed), Localization in Neuropsychology. New York: Academic Press, 1983, pp. 429–454.

Stuss DT, Benson DF, Kaplan EF, Weir WS, Della Malva C. Leucotomized and nonleucotomized schizophrenics: Comparison on tests of attention. Biol Psychiatry 16:1085–1100, 1981a.

Stuss DT, Kaplan EF, Benson DF, Weir WS, Naeser MA, Levine H. Long-term effects of prefrontal leucotomy. An overview of neuropsychologic residuals. J Clin Neuropsychol 3:13–32, 1981b.

Stuss DT, Gow CA. Frontal lobe dysfunction after traumatic brain injury. Neuropsychiat Neuropsychol Beh Neurol: in press.

Stuss DT, Kaplan EF, Benson DF, Weir WS, Chiulli S, Sarazin FF. Evidence for the involvement of orbito-frontal cortex in memory functions: An interference effect. J Comp Physiol Psychiat 96:913–925, 1982.

Stuss DT, Stethem LL, Hugenholtz H, Picton T, Pivik J, Richard MT. Reaction time after head injury: Fatigue, divided and focused attention and consistency of performance. J Neurol Neurosurg Psychiatry 52:742–748, 1989.

Teuber HL. The riddle of frontal lobe function in man. In Warren JM, Akert K (eds), The Frontal Granular Cortex and Behavior. New York: McGraw-Hill, 1964, pp. 410–444.

Wechsler D. A standardized memory scale for clinical use. J Psychol 19:87–95, 1945.

Wechsler D. Manual for the Wechsler Adult Intelligence Scale. New York: Psychological Corporation, 1955.

9

What Is the Role of Frontal Lobe Damage in Memory Disorders?

ARTHUR P. SHIMAMURA,
JERI S. JANOWSKY,
AND LARRY R. SQUIRE

The prefrontal cortex comprises over 29% of the cortical mantle in humans (see Fuster, 1989). It is richly connected to other cortical regions (e.g., association areas, limbic structures) as well as to various subcortical structures (e.g., the mediodorsal nucleus of the thalamus) (Barbas and Pandya, Chapter 2, this volume; Goldman-Rakic, 1987, Chapter 4, this volume; Fuster, 1989). Thus, it is not surprising that damage to the prefrontal cortex can cause a variety of dysfunctions in humans—including disorders of affect, motor control, language, problem solving, and memory (for reviews: Hécaen and Albert, 1978; Luria, 1966; Milner, 1964; Milner et al., 1985; Schacter, 1987; Stuss and Benson, 1986). In this chapter, we describe the memory disorders observed in a group of patients with frontal lobe lesions. In addition, we contrast these disorders with the amnesic syndrome observed in patients with bilateral damage to the medial temporal lobe (including hippocampus) or to the diencephalic midline (thalamic nuclei and mammillary nuclei).

The significance of the frontal lobes to memory functions has been a rather controversial issue. It has been suggested that memory functions per se are not impaired in patients with frontal lobe damage and that decrements in performance on memory tests are secondary to disorders of on-line processes, such as encoding, attention, problem solving, and disinhibition (Hécaen and Albert, 1978; Luria, 1973). Others, however, have emphasized the primary role of the frontal lobes on memory tests such as delayed response, conditioned associative learning, and memory for temporal order (Jacobsen, 1935; Milner, 1971; Petrides, 1985; for review: Petrides, 1989; Schacter, 1987b). Although we do not propose a resolution of this issue, we suggest that the cognitive and memory dysfunctions associated with frontal lobe lesions are quite distinct from the memory dysfunctions associated with bilateral damage to the medial temporal lobe or to the diencephalic midline.

The outstanding feature of medial temporal lobe or diencephalic amnesia is an impairment in new learning ability (i.e., anterograde amnesia). That is, patients with damage to these areas have difficulty remembering information and events experienced after the onset of amnesia (for review: Mayes, 1988; Shimamura, 1989; Squire, 1987). Retrograde amnesia (i.e., impaired memory for events that occurred prior to the onset of amnesia) typically accompanies antero-grade amnesia. Various neurologic disorders, such as anoxia, ischemia, viral encephalitis, and Alzheimer's disease, can damage the medial temporal lobe and thereby produce amnesia. In addition, damage to diencephalic structures has been implicated in the amnesic disorder associated with Korsakoff's syndrome. It should be noted that some of these neurologic disorders (e.g., Alzheimer's disease, Korsakoff's syndrome) also involve other brain structures, thus producing more widespread cognitive disorders, such as disorders of attention and response initiation. For example, patients with amnesia resulting from Korsakoff's syndrome, viral encephalitis, or an anterior communicating artery aneurysm often exhibit signs of frontal lobe impairment in addition to anterograde amnesia (see Shimamura, 1989). Yet, when medial temporal lobe or diencephalic damage occurs in the absence of other outstanding neurologic damage, anterograde amnesia can occur as a relatively circumscribed disorder.

This chapter reviews experimental findings from a group of patients with frontal lobe lesions, some of which have been published elsewhere (Janowsky et al., 1989; 1989a,b; Shimamura et al., 1990). These findings help to characterize the role of the frontal lobes in normal memory performance. We also contrast performance by patients with frontal lobe lesions with performance by patients with anterograde amnesia. In this way, we attempt to define more specifically the contribution of frontal lobe damage to memory disorders, such as the memory disorder associated with Korsakoff's syndrome.

NEUROPSYCHOLOGIC ASSESSMENT OF PATIENTS WITH FRONTAL LESIONS

Patient Characteristics

Seven patients with lesions of the frontal lobes were identified by an extensive review of medical records and computed tomography (CT) scans at the VA Medical Center, San Diego, and the University of California, San Diego Medical Center (for details, see Janowsky et al., 1989). Patients were included who had a lesion restricted to the frontal lobes—as observed on CT or magnetic resonance (MR) scans—and who had no other diagnosis likely to affect cognition or interfere with participation in the study (e.g., significant psychiatric disease, alcoholism). In no case did the patients selected for study have lesions extending into the basal forebrain. Figure 9–1 illustrates the lesion site of each patient, as reconstructed by CT or MR scans. The seven patients averaged 63.9 years of age and 13.0 years of education.

Five patients had unilateral frontal lobe lesions (two left, three right), and two patients had bilaterial lesions. Figure 9–1 shows the variable extent and loca-

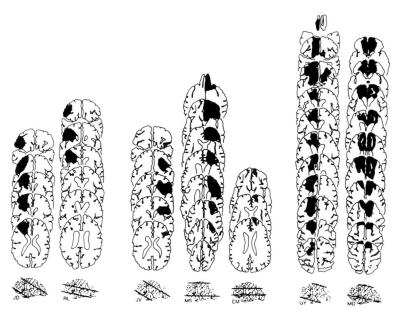

Figure 9-1   Reconstructions from CT or MR brain scans of the frontal lobes damage (in black) for each study patient, using the method of H. Damasio (1983, and personal communication). The most ventral section is shown at the top. The lateral view below each reconstruction shows the angle of the horizontal sections and the locations of the most dorsal and ventral sections. (From Janowsky et al., 1989.)

tion of the frontal lobe lesions among these patients. Four of the patients (R.L., J.V., G.Y., and M.D.) had suffered cerebral vascular accidents. Of the other three patients, J.D. had a brain abcess surgically removed in 1973; M.S. suffered damage to the right frontal lobe in conjunction with surgery to remove a tumor of the right optic nerve; and E.M. had a small unilateral lesion of the right frontal pole (area 10) of unknown etiology. Eleven healthy subjects (seven men, four women) served as control subjects for the patients with frontal lobe lesions. These control subjects matched the patients with respect to average age (60.8 years) and education (14.0 years).

The patients with frontal lobe lesions had Wechsler Adult Intelligence Scale-Revised (WAIS-R) IQ Full-Scale scores within the normal range, and these Full-Scale scores were not significantly different from the scores obtained by the control subjects (t[16] = 1.58, $p > .10$) (Table 9–1). In addition, the control subjects were specifically matched to the study patients on the basis of two WAIS-R subtest scores, information and vocabulary. These two subtests are considered to assess premorbid knowledge and are relatively resistant to impairment after focal brain injury. As a group, the patients did perform significantly worse than the control subjects on three subtests: Digit Span (t[16] = 3.04, $p < .01$), Picture Arrangement (t[16] = 2.8, $p < .01$), and Block Design (t[16] = 2.3, $p < 0.5$) (Table 9–1). The finding of relatively preserved Full-Scale IQ in the pres-

Table 9–1 Performance on the Wechsler Adult
Intelligence Scale-Revised

	Control subjects	Frontal patients
Full Scale IQ		
Verbal IQ		
Information	22.5	21.9
Digit Span	17.4	12.4**
Vocabulary	55.5	53.7
Arithmetic	13.1	10.4
Comprehension	23.7	21.1
Similarities	20.0	17.7
Performance IQ		
Picture Completion	14.2	11.9
Picture Arrangement	12.3	6.5**
Block Design	31.4	21.0*
Object Assembly	28.5	25.3
Digit Symbol	48.0	37.6

Note: All subtest scores are raw scores
*$p < .05$
**$p < .01$

ence of deficits on specific subtests of the WAIS-R is consistent with previous studies of patients with frontal lobe lesions (Drewe, 1974; McFie and Thompson, 1972; Stuss and Benson, 1986).

The neuropsychological profile of patients with frontal lobe lesions was compared with the profile of seven patients with Korsakoff's syndrome and five other amnesic patients. These memory-impaired patients have been assessed on a variety of neuropsychological tests as part of an ongoing research program on amnesia (see Squire, 1982; Squire et al., 1989; Squire and Shimamura, 1986). The seven patients with Korsakoff's syndrome averaged 54.6 years of age and had an average educational level of 11.4 years. Their average WAIS-R Full Scale IQ was 97.1. Of the five other amnesic patients, three patients (A.B., G.D., and L.M.) became amnesic after an episode of anoxia or ischemia. Another amnesic patient (W.H.) became amnesic in 1986 without a known precipitating event. His amnesia occurred without head trauma or a known episode of unconsciousness and developed during a period of at most 3 days. MR scans have identified bilateral medial temporal pathology in L.M. and W.H. (Press et al., 1989). The fifth amnesic patient (M.G.) became amnesic in 1986 following a bilateral thalamic infarction, as confirmed by MR scan. As a group, the five patients averaged 55.8 years of age and had an average educational level of 15.6 years. Their average WAIS-R Full Scale IQ was 109.2. Additional neuropsychologic data for these amnesic patients can be found elsewhere (Janowsky et al., 1989; Squire and Shimamura, 1986; Squire et al., 1989).

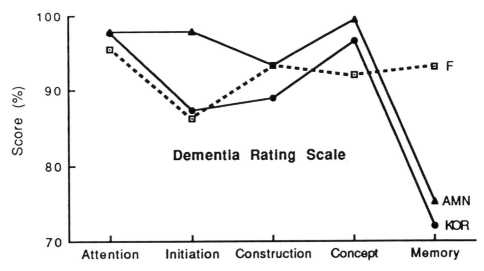

Figure 9–2 Performance on the Dementia Rating Scale by patients with frontal lobe lesions (F) and amnesic patients (KOR, patients with Korsakoff's syndrome; AMN, five other patients with amnesia). Patients with frontal lobe lesions and patients with Korsakoff's syndrome exhibited impaired performance on the Initiation Index, whereas amnesic patients (Korsakoff and non-Korsakoff patients) exhibited impaired performance on the Memory Index.

Cognitive Impairment: Fluency and Problem Solving

The seven patients with frontal lobe lesions exhibited cognitive impairment on tests of fluency, initiation, perseveration, and problem solving. Most of the data reported in this section are presented in Janowsky et al. (1989). For example, cognitive impairment was observed on the Initiation-Perseveration index of the Dementia Rating Scale (DRS, Mattis, 1976). This index assesses performance on a variety of cognitive and motor initiation tasks, including the Supermarket fluency test, in which subjects are asked to name as many items that they can think of that could be purchased at a supermarket. Patients with frontal lobe lesions exhibited lower scores than control subjects on this index, yet they exhibited normal performance on the other four indices (Attention, Construction, Conceptualization, and Memory). In fact, a double dissociation of function was noted between the patients with frontal lobe lesions and the five non-Korsakoff amnesic patients (Fig. 9–2). That is, the patients with frontal lobe lesions exhibited significantly poorer scores on the Initiation-Perseveration index compared to the five non-Korsakoff amnesic patients but exhibited significantly better scores on the memory index ($F[1,10] = 10.6, p < .01$).

Interestingly, patients with Korsakoff's syndrome exhibited deficits on the Memory index of the DRS and, like the patients with frontal lobe lesions, were also impaired on the Initiation-Perseveration index (see Fig. 9–2). This finding shows that patients with Korsakoff's syndrome exhibit some cognitive deficits in addition to deficits in memory. Indeed, there are several disorders (some of which will be described later) that are observed both in patients with frontal lobe lesions and in patients with Korsakoff's syndrome. These findings suggest that patients with Korsakoff's syndrome have frontal lobe damage in addition to diencephalic damage. This hypothesis has been confirmed in a radiological study of patients with Korsakoff's syndrome, which included six of the seven patients whose neuropsychological data are being presented here (Shimamura et al., 1988). In that study, evidence for both frontal lobe atrophy and thalamic damage was obtained in quantitative analyses of CT scans.

Impairment on tests of initiation and perseveration, which is exemplified by poor performance on the Supermarket task from the DRS, may be related to difficulties in organizing and searching information (e.g., words) in semantic memory. A similar impairment has been observed on another fluency test (Benton and Hamsher, 1976), in which subjects are given 1 minute to produce words beginning with the letter F. The same task is then repeated for the letters A and S, and performance is based on the total number of words produced for the three letters (F, A, S). We found that patients with left or bilateral frontal lobe lesions produced significantly fewer words on this task (21.5 words produced) than control subjects (37.5 words produced) (Janowsky et al., 1989). Patients with right frontal lesions, however, were unimpaired (40.7 words produced). Although a nonverbal fluency task was not administered, patients with right frontal lobe lesions have previously been found to be impaired on a nonverbal version of the fluency test (Jones-Gotman and Milner, 1977).

The patients with frontal lobe lesions were also impaired on the Wisconsin Card Sorting Test (Heaton, 1981; Milner, 1964). This problem-solving test measures the ability to identify the relevant dimension or category for a series of stimulus cards that vary in three dimensions (shape, color, number). The relevant category switches across trials, and performance therefore depends on flexible thinking and the ability to inhibit previously correct responses. The patients with frontal lobe lesions averaged only 2.1 correct categories (perfect performance = 6 categories) and committed 41.6% perseveration errors, whereas control subjects averaged 4.0 correct categories and 20% perseveration errors (Janowsky et al., 1989). Patients with Korsakoff's syndrome were also impaired on this task. They achieved fewer categories than alcoholic control subjects (3.3 vs. 4.8 categories) and made more perseverative errors (25% vs. 16.9% errors).

A new sorting test was designed to analyze the nature of the impairment observed on problem-solving tasks such as the Wisconsin Card Sorting Test (Delis et al., 1989). In this sorting test, each set of stimuli consisted of six cards, and each card had multiple features (e.g., a yellow oval card with a blue rectangle inside it and the word "butterfly" printed within the rectangle). There were eight possible ways in which the cards could be sorted into two piles on the basis of their stimulus features. Several sorts were based on the physical features of the cards—for example, card shape (three rounded versus three edged cards); card color (three yellow versus three green cards); or rectangle color (three blue versus three red rectangles). Other sorts were based on the semantic nature of the words that appeared on each card—for example, living things versus vehicles, things that fly versus things that move on the ground.

Table 9-2 Performance on the Card Sorting Test Developed by Delis et al. (1989)

	Control subjects	Frontal patients
Free sorting condition		
Percentage of correct sorts	87.6%	66.7%*
Rule identification condition		
Correct rule naming	14.88	7.75**
Cued sorting condition		
Correct sorts	22.00	17.38**

*$p < .05$
**$p < .01$

In the first condition *(free sorting condition),* subjects were shown the cards in a random order and were given 5 minutes to generate as many different ways as possible to sort the cards into two equal piles. For each sort, the subjects were also asked to name the sorting rule. In a second condition *(rule identification condition),* the experimenter sorted the cards into each of the eight correct sorts by placing three cards in one pile and three cards in another pile. Subjects were then asked to identify the sorting rule. In the third condition *(cued sorting condition),* the experimenter asked the subjects to sort the cards on the basis of cues presented by the experimenter (e.g., "has to do with the outer edges of the shapes"). All three conditions were administered for each of three different sets of cards. Thus for each condition, the total number of correct sorts was 24 (eight correct sorts for each of the three different card sets).

Table 9-2 shows the data from the three sorting conditions (Delis et al., 1989). In the free sorting condition, the patients with frontal lobe lesions were not significantly impaired in the percentage of correct sorts (see Table 9-2). This impairment was also evident in the rule identification condition. That is, when the experimenter generated the sort, patients with frontal lobe lesions had difficulty identifying the sorting rule. Moreover, as indicated by the cued sorting condition, patients with frontal lobe lesions were impaired in the apparently straightforward task of constructing the sort when given a cue. These findings demonstrated that impaired performance by patients with frontal lobe lesions is, at least in part, a failure to discriminate or attend to relevant stimulus information.

ASSESSMENT OF MEMORY FUNCTIONS

Short-term Memory

Short-term memory refers to information that is stored momentarily or "kept in mind." It is short lasting and thus can be contrasted with long-term memory—that is, the permanent storehouse of knowledge (Baddeley, 1986). One hallmark test of short-term memory is the digit span test in which subjects are

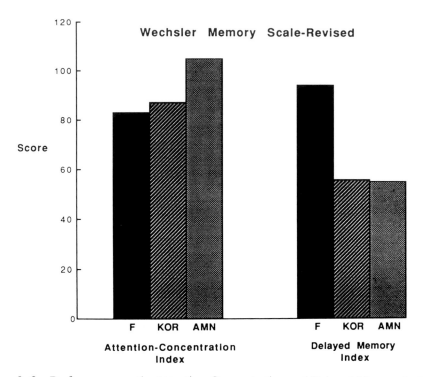

Figure 9–3   Performance on the Attention-Concentration and Delayed Memory Indices of the Wechsler Memory Scale-Revised (WMS-R) by patients with frontal lobe lesions (F) and amnesic patients (KOR, patients with Korsakoff's syndrome; AMN, five other patients with amnesia). Patients with frontal lobe lesions and patients with Korsakoff's syndrome exhibited impaired performance on the Attention-Concentration Index, whereas amnesic patients (Korsakoff and non-Korsakoff patients) exhibited impaired performance on the Delayed Memory Index.

asked to report a series of digits immediately following presentation. Although extensive analyses of short-term memory in patients with frontal lobe lesions have not been performed, there is evidence to suggest that the frontal lobes contribute to this form of memory. As cited earlier, patients with frontal lobe lesions exhibit significant impairment on the digit span test of the WAIS-R compared with control subjects ($t[16] = 3.04$, $p < .01$). This impairment occurred when patients with frontal lobe lesions were asked to report the digits in the same order as they were presented as well as when the patients were required to report the digits in the reverse order. Patients with amnesia resulting from medial temporal lobe or diencephalic damage exhibit normal performance on this and other tests of short-term memory (for review: Shimamura, 1989).

New Learning Ability

Despite disorders of response fluency, problem solving, and short-term memory, patients with frontal lobe lesions do not exhibit significant impairment on most tests of new learning ability. That is, patients with frontal lobe lesions do not exhibit anterograde amnesia. For example, the patients with frontal lobe lesions scored within the normal range on all four of the indices of the Wechsler Memory Scale-Revised (WMS-R) that measure new learning ability (Fig. 9–3). They did, however, exhibit poor performance on the Attention-Concentration index of the WMS-R. An interesting double dissociation was observed between the patients with frontal lobe lesions and non-Korsakoff amnesic patients (see Fig. 9–3). That is, patients with frontal lobe lesions exhibited better performance than non-Korsakoff amnesic patients on the Delayed Memory index but poorer performance on the Attention-Concentration index ($F[1,9] = 79$, $p < .01$). Patients with Korsakoff's syndrome exhibited low scores on both WMS-R indices. These findings are consistent with the findings from the Memory and Initiation-Perseveration indices from DRS that were described before and illustrated in Figure 9–2.

Other analyses of new learning ability confirmed the good memory abilities of patients with frontal lobe lesions. Figure 9–4 illustrates performance on three tests of new learning ability by patients with frontal lobe lesions, patients with

Figure 9–4 Performance of patients with frontal lobe lesions, amnesic patients, and control subjects on three tests sensitive to anterograde amnesia (KOR, patients with Korsakoff's syndrome; AMN, five other patients with amnesia; F, seven patients with frontal lobe lesions; ALC, alcoholic control subjects matched to the Korsakoff patients; CON, healthy control subjects matched to the five other amnesic patients; F-CON, control subjects matched to the patients with frontal lobe lesions. Brackets show standard error of the mean.) (From Janowsky et al., 1989.)

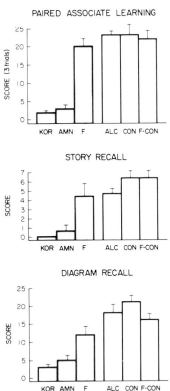

Korsakoff's syndrome, the five other amnesic patients, and respective control subjects. On the paired-associate learning test, subjects were presented 10 unrelated noun–noun pairs on each of three successive study-test trials. On each test trial, subjects were asked to try to recall the second word in each pair when the first word was given as a cue. On the story recall test, a short prose passage consisting of 21 segments was presented, and subjects were asked to recall as much information about the story as possible after a 12-minute delay. On the diagram recall test, subjects copied a complex diagram (Rey-Osterreith figure) and then were asked to draw the diagram from memory after a 12-minute delay. Although amnesic patients were severely impaired on these three tests of new learning ability, the patients with frontal lobe lesions performed normally.

Recall Versus Recognition

On one sensitive measure of long-term memory—multiple trials of free recall for unrelated words—patients with frontal lobe lesions did exhibit significant impairment. Figure 9–5A shows free recall performance for a 15-word list across five study-test trials (Janowsky et al., 1989). Patients with frontal lobe lesions exhibited significant impairment on this test, despite good performance on a comparable test of yes/no recognition memory (Fig. 9–B). Interestingly, patients with Korsakoff's syndrome exhibited a disproportionate recall impairment across study-test learning trials compared to other non-Korsakoff amnesic patients (Fig. 9–5C). This finding may be indicative of additional frontal lobe pathology in patients with Korsakoff's syndrome. However, note that patients with Korsakoff's syndrome showed disproportionately impaired recall only during trials 2–5, not on trial 1. Thus, the interfering effects of multiple learning trials may be necessary to demonstrate differences between recall and recognition performance related to frontal lobe dysfunction. Other findings confirm that this disproportionate impairment of free recall in patients with Korsakoff's need not be observed in studies that use single study-test trials (Haist et al., 1989).

One possibility for the deficit on this sensitive test of free recall is that such tests require extensive use of retrieval strategies and planning. Patients with frontal lobe lesions may exhibit impairment on some tests of free recall as a result of cognitive deficits in fluency, problem solving, and planning (Milner et al., 1985). Significant impairment of free recall in patients with frontal lobe lesions has been reported by other investigators (Jetter et al., 1986; Smith and Milner, 1984). One possibility is that this deficit is related to problems in retrieval and thus can be contrasted with storage or consolidation deficits, which occur in patients with damage to medial temporal lobe and diencephalic areas.

Semantic Encoding and Release from Proactive Interference

It has been suggested that one aspect of frontal lobe dysfunction is a failure to encode information semantically (Moscovitch, 1982). This suggestion was derived from a test of the "release from proactive interference" (Wickens, 1970). In this test, subjects are presented three words and then asked to recall the words following a 15- to 20-second distraction task. For the first four trials, words from

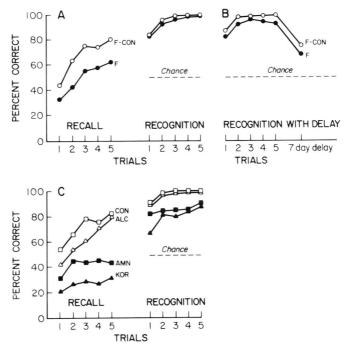

Figure 9-5 Performance by patients with frontal lobe lesions, amnesic patients, and control subjects on the Rey Auditory Verbal Learning Test. **A:** Recall performance for 15 words during five study-test trials and yes-no recognition performance for 15 study words and 15 distractor words during five study-test trials. (F, patients with frontal lobe lesions; F-CON, control subjects). **B:** A second test of yes-no recognition performance by patients with frontal lobe lesions and control subjects for 15 study words and 15 distractor words. The delayed test trial was given 7 days after the five study-test trials. **C:** Recall and recognition performance as in A. (KOR, patients with Korsakoff's syndrome; AMN, five other patients with amnesia; ALC, alcoholic control subjects; CON, healthy control subjects.) (From Janowsky et al., 1989.)

the same semantic category are presented (e.g., clothing articles). Normal subjects typically exhibit a decline in recall performance across the four trials as a result of interference from previous trials (i.e., proactive interference). On the fifth trial, words from a different semantic category (e.g., bird names) are presented for study, and on this trial normal subjects perform as well as they did on the first trial (Wickens, 1970). This "release from proactive interference" indicates that subjects can improve their performance by noticing (encoding) the shift in the meaning of the word stimuli.

Neuropsychologic findings have shown that patients with Korsakoff's syndrome do not exhibit this release from proactive interference (Cermak et al., 1974; Squire, 1982). Presumably, these patients do not adequately encode information in a semantic manner and thus fail to benefit from a shift in semantic categories. Yet, normal release from proactive interference can be observed in

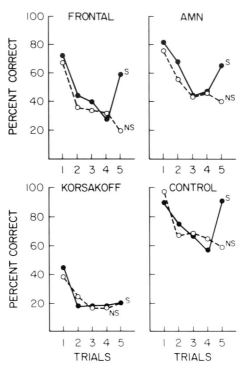

Figure 9–6 Release from proactive interference by patients with frontal lobe lesions, patients with Korsakoff's syndrome, five other patients with amnesia (AMN, N = 5), and healthy control subjects. (From Janowsky et al., 1989.)

other amnesic patients, such as patients with amensia due to an anoxic or ischemic episode, patients with viral encephalitis, and psychiatric patients prescribed electroconvulsive therapy (ECT) (Cermak, 1976; Janowsky et al., 1989; Squire, 1982). Moscovitch (1982) suggested that failure to release from proactive interference, as observed in patients with Korsakoff's syndrome, was mediated by frontal lobe damage. To substantiate this hypothesis, Moscovitch (1982) reported that patients with left frontal lobe lesions did not exhibit release from proactive interference.

In our sample of patients with frontal lobe lesions (two left, three right, and two bilateral frontal patients), release from proactive interference was comparable to that of normal subjects (Fig. 9–6). In contrast, patients with Korsakoff's syndrome (but not other amnesic patients) failed to release from proactive interference on the same test. This finding suggests the possibility that combined frontal lobe dysfunction and amnesia is needed for the semantic encoding impairment observed in patients with Korsakoff's syndrome. In agreement with this idea, Freedman and Cermak (1986) showed that failure to release from proactive interference in patients with frontal lobe lesions was correlated with performance on tests of anterograde amnesia.

Metamemory

Metamemory refers to knowledge about one's memory capabilities and knowledge about strategies that can aid memory (see Flavell and Wellman, 1977; Gruneberg, 1983). Metamemory is an important memory function, because an awareness of one's memory capabilities and knowledge about mnemonic techniques can facilitate memory organization and retrieval, especially when the demands on memory are large. That is, in order to retrieve information efficiently, it is necessary to plan, monitor, and organize appropriate memory strategies. An everyday manifestation of metamemory is the "tip-of-the-tongue" experience—that is, the feeling of having available some knowledge about what one is trying to remember, such as the initial letter of a to-be-remembered word, though complete recall is not possible. In order to overcome these experiences it is necessary to develop appropriate memory strategies.

Some of the components of metamemory are similar to functions that have been attributed to the frontal lobes, such as planning, monitoring, and organizing motor and cognitive functions. Alternatively, it is possible that metamemory is directly related to memory ability. Shimamura and Squire (1986) tested the accuracy of metamemory of *feeling-of-knowing* judgments in patients with Korsakoff's syndrome and other amnesic patients (e.g., patients prescribed ECT, patients with amnesia due to an anoxic or ischemic event, and patient N.A). Subjects were given 24 sentences to learn (e.g., Patty's garden was full of marigolds). After a 5-minute delay, cued recall was assessed for the last word in each sentence (e.g., Patty's garden was full of _____). If the correct answer to a question could not be recalled, then subjects rated their feeling of knowing—that is, they rated on a four-point scale how likely they would be able to recognize the answer if some choices were given. To verify the accuracy of feeling-of-knowing judgments, the judgments were correlated with performance on a subsequent recognition test. Of all the amnesic patients tested, only patients with Korsakoff's syndrome exhibited deficits in feeling-of-knowing accuracy. That is, these patients were poor at predicting whether they would be able to answer an item correctly in a subsequent recognition test. Other amnesic patients were as accurate as control subjects in their ability to predict subsequent recognition memory performance.

The findings from amnesic patients show that metamemory impairment is not an obligatory feature of amnesia. That is, some amnesic patients can express knowledge about what they know and what they do not know, despite having severe impairment in the ability to acquire new knowledge. Patients with Korsakoff's syndrome, however, exhibited impaired metamemory in addition to impaired new learning ability. The deficit in metamemory observed in patients with Korsakoff's syndrome suggested that frontal lobe dysfunction was involved. This conjecture was supported in a subsequent study in which patients with frontal lobe lesions exhibited deficits in feeling-of-knowing accuracy, despite normal cued recall performance (Janowsky et al., 1989a). In that study, patients with frontal lobe lesions were tested after two different delays (5 minutes and 1–3 days, each delay condition involving different study items). The longer delay was used to match cued recall performance of the patients with frontal lobe lesions

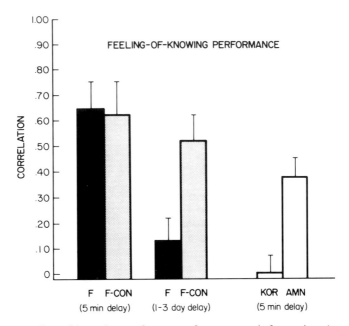

Figure 9–7 Feeling-of-knowing performance for sentence information that could not be recalled. Recall was tested after a 5-minute interval for all subjects (F, patients with frontal lobe lesions; F-CON, control subjects; KOR, patients with Korsakoff's syndrome; AMN, five other patients with amnesia). For a different set of sentences, performance was tested after a 1–3-day retention interval for patients with frontal lobe lesions and control subjects. At this delay, recall performance was comparable with the performance of amnesic patients tested after a 5-minute delay. Feeling-of-knowing accuracy was calculated by correlating feeling-of-knowing ranking with subsequent recognition performance. Patients with frontal lobe lesions and patients with Korsakoff's syndrome exhibited impaired feeling-of-knowing accuracy. (Bars show standard error of the mean.) (From Janowsky et al., 1989.)

with cued recall performance of amnesic patients (both Korsakoff patients), who were tested after a 5-minute delay. Despite matched levels of cued recall performance, patients with frontal lobe lesions and patients with Korsakoff's syndrome exhibited impaired feeling-of-knowing ability. The other amnesic patients performed normally (Fig. 9–7).

It should be noted that the feeling-of-knowing impairment observed in patients with frontal lobe lesions was not identical to the impairment observed in patients with Korsakoff's syndrome. For example, patients with frontal lobe lesions did not exhibit a feeling-of-knowing impairment when performance was assessed after a short (5 minute) delay—the same delay at which patients with Korsakoff's syndrome did exhibit significant impairment (see Fig. 9–7). Also, patients with frontal lobe lesions were not impaired on a feeling-of-knowing task involving general information questions, whereas patients with Korsakoff's syndrome were impaired on this task. In that study (Janowsky et al., 1989b), subjects were presented factual questions (e.g., *"Who invented the wireless radio?"*

[Marconi]) and were asked to make feeling-of-knowing judgments for nonrecalled questions (i.e., to judge how likely they would be able to answer the questions that they failed to recall if they were provided some choices). One possibility is that the metamemory impairment in patients with Korsakoff's syndrome is more severe, perhaps as a result of both memory and metamemory deficits. Another possibility is that the 5 minute retention test and the general information test were too easy and may not have taxed metamemory functions enough to observe impaired feeling-of-knowing ability in patients with frontal lobe lesions.

The feeling-of-knowing impairment exhibited by patients with frontal lobe lesions may be related to deficits in other tasks that involve inferential judgments. One such example is the finding that patients with frontal lobe lesions have difficulty making estimates or inferences from everyday experiences (e.g., How tall is the average English woman?; Shallice and Evans, 1978). Similarly, patients with frontal lobe lesions have difficulty estimating the price of objects (Smith and Milner, 1984). Deficits in cognitive estimation as well as the deficit in feeling-of-knowing accuracy just described (estimating the contents of memory) can be construed as deficits in metamemory (i.e., knowing about what is stored in memory). These findings of impaired metamemory, in conjunction with preserved new learning ability, suggest that the frontal lobes are critically involved in the manipulation and organization of information, including information already in storage, but are not critically involved in establishing new information in memory.

Memory for the Temporal Order of Events

Another aspect of memory that appears to be related to frontal lobe function is memory for temporal order. For example, in studies of recency judgment, subjects are shown a series of stimuli (e.g, words, pictures) and then asked to judge which one of two stimuli was presented more recently. Corsi (as cited by Milner, 1971; see also Milner, this volume) showed that patients with frontal lobe lesions exhibit poor recency memory but are not impaired on tests of item recognition memory (i.e., whether a stimuli was previously presented or was never presented).

Patients with Korsakoff's syndrome also exhibit severe impairment on tests of recency (Huppert and Piercy, 1976; Meudell et al., 1985; Squire, 1982). Specifically, their impairment was larger than the impairment of control subjects who were tested after a long retention interval, and who therefore exhibited comparable levels of item recognition memory (Meudell et al., 1985). Moreover, their impairment was larger than the impairment exhibited by non-Korsakoff amnesic patients, despite comparable impairment of item memory (Squire, 1982). Finally, in patients with Korsakoff's syndrome, impaired performance on recency tests was correlated with performance on tests sensitive to frontal lobe dysfunction (e.g., Wisconsin Card Sort Test, Verbal Fluency Test) (Squire, 1982).

More recently, performance on tests of temporal order memory was compared directly in patients with frontal lobe lesions, patients with Korsakoff's syn-

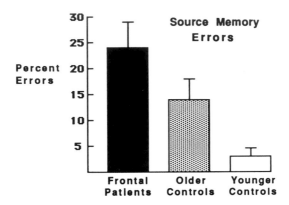

Figure 9–8 Following the presentation of 15 words, subjects were asked to recall and recognize the words on the list or, on a different occasion, to reconstruct the order in which the words were presented. Word sequencing performance was based on the correlation of the judged order of the words with the actual list order. (F, patients with frontal lobe lesions; F-CON, control subjects for patients with frontal lobe lesions.) (From Shimamura et al., 1990.)

drome, and non-Korsakoff amnesic patients (Shimamura et al., 1990). Rather than making two-choice recency judgments, subjects were presented a list of 15 words and then asked to reproduce the list order from a random array of the words. Memory for temporal order was assessed by correlating for each subject the judged order with the actual presentation order of the words. On another occasion, subjects were given tests of word recall and recognition memory. Patients with frontal lobe lesions exhibited significant impairment on this "word sequencing" test, despite good performance on tests of word recall and recognition (Fig. 9–8). As expected by their general amnesic disorder, Korsakoff and non-Korsakoff amnesic patients exhibited both impaired item memory and impaired memory for temporal order. In addition, patients with Korsakoff's syndrome exhibited somewhat greater impairment on the word sequencing test, though this difference was only marginally significant.

In a second study, patients with frontal lobe lesions, patients with Korsakoff's syndrome, and non-Korsakoff amnesic patients were asked to reproduce the chronological order of 15 factual events that occurred between 1940 and 1985 (e.g., *Jonas Salk discovered the first polio vaccine; The name of the Polish Labor Movement led by Lech Walesa was Solidarity*). The findings from this "fact sequencing" test corroborated the findings obtained from the word sequencing test. Specifically, patients with frontal lobe lesions exhibited significant impairment on the fact sequencing test but were not significantly impaired on recall or recognition tests about the facts themselves. Also, as expected, both groups of amnesic patients exhibited impaired performance on tests of fact sequencing, fact recall, and fact recognition. However, the patients with Korsakoff's syndrome were more impaired on the fact sequencing test than non-Korsakoff amnesic patients. This study demonstrated that impaired memory for temporal order can occur in patients with frontal lobe lesions, even when the memory for the items is good and when the items are distributed across a 45-year period.

Disorders of Source Memory

In everyday experiences, one often remembers some factual information (e.g., an experimental finding, a news item) but forgets when and where the information was encountered. Such instances represent a loss of source or contextual memory. Several theoretical accounts of memory have distinguished between memory for factual or semantic information and memory for contextual or episodic memory (Hirst, 1982; Jacoby and Dallas, 1981; Tulving, 1972; 1983). Neuropsychological studies suggest that disorders of source memory may be mediated by at least two factors (Schacter et al., 1984; Shimamura and Squire, 1987; in press). One factor is the pervasive new learning impairment exhibited by amnesic patients which affects many forms of memory including source memory. Another factor is the impairment of memory for spatial-temporal context observed in patients with frontal lobe lesions. In fact, disorders of source memory may be related to impaired memory for the temporal order of events. That is, it seems likely that failure to judge temporal order accurately is related to a disconnection between factual information and the context in which it was encountered.

To test whether patients with frontal lobe lesions exhibit source memory impairment, Janowsky and colleagues (1989b) asked patients with frontal lobe lesions, age-matched control subjects, and younger control subjects to learn a set of 20 trivia facts that could not be previously recalled (e.g., *The last name of the actor who portrayed Dr. Watson in the Sherlock Holmes series was Bruce; The name of the dog on the Cracker Jacks box is Bingo*). After a 6–8 day retention interval, fact recall was tested for the 20 learned facts (e.g., *What was the last name of the actor who portrayed Dr. Watson in the Sherlock Holmes series?*) and for 20 new facts. When subjects correctly answered a fact question, they were asked to recollect the source of the information ("Can you tell me where you learned the answer?"; "When was the most recent time you heard that information?"). Two kinds of source errors were scored: (1) When subjects correctly recalled any of the 20 learned facts but reported that the most recent time the fact was heard was at some other time prior to the learning session, and (2) when subjects correctly recalled any of the 20 new facts but reported incorrectly that the fact was encountered during the learning session.

Source memory ability was significantly impaired in patients with frontal lobe lesions, even though recall memory for the facts themselves was normal (Fig. 9–9). This rather selective memory impairment suggests that the frontal lobes contribute specifically to contextual memory.

Source memory impairment can be severely impaired in some amnesic patients (Shimamura and Squire, in press). In a previous study (Shimamura and Squire, 1987), about half of the amnesic patients tested exhibited *source amnesia*—that is, they never mentioned the prior learning session as the source of presented facts. The other amnesic patients exhibit source memory impairment but it was commensurate with their fact learning impairment. Interestingly, fact

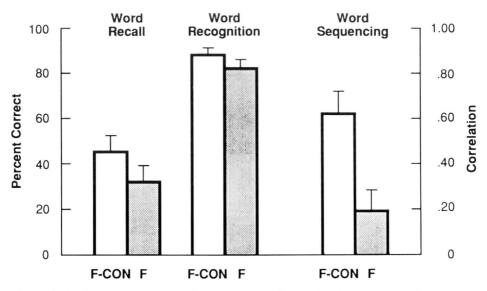

Figure 9–9   Source memory performance by patients with frontal lobe lesions (mean age = 64 years), age-matched control subjects (mean age = 62 years), and younger control subjects (mean age = 49 years). Source errors represent instances when a subject failed to recall the time and place a fact was presented. (Data from Janowsky et al., 1989b, Experiment 2.)

memory performance by the patients who exhibited source amnesia was at the same level as the performance by patients who did not exhibit source amnesia.

Source memory impairment can also occur with normal aging, as indicated by the finding that older control subjects (mean age = 63.9 years) made more source errors than younger control subjects (mean age = 49.4 years) (Fig. 9–9; see also McIntyre and Craik, 1987). Interestingly, neuronal cell loss associated with aging occurs prominently in the frontal lobes (see Haug et al., 1983), which suggests that source memory impairment in normal aging may also be related to subtle frontal lobe dysfunction.

WHAT IS THE ROLE OF FRONTAL LOBES IN MEMORY FUNCTIONS?

Table 9–3 summarizes the memory and cognitive disorders that occur in patients with frontal lobe damage. The memory disorders include impairment of short-term memory (e.g., digit span), free recall, metamemory, memory for temporal order, and source memory. Interestingly, new learning ability is *not* severely affected in patients with frontal lobe lesions (see Figs. 9–2–9–5). The only exception appears to be impairment on sensitive tests of free recall (e.g., multiple study-test trials). Cognitive disorders include problems in planning, problem solving, initiation, perseveration, fluency, cognitive estimation, and disinhibition. Baddeley (1986) refers to these cognitive disorders as *dysexecutive* syndrome. He views the frontal lobes as having the function of coordinating,

Table 9-3 Memory and Cognitive Disorders that Occur in Patients with Frontal Lobe Lesions

Memory disorders ("prospective" memory deficits)	Cognitive disorders ("dysexecutive" syndrome)
Short-term memory	Planning
Free recall	Problem solving
Metamemory	Initiation
Memory for temporal order	Perseveration
Source memory	Fluency
	Cognitive estimation
	Disinhibition

monitoring, and organizing on-line information or information in working memory (see also, Goldman-Rakic, 1987). Another view of the disorder concerns the role of the prefrontal cortex in regulating inhibitory control. Thus, some have suggested that frontal lobe dysfunction reflects a failure to inhibit irrelevant responses (i.e., *disinhibition*) (Luria, 1966; Rosvold and Mishkin, 1961). Similarly, the memory disorders observed in patients with frontal lobe lesions have been referred to as deficits in *prospective* memory (Shimamura, 1990). Prospective memory reflects processes involved in planning, organization, and other strategic aspects of learning and memory that may facilitate encoding and retrieval of information.

Previously, the term "prospective memory" has been used to characterize the processes and strategies by which one remembers to perform and monitor future actions (Dobbs and Rule, 1987; Meacham and Leiman, 1982). For example, remembering to take pills or to make appointments requires prospective memory. The definition of prospective memory could usefully be broadened to include processes and strategies involved in planning, monitoring, and organizing *memory,* not just actions. Like a prospector searching for gold, prospective memory concerns self-initiated searches and retrieval of information in memory. For example, a tortuous search of memory—such as remembering what you had for dinner 7 days ago—will likely require prospective memory, because it is necessary to plan and develop strategies that will help retrieve a memory that is embedded within a particular context.

Prospective memory impairment, the dysexecutive syndrome, and the notion of disinhibition share many features in common. For example, prospective memory involves the ability to access, monitor, and manipulate associations within a temporal/spatial context as well as within a semantic context. In many ways, memory searches are like problem-solving tasks in that they require cognitive fluency, initiation, and flexible thinking. For memory, the problem-solving task is to develop, plan, and initiate efficient encoding and retrieval strategies for accessing knowledge systems. One might suppose that such strategies involve discrimination and inhibition of irrelevant information. Thus, an impairment of inhibitory control would likely translate into a dysexecutive or prospective memory impairment, because appropriate (relevant) strategies or plans may not be discriminated from inappropriate ones. By this view, an impairment of prospective memory would especially affect self-initiated memory tasks such as free recall and judging the temporal order of learned events (e.g., recency/sequencing judgments, source memory).

Prospective memory differs from the kind of memory that is dependent on the integrity of the medial temporal lobe or diencephalic midline in that the former is needed to manipulate and organize memory, whereas the latter is needed to store and consolidate new memories. Another way to view the distinction is to consider the role of the frontal lobes in terms of an executive or "working memory" system and the medial temporal lobe and diencephalic regions in terms of a long-term (declarative) memory storage system. Thus, the executive memory system has the function of coordinating various cognitive and memory processes for the purpose of manipulating news material as well as material already in storage (Baddeley, 1986). The declarative memory system is essential for the storage of new information in such a way that it can be accessed in a conscious or explicit manner (Squire, 1987).

As evident by the findings reviewed here, a deficit in prospective memory does not necessarily imply a deficit in declarative memory, and vice versa. Specifically, patients with frontal lobe lesions have impaired prospective memory, despite normal performance on many tests of new learning capacity (i.e., declarative memory). Conversely, amnesic patients can perform well on many tests of prospective memory but still fail on tests of new learning. Finally, for normal individuals performance on prospective memory tasks is not correlated with performance on long-term, declarative memory tests (Meacham and Leiman, 1982; Wilkins and Baddeley, 1978). Taken together, these findings provide strong evidence that these two memory functions can be dissociated from one another and are separately organized. One important finding is that patients with Korsakoff's syndrome appear to exhibit both prospective memory and declarative memory impairment, presumably as a result of their combined frontal and diencephalic neuropathology.

In summary, patients with frontal lobe lesions exhibit deficits on a variety of memory and cognitive functions, though new learning capacity is relatively preserved. Terms such as "dysexecutive syndrome," "loss of inhibitory control," and "prospective memory impairment" have been used to describe these deficits of planning, monitoring, organization, and initiation. The impairment exhibited by these patients is markedly different from that observed in patients with damage to medial temporal lobe or diencephalic areas, where the prominent impairment is a failure of the ability to establish usable declarative memory.

REFERENCES

Baddeley A. Working memory. Oxford: Oxford University Press, 1986.
Barbas H, Pandya DN. Patterns of connections of the prefrontal cortex in the rhesus monkey associated with cortical architecture. *In* Levin HS, Eisenberg HM, Benton AL (eds) Frontal Lobe Function and Dysfunction. New York: Oxford University Press, 1990.

Benton AL, Hamsher KD. Multilingual asphasia examination. Iowa City: University of Iowa Press, 1976.

Cermak LS. The encoding capacity of a patient with amnesia due to encephalitis. Neuropsychologia 14:311–326, 1976.

Cermak LS, Butters N, Moreines J. Some analyses of the verbal encoding deficit of alcoholic Korsakoff patients. Brain and Language 1:141–150, 1974.

Damasio H. A computed tomographic guide to the indentification of cerebral vascular territories. Archives of Neurology 40:138–142, 1983.

Delis DC, Bihrle AM, Janowsky JS, et al. Mechanisms of problem-solving impairment in frontal lobe patients. Journal of Clinical and Experimental Neuropsychology 11:65, 1989.

Drewe EA. The effect of type and area of brain lesion on Wisconsin Card Sorting Test performance. Cortex 10:159–170, 1974.

Dobbs AR, Rule BG. Prospective memory and self-reports of memory abilities. Canadian Journal of Psychology 41:209–222, 1987.

Flavell JH, Wellman HM, Kail RV, Hagen JW. Perspectives on the Development of Memory and Cognition. Hillsdale, NJ: Earlbaum, 1977, pp. 3–33.

Freedman M, Cermak LS. Semantic encoding deficits in frontal lobe disease and amnesia. Brain and Cognition 5:108–114, 1986.

Fuster JM. The Prefrontal Cortex, 2nd Ed. New York: Raven Press, 1989.

Goldman-Rakic PS. Circuitry of primate prefrontal cortex and regulation of behavior by representational memory. In Plum F (ed), Handbook of Physiology: The Nervous System. Vol. 5. Bethesda, MD: American Physiological Society, 1987, pp. 373–417.

Goldman-Rakic PS. Relationship of circuitry of primate prefrontal cortex to working functional memory. In Levin HS, Eisenberg HM, Benton AL (eds), Frontal Lobe Function and Dysfunction. New York: Oxford University Press, 1991.

Gruneberg MM. Memory processes unique to humans, Mayes A: Memory in Animals and Man. London: Van Nostrand, 1983, pp. 253–281.

Haist, F, Shimamura AP, Squire LR. The structures damaged in amnesia contribute similarly to recall and recognition memory. Society for Neuroscience Abstracts 15:341, 1989.

Haug H, Barmwater U, Eggers R, et al. Anatomical changes in aging brain: Morphometric analysis of the human prosencephalon. In Cervos-Navarro J, Sarkander HI (eds), Brain Aging: Neuropathology and Neuropharmacology. New York: Raven Press 21:1–12, 1983.

Heaton RK. Wisconsin Card Sorting Test Manual. Odessa, FL: Psychology Assessment Resources, 1981.

Hécaen H, Albert ML. Human Neuropsychology. New York: John Wiley & Sons, 1978.

Hirst W. The amnesic syndrome: Descriptions and explanations. Psychological Bulletin 91:435–460, 1982.

Huppert FA, Piercy M. Recognition memory in amnesic patients: Effect of temporal context and familiarity of material. Cortex 12:3–20, 1976.

Jacobsen CF. Functions of the frontal association area in primates. Arch. Neurol. Psychiatry 33:558–569, 1935.

Jacoby LL, Dallas M. On the relationship between autobiographical memory and perceptual learning. Journal of Experimental Psychology: General 110:306–340, 1981.

Janowsky JS, Shimamura AP, Kritchevsky M, et al. Cognitive impairment following frontal lobe damage and its relevance to human amnesia. Behavioral Neuroscience 103:548–560, 1989.

Janowsky JS, Shimamura AP, Squire LR. Memory and metamemory: Comparisons between patients with frontal lobe lesions and amnesic patients. Psychobiology 17:3–11, 1989a.

Janowsky JS, Shimamura AP, Squire LR. Source memory impairment in patients with frontal lobe lesions, Neuropsychologia 27:1043–1056, 1989b.

Jetter W, Poser U, Freeman RB, et al. A verbal long term memory deficit in frontal lobe damaged patients. Cortex 22:229–242, 1986.

Jones-Gotman M, Milner B. Design fluency: The invention of nonsense drawings after focal cortical lesions. Neuropsychologia 15:653–674, 1977.

Luria AR. Higher Cortical Functions in Man. New York: Basic Books, 1966.

Luria AR. The Working Brain. New York: Basic Books, 1973.

Mattis S. Dementia rating scale. In Bellack R, Karasu B (eds), Geriatric Psychiatry 1. New York: Grune & Stratton, 1976, pp. 77–121.

Mayes AR. Human Organic Memory Disorders. Cambridge: Cambridge University Press, 1988.

Mayes AR, Meudell PR, Pickering A. Is organic amnesia caused by a selective deficit in remembering contextual information? Cortex 21:167–202, 1985.

McFie J, Thompson JA. Picture arrangement: A measure of frontal lobe function? British Journal of Psychiatry 121:547–552, 1972.

McIntyre JS, Craik FIM. Age differences in memory for item and source information. Canadian Journal of Psychology 42:175–192, 1987.

McKoon G, Ratcliff R, Dell GS. A critical evaluation of the semantic-episodic distinction. Journal of Experimental Psychology: Learning Memory and Cognition 12:295–306, 1986.

Meacham JA, Leiman B. Remembering to perform future actions. In Neisser U (ed), Memory Observed: Remembering in Natural Contexts. San Francisco: W.H. Freeman & Co., 1982, pp. 327–336.

Meudell PR, Mayer AR, Ostergaard A, et al. Recency and frequency judgments in alcoholic amnesics and normal people with poor memory. Cortex 21:487–511, 1985.

Milner B. Some effects of frontal lobectomy in man. In Warren JM, Akert K (eds), The Frontal Granular Cortex and Behavior. New York: McGraw-Hill, 1964, pp. 313–334.

Milner B. Interhemispheric differences in the localization of psychological processes in man. British Medical Bulletin 127:272–277, 1971.

Milner B. Cognition and memory following frontal lobectomy. In Levin HS, Eisenberg HM, Benton AL (eds), Frontal Lobe Function and Injury. New York: Oxford University Press, 1990.

Milner B, Petrides M, Smith ML. Frontal lobes and the temporal organization of memory. Human Neurobiology 4:137–142, 1985.

Moscovitch M. Multiple dissociations of function in amnesia. In Cermak L (ed), Human Memory and Amnesia. Hillsdale, NJ: Earlbaum, 1982, pp. 337–370.

Petrides M. Deficits on conditional associative-learning tasks after frontal- and temporal-lobe lesions in man. Neuropsychologia 23:601–614, 1985.

Petrides M. Frontal lobes and memory. In Boller F, Grafman J (eds), Handbook of Neuropsychology. The Netherlands: Elsevier, 1989, pp. 75–90.

Press GA, Amaral DG, Squire, LR. Hippocampal abnormalities in amnesic patients revealed by high-resolution magnetic resonance imaging. Nature 341:54–57, 1989.

Rosvold HE, Mishkin M. Non-sensory effects of frontal lesions on discrimination learning and performance. In Delafresnaye, JF (ed), Brain Mechanisms and Learning. Oxford: Blackwell, 1961, pp. 555–576.

Schacter DL. Memory, amnesia, and frontal lobe dysfunction. Psychobiology 15:21–36, 1987.

Schacter DL, Harbluck J, McLaughlin D. Retrieval without recollection: An experimental analysis of source amnesia. Journal of Verbal Learning and Verbal Behavior 23:593–611, 1984.

Shallice T, Evans ME. The involvement of the frontal lobes in cognitive estimation. Cortex 14:294–303, 1978.

Shimamura AP. Disorders of memory: The cognitive science perspective. *In* Boller F, Grafman J (eds), Handbook of Neuropsychology. Amsterdam, The Netherland: Elsevier, 1989, pp. 35–73.

Shimamura AP, Janowsky JS, Squire LR. Memory for the temporal order of events in patients with frontal lobe lesions and amnesic patients. Neuropsychologia 28(8):803–14, 1990.

Shimamura AP, Jernigan TL, Squire LR. Korsakoff's syndrome: Radiological (CT) findings and neuropsychological correlates. Journal of Neuroscience 8:4400–4410, 1988.

Shimamura AP, Squire, LR. Korsakoff syndrome: A study of the relation between anterograde amnesia and remote memory impairment. Behavioral Neuroscience 100:165–170, 1986.

Shimamura AP, Squire LR. A neuropsychological study of fact memory and source amnesia. Journal of Experimental Psychology: Learning, Memory and Cognition 13:464–473, 1987.

Shimamura AP, Squire, LR. The relationship between fact and source memory: Findings from amnesic patients and normal subjects. Psychobiology (in press).

Smith ML, Milner B. Differential effects of frontal-lobe lesions on cognitive estimation and spatial memory. Neuropsychologia 22:697–705, 1984.

Squire LR. Comparisions between forms of amnesia: Some deficits are unique to Korsakoff's syndrome. Journal of Experimental Psychology: Learning Memory and Cognition 8:560–571, 1982.

Squire LR. Memory and Brain. New York: Oxford University Press, 1987.

Squire LR, Haist F, Shimamura AP. The neurology of memory: Quantitative assessment of retrograde amnesia in two groups of amnesic patients. Journal of Neuroscience 9:828–839, 1989.

Squire LR, Shimamura AP. Characterizing amnesic patients for neurobehavioral study. Behavioral Neuroscience 100:866–877, 1986.

Stuss DT, Benson DF (eds). The Frontal Lobes, New York: Raven Press, 1986.

Tulving E. Episodic and semantic memory. *In* Tulving E, Donaldson W (eds), Organization of Memory. New York: Academic Press, 1972.

Tulving E. Elements of Episodic Memory. Oxford: Clarendon Press, 1983.

Tulving E. What kind of hypothesis is the distinction between episodic and semantic memory? Journal of Experimental Psychology: Learning, Memory, and Cognition 12:307–311, 1986.

Wickens DD. Encoding strategies of words: An empirical approach to meaning. Psychological Review 22:1–15, 1970.

Wilkins AJ, Baddeley AD. Remembering to recall in everyday life: An approach to absentmindedness. *In* Gruneberg MM, Morris PE, Sykes RN (eds), Practical Aspects of Memory. New York: Academic Press, 1978, pp. 27–34.

V
Response Preparation and Motor Functioning

10
Intentional Motor Disorders

KENNETH M. HEILMAN
AND ROBERT T. WATSON

The major efferent pathway from the brain that activates motor units in the brain stem and spinal cord is the *corticospinal or pyramidal motor system.* For the most part the cell bodies of the neurons in this system can be found in the precentral frontal areas or Brodmann's area 4. This system can mediate an almost infinite number of movements. However, since the purpose of motor systems is to interact with the environment, the pyramidal motor neurons need to be guided by instructions or programs. Luria (1966) posited that four systems are important in the control of movement: (1) Kinesthetic afferent impulses to direct the motor output in the correct direction, (2) optic-spatial systems to construct movement in external space, (3) premotor systems that link the chain individualize movement for complex movement, (4) the prefrontal area for linking goals with actions. While Luria's classification overlaps with ours, we believe that in order for the motor system to deal effectively with the environment it needs at least two major types of programs, which we term *praxic programs* and *intentional programs.*

The interrogative pronouns used by humans may reflect the major components of human brain organization. For example, in discussing the organization of the visual system Mishkin and colleagues (1983) describe a dorsal "where" system and a ventral "what" system. Animals or patients with dorsal disease can recognize objects but may have trouble locating them in space, and animals or patients with ventral lesions may be able to locate an object in space but not recognize the object. In regard to the motor system we may also term praxic systems as "how" systems and the intentional systems as "when" systems. The "how," or praxic, programs provide three types of instructions: (1) "How" to move in space. That is the nature of the spatial trajectory. This program may contain both allocentric and egocentric information; (2) "how" rapidly to move in space or the timing of movement; (3) "how" to order components of an act. Disorders of this "how," or praxic, system are called apraxias, and patients with apraxia make spatial and temporal errors. The systems that mediate praxis are similar to the first three systems described by Luria. For a further discussion of apraxia, see Heilman and coworkers (1989).

Unlike the praxis, or "how," systems that program the temporospatial aspects of a movement the "when," or intentional, systems provide, as Luria suggested, instructions about goals. There are at least four different types of intentional instructions: (1) "When" to start a movement; (2) "when" not to start a movement; (3) "when" to continue or sustain a movement or posture; (4) "when" to stop a movement.

The inability to initiate a movement in the absence of a corticospinal or motor unit lesion is termed *akinesia.* Hypokinesia is a delay in initiating a response. The inability to withhold a response to a sensory stimulus we term *defective response inhibition.* The inability to sustain a movement or posture is called *motor impersistence,* and the inability to stop a movement or an action program is termed *motor perseveration.*

In this summary of intentional disorders we will first describe each of these intentional disorders in more detail including subtypes of each category. In this initial discussion we will also discuss how to examine patients for these disorders. In a subsequent section we will discuss the pathophysiologic and neuropsychologic mechanisms that may be associated with these disorders. Our discussion will focus on the special pole of the right hemisphere in the control of these "when," or intentional, systems. While the networks that mediate the intentional systems are widely distributed, the frontal lobes, as Luria suggests, play a critical role.

THE AKINESIAS

Definition

There are many causes of an inability of an organism to initiate a movement. Comprehension, attentional, perceptual, and sensory disorders that lead to a failure of movement should not be termed "akinesia." Dysfunction of the motor system, including the motor unit (lower motor neuron, myoneural junction, and muscle) and the upper motor neuron (pyramidal or corticospinal system) may be associated with an initiation failure. Akinesia is defined by an initiation failure that cannot be attributed to dysfunction in these upper and lower motor systems. Akinesia is caused by a failure of the systems necessary to activate these motor neurons.

There are two major methods by which a clinician can distinguish an akinesia from dysfunction of the motor systems. One is behavioral and the other depends on the pathologic locus of a lesion. Certain types of akinesia are present under certain sets of circumstances and absent in others. If one can demonstrate that a patient may make a movement in one set of circumstances and not in the other, then one cannot attribute this failure to move purely to dysfunction in the motor system. However, if the akinesia is not limited to a set of circumstances but is global, then one may have to depend upon brain imaging (e.g., computerized tomography (CT) or magnetic resonance imaging (MRI) or pathology to demonstrate that the brain lesion did not involve the motor system.

Types of Akinesia

There are many forms of akinesia. For ease of discussion we have divided them into four major categories: (1) Body part; (2) action space; (3) stimulus-response conditions; and (4) special acts. As will be seen, these categories may be interactive.

1. Akinesia may involve the eyes, the head, a limb, or the total body.
2. Akinesia of the limbs, eyes, or head may depend upon where in space the body part is moved, or in what direction it is moved, or there may be a hemispatial or directional component to the akinesia. In *directional akinesia* there is a reluctance to move in a specific spatial direction usually contralateral to the lesion. For example, certain forms of gaze palsy are directional akinesias. Similarly, there may be directional akinesias of both head and even arms such that there is a reluctance to move these away from the side of a lesion. *Spatial akinesia* has been described for the arm (Meador et al., 1986) such that, independent of direction, an arm that fails to move in one hemispace or has decreased movements moves better in the opposite hemispace. We do not know if hemispatial akinesia that is totally independent of direction has been described for the eyes or head.
3. Movements can be produced in response to an external stimulus or they can occur in the absence of an external stimulus. We term those movements that are in response to a stimulus exogenously evoked motor activation (exo-evoked), and those that appear to be spontaneous endogenously evoked activation (endo-evoked). A patient may have both exo- and endo-evoked akinesia, which we term *mixed akinesia.*
4. In the absence of an akinesia of the buccofacial and laryngeal muscles, patients may have a reluctance to speak; in spite of an akinesia of the hand they may have a reluctance to write. This reluctance to speak or write may be primarily endo-evoked. That is, patients with a language akinesia often repeat, copy, and name better than they communicate spontaneously. Aphasiologists term this disorder transcortical motor aphasia (Benson, 1985).

Testing for Akinesia

When testing for akinesia one may want to assess the various body parts discussed. To determine if someone has endo-evoked akinesia, one has to observe spontaneous behavior or the lack of it, as well as obtain a history. Patients with endo-evoked akinesia often have symptoms of abulia. Patients with endo-evoked akinesia, in spite of having reduced spontaneous activity, may respond normally to external stimuli. For example, endo-evoked akinesia is frequently associated with Parkinson's disease. Patients with severe Parkinson's disease will often fail to move spontaneously; however, when stimulated they may show almost normal movements (akinesia paradoxica).

When a patient has good strength and spontaneously moves but fails to move to a specific stimulus, the failure to move in response to a stimulus is often attributed either to an elemental sensory defect or to sensory inattention or sensory neglect. While sensory defects and sensory neglect may be responsible for a lack of responsivity, exo-evoked akinesia is often confused with sensory defects and sensory neglect. The basic testing method used for dissociating sensory defects and sensory neglect from exo-evoked akinesia (motor neglect) is the *cross response task* (Watson et al., 1978).

Watson and colleagues had monkeys respond with the right arm to a left-sided stimulus and with their left arm to a right-sided stimulus. If the animal failed to respond to a contralesional stimulus using the ipsilesional arm it was considered to have sensory neglect. However, if the animal demonstrated good strength of the contralesional extremity and moved it spontaneously but failed to move the contralesional extremity in response to ipsilesional stimuli it was considered to have exo-evoked akinesia or motor neglect.

If a patient fails to move both spontaneously and in response to a stimulus as previously discussed he has a mixed akinesia. One can use the test described to test the limbs, the eyes, the head, or the whole body.

When assessing action space one needs to test both directional and hemispatial movements of both the eyes and the limbs. When possible one needs to determine if the directional or hemispatial movements are endo- or exo-evoked. When attempting to determine if there is an endo-evoked directional akinesia of the eyes one should observe the spontaneous eye movements of a patient and see if there is a deviation of the eyes or a gaze paresis toward the ipsilateral side and a failure of the patient to spontaneously look into contralesional space. To determine if a patient has an exo-evoked directional akinesia of the eyes one can use a modification of the Watson and coworkers (1978) paradigm where the patient must look both toward (ipsilesional direction) and away (contralesional direction) from an ipsi- and contralesional stimulus. For example, the examiner stands directly in front of a patient and asks the patient to fixate on the examiner's nose. The examiner raises both hands to eye level and keeps one hand in the patient's right visual field and the other in the left visual field. The patient is instructed to look away from the moving finger if the finger moves downward and toward the moving finger if it moves upward. When the contralesional finger is moved upward, a failure to look at the contralesional finger (moving in a contralesional direction) may be related to a sensory defect (e.g., hemianopsia), sensory neglect, or a directional akinesia. However, when the ipsilesional finger moves downward, a failure to look toward the contralesional finger suggests an exo-evoked directional akinesia of the eyes.

An exo-evoked hemispatial akinesia of the eyes could be detected by using a similar paradigm. However, in this test the eyes should be initially directed into either right or left hemispace and the finger placed in a vertical (one in the inferior field and one in the superior field) position. A failure to look up and down in one hemispace but not the other would suggest hemispatial akinesia of the eyes. To our knowledge this has never been described (perhaps because it has never been assessed).

In order to test for directional and hemispatial akinesia of the head or an arm one can use similar tests. To test for a directional bias of an arm (similar to eye deviation) one can ask a patient to close his eyes and point to his sternum (breast bone). If he is able to do this, one then asks him to point with his index finger to a point in space perpendicular to his sternum (e.g., the midsagittal plane). Patients with a motor (intentional) bias will point toward their lesioned hemisphere (Heilman et al., 1983).

De Renzi and coworkers (1970) developed a task that can be used to test for endo-evoked directional limb akinesia. In our modification, a patient is blindfolded and small objects such as pennies are randomly scattered on a table in both body hemispatial fields within arm's reach. The patient is asked to retrieve as many pennies as possible. The task is considered endo-evoked because the patient cannot see the pennies and must initiate exploratory behavior in the absence of an external stimulus. Patients with an endo-evoked directional akinesia of the arm may fail to move their arm fully into contralateral hemispace and explore for pennies.

One can also use the paradigm used by Coslett and associates (1990) to test for directional akinesia where the stimulus feedback and hand action can be dissociated by using a technique in which patients can see their hand bisecting a line only through a TV monitor. The line (where the action takes place) can be positioned in contra- or ipsilesional hemispace and the TV monitor can also be independently placed in either hemispace. If, as demonstrated by Coslett and colleagues, line bisection is not affected by the spatial position of the monitor but misbisection of the line toward ipsilesional hemispace increases as the line is brought into contralesional hemispace, it would suggest that the patient has a directional akinesia of the arm.

Although directional akinesia has been best described in horizontal hemispace, there are three planes of action. In addition to horizontal, there is also vertical and radial. Neglect of lower (Rapcsak et al., 1988) and upper (Shelton et al., 1990) vertical as well as radial space (Shelton et al., 1990) has been reported. Although the nature of neglect in these other planes has not been fully elucidated, one case of upper vertical neglect was noted to have a directional akinesia, and directional akinesia may also be associated with these other forms of neglect.

To test for hemispatial akinesia of the arm two marks are made on a table top each about 7 inches from the midsagittal plane. In uncrossed conditions each hand is placed on the mark in compatible hemispace. In the crossed condition each hand is placed on the mark in the opposite hemispace. The patient is instructed to lift the hand on the same side if he sees the examiner's finger move up and to move the hand on the opposite side if he sees the examiner's finger move down. The examiner randomly moves his right or left index finger up or down. If a patient fails to move the contralesional arm when it is in contralesional hemispace but moves the arm when it crossed over into ipsilesional hemispace, the patient is considered to have hemispatial limb akinesia (Meador et al., 1986).

HYPOKINESIA

Definition

Many patients with defects in their intentional ("when") systems may have a mild defect and not demonstrate a total inability to initiate a response (e.g., akinesia), but, instead, their intention disorder may only become manifest by a delay in initiating a response. We have termed this delay *hypokinesia*. This hypokinesia may be defined in a manner similar to the akinesia. Since the reaction time paradigm is required to detect hypokinesia, we cannot divide hypokinesia into exo- and endo-evoked.

The same paradigms that are used to test for akinesia of the eye and limbs can be used to test for hypokinesia. While some patients with hypokinesia have such markedly slowed initiation times that hypokinesia can easily be detected, others have more subtle defects, and reaction time paradigms may be needed to observe their defects. Reaction times can be slowed for a variety of reasons including impaired attention, bradyphrenia, or hypokinesia. To detect hypokinesia one should use simple reaction times that do not require cognition and, therefore, cannot be impaired by bradyphrenia. Similarly, in order to test for hypokinesia, one has to use stimulus parameters that ensure that inattention cannot masquerade as hypokinesia.

Hypokinesia can be seen both in the limbs and eyes and may be independent of direction or directionally specific such that when making directional movements there is a greater delay initiating movements in a contralesional direction than there is initiating movements in an ipsilesional direction (Heilman et al., 1985). Hypokinesia can also be hemispatial such that movements with the same limb may be slower in one hemispace than they are in the other hemispace (Meador et al., 1986).

MOTOR IMPERSISTENCE

Definition

Motor impersistence is the inability to sustain an act. It is the intentional equivalent to the attentional disorder termed distractibility. Like akinesia it can be associated with a variety of body parts including the limbs and eyes. However, it may include other body parts including the eye lids, jaw, and tongue. Like akinesia it may also be directional (Kertesz et al., 1985) or hemispatial (Roeltgen et al., 1989). While impersistence cannot be entirely endo-evoked, the stimulus that induces the initial movement can rapidly terminate or persist such that the stimulus remains present throughout the period action is required. We shall call the former *endo-evoked persistence* and the latter *exo-evoked persistence.*

Testing

When testing for impersistence of midline one can ask the patient to keep his eyes closed for 20 seconds. Alternatively, one can ask a patient to keep his mouth open or protrude his tongue for 20 seconds. Patients who can successfully persist at these acts may be further taxed by asking them to persist at two movements simultaneously. For example, they may be asked to both keep their eyes closed and their mouth open for 20 seconds.

Limb impersistence can be tested for by asking a patient to maintain a posture such as keeping an arm extended for 20 seconds. Since limb impersistence can be hemispatial (Roeltgen et al., 1989) one may want to test each limb in its own and opposite hemispace. Hemispatial impersistence, in the absence of directional impersistence, has not been reported for the head or eyes, but this may be because it has never been tested in patients. One could ask a patient to sustain up (or down) gaze for 20 seconds while the eyes are directed either toward the right or left. If the patient could maintain gaze in one hemispace (e.g., the right) but could not in the other (e.g., left) it would suggest that the patient has hemispatial impersistence of the eyes. If a patient has a directional impersistence of the eyes we may be unable to maintain his or her eyes directed to either the right or left hemispace and, therefore, one may not be able to test for hemispatial impersistence. To test for directional impersistence of the eyes one requests the patient to look either to the left or right for 20 seconds. A similar procedure can also be used to test the head for directional impersistence. Directional impersistence may be influenced by hemispatial factors such that directional impersistence is worse in one hemispace than the other. Directional impersistence has not been described with the arm.

Patients with directional impersistence usually have more difficulty in maintaining motor activation in contralesional hemispace or in the contralesional direction. While all persistence tasks are exo-evoked, as stated earlier, one can use a signal or instructions to initiate the activity and then withdraw the stimulus or one can let the stimulus persist throughout the trial. Except for one circumstance, patients' performance is better in the latter condition than it is in the former condition. The exception is when the stimulus and persistent action take place in opposite directions. However, these errors may be related to defective response inhibition rather than motor impersistence.

DEFECTIVE RESPONSE INHIBITION: MOTOR ALLOCHIRIA AND HYPERKINESIA

Definition

Defective response inhibition is responding when either no response is called for or a response of the opposite limb is called for. Defective response inhibition can be seen in the eyes, head, or limbs. Directional defective response inhibition has been reported for the eyes but not for the limbs or head, however, it may never have been tested. Similarly, hemispatial defective response inhibition has not been reported; however, it, too, may never have been tested. There are, in general, two forms of defective response inhibitions. In one form the ipsilesional limb moves when the correct response was a movement of the contralesional limb, or the eyes or head moved in an ipsilesional direction when the correct response was a movement in the contralesional direction. This type of defective response inhibition may be termed *motor (limb or directional) allochiria* (Jones, 1907). However, before one terms such a condition motor allochiria one must be certain a perceptual problem has not induced the disorder (see later), in which case it is not defective response inhibition but is true *allochiria* or *allesthesia*. In the second form of defective response inhibition, it is the contralesional limb that moves when it should not move or movement is in a contralesional direction when there should be either no movement or movement should have been in an ipsilesional direction. We will term this form of defective response inhibition *hyperkinesia*. Whereas by definition motor allochiria can only be with one limb or unidirectional, the hyperkinetic response disinhibition can be bilateral or bidirectional. Hyperkinesia can also be exo-evoked or endo-evoked and the latter, when bilateral, can be synonymous with akathesia.

Testing

If a patient is able to understand complex instructions, the best way to test for both motor allochiria and exo-evoked hyperkinesia of the limbs is to instruct the patient to) move or lift the opposite hand (off a table) when a hand is stroked downward and to move the same hand as touched when it is stroked upward. Prior to testing for the different forms of defective response inhibition it is important to establish that the patient does not have a perceptual disorder and can correctly detect stimuli and can recall instructions. If, when the contralesional hand is brushed up, the patient moves the ipsilesional arm rather than the contralesional the patient has motor allochiria. If when the contralesional arm is brushed downward (which is a signal to move the ipsilesional arm) the contralesional arm is moved instead of the ipsilesional arm, the patient has a contralesional exo-evoked limb hyperkinesia. If this happens with both arms the patient has bilateral exo-evoked hyperkinesia. Patients with exo-evoked limb hyperkinesia may also fail on the type of go–no-go tasks described by Luria. For example, the subject may be instructed to put up two fingers when the examiner puts up one finger and to put up no fingers if the examiner puts up two fingers. If the patient mimics the examiner such that when the examiner puts up one finger the patient puts up one finger and when the examiner puts up two fingers the patient puts up two fingers the patient has echopraxia (a third form of defective response inhibition). However, if the patient responds when the examiner puts up two fingers this is also a form of limb hyperkinesia.

A paradigm similar to that used for directional akinesia of the eyes can be used to determine if there is a directional motor allochiria or a directional hyperkinesia of the eyes or head. The subjects are told to fix their eyes on the examiner's nose. If the index finger of either hand moves down they are to direct their eyes to the opposite finger and if the finger moves up they are to direct their eyes to the finger that moved. When the finger in the patient's contralesional visual field moves up and, instead of looking at that finger, the patient looks at the opposite finger the patient has a directional motor allochiria. If when the contralesional finger moves down the patient looks at the finger rather than looking in the opposite direction the patient has a contralesional directional hyperkinesia (or visual grasp). This directional hyperkinesia (visual grasp) may be bilateral.

MOTOR PERSEVERATION

Definition

Perseveration is when a patient incorrectly repeats a prior response. While there are many classification systems (Sandson and Albert, 1987), there seems to be a spectrum between cognitive and motor perseveration. Cognitive perseveration is when one uses a previously used cognitive strategy inappropriately for a new or different task. Sandson and Albert call this "stuck in set" perseveration. Luria (1965) discussed two types of motor perseveration. In one type of motor perseveration the patient is unable to switch to a different motor program and repeats the prior program even though the task requirements have changed. Luria calls this *inertia of program action,* and Sandson and Albert call this *recurrent perseveration.* In the second type the patient continues to perform a movement even though the task is completed, but when instructed can switch to other movements. Luria called this *efferent perseveration.* This is similar to Sandson and Albert's *continuous perseveration.*

Both continuous and recurrent perseveration are forms of motor perseveration and may represent defects in the "when," or intentional, system. This is a defect of "when" to stop a motor program.

Testing for Motor (Efferent) Perseveration

Patients may show motor (efferent) perseveration on drawing and copying tasks. For example, a patient can be asked to draw or copy a cube. Patients with motor perseveration will repeatedly draw over lines.

When performing a cancellation task patients with motor perseveration will perform multiple cancellations of the same target. When asked to draw or copy a double loop, patients with motor (efferent) perseveration will draw more than two loops.

PATHOPHYSIOLOGY OF INTENTION ACTIVATION DISORDERS

Right-Left Dichotomies

In our introductory discussion we advanced the hypothesis that there are, in general, two major types of programs that control the motor system, the "how," or praxis, system and the "when," or intentional, system. In right-handers disorders of the praxis production system, as evidenced by ideomotor apraxia, are almost always associated with left hemisphere dysfunction (Heilman and Rothi, 1985). While intentional disorders are frequently associated with bilateral hemispheric lesions, when the lesions that induce intentional disorders are unilateral they are most commonly associated with right hemisphere lesions. For example, Coslett and Heilman (1989) show that limb akinesia is more frequently associated with right hemisphere lesions than left hemisphere lesions. However, the intentional defect associated with right hemisphere dysfunction is not limited to the left limb. Howes and Boller (1975), using a reaction time paradigm, reported that right hemisphere infarctions are associated with a greater slowing of reaction times (hypokinesia) than are left hemisphere infarctions even when the ipsilesional arm is used and lesions are matched for size. Rehabilitation specialists have noted that it is more difficult to rehabilitate patients with left hemiplegia than right. In addition, patients with left hemiplegia are more likely to develop decubiti and pulmonary emboli. Both of these conditions may be related to a global akinesia associated with right hemisphere dysfunction. Directional akinesia of the limbs as determined by tasks such as those used by De Renzi and associates (1970), Coslett and coworkers (1990), and Heilman and colleagues (1985) was also more frequently reported with right hemispheric lesions. The case of hemispatial limb akinesia reported by Meador and associates (1986) had a right hemisphere lesion. Although impersistence is often associated with bilateral hemispheric dysfunction, when it is associated with unilateral hemispheric disease it most commonly occurs with right hemisphere lesions (Kertesz et al., 1985).

Defective response inhibition of the eyes or arms may be seen with bilateral hemispheric dysfunction. However, when it is seen with unilateral hemispheric disease it has been associated with right hemispheric dysfunction (Verfaellie and Heilman, 1987). Lastly, motor (or continuous) perseveration has also been reported to be associated with right hemisphere dysfunction (Sandson and Albert, 1987).

The term "dominance" implies that one hemisphere contains specialized processing systems or representations (programs) such that the nondominant hemisphere is not, by itself, competent to fully process and program afferent and efferent information. While our discussion has provided evidence that right hemisphere damage may be dominant for intentional control of the motor systems this evidence is indirect. However, two studies in normal controls provide further evidence for right hemisphere intentional dominance (Heilman and Van Den Abell, 1979; Verfaellie et al., 1988). Warning stimuli reduce reaction times because they either direct the subject's attention to the location of the imperative stimulus (Posner et al., 1984) or because they activate motor systems in preparation for a movement. Using a reaction time paradigm, Heilman and Van Den Abell (1979) demonstrated in normal subjects that warning stimuli projected to the right hemisphere reduce reaction times more than warning stimuli projected to the left. Verfaellie and associates (1988) used a reaction time paradigm that was capable of fully dissociating attention from intention and also showed that the right hemisphere was dominant for intention.

While these studies demonstrate right hemisphere superiority for intentional processes, we do not know what anatomic or physiologic asymmetries may underlie this functional asymmetry. Intention would appear to be closely linked to motivation. Herbert Spencer's biologic theory of hedonism is perhaps still the best guide for understanding motivation. According to Spencer's theory, every animal seeks pleasure and avoids pain where pain is the correlative of actions that are injurious to the organism and pleasure is the correlative of actions that are conducive to the organism's welfare. In humans there are at least three major motivational systems: The primary drive systems, the emotional systems, and the cognitive systems.

The primary drive systems monitor the internal milieu, and when there is a deficiency state or an absence of homeostasis the organism has unpleasant or painful sensations that induce goal-oriented behavior. When the goal is achieved and homeostasis is reestablished, there are pleasant internal sensations. In normal circumstances the emotional systems are activated by external stimuli. Based on either the nature of the stimulus or the interpretation of stimulus significance, positive or negative emotions are evoked. Positive emotions (e.g., happiness, satisfaction) are internal sensations or feelings that are associated with stimuli that are conducive to the organism's welfare, and negative emotions (e.g., fear and anger) are associated with stimuli that are either directly injurious to the organism or foretell possible injury. These positive or negative feelings provide the organism with goals.

The cognitive systems contain knowledge of the environmental circumstances that may be either conducive or injurious to the welfare of the organism and, hence, may produce future pain or pleasure through the primary drive or emotional systems. Therefore, even in the absence of a primary drive or emotion that induces pain or pleasure, the organism's desire to avoid pain and seek pleasure ensures that its action is directed toward the appropriate goals.

While there has been much written about motivational systems, knowledge of their anatomic and physiologic bases is far from complete. Since the primary purpose of this chapter is to discuss intentional systems we will not fully review this work. However, it is important to note that motivational behavior appears to be mediated by diencephalic limbic-cortical networks.

Although the anatomic and physiologic basis for the right hemisphere's special role in intentional activity is unknown, the limbic system, which plays a critical role in motivation, has two major outputs to the cortex, one from the hippocampus and the other via the cingulate gyrus. While bilateral medial temporal lobe lesions are associated with profound amnesia, severe motivational or intentional disorders have not been associated with these lesions. However, bilateral medial hemispheric lesions that involve the cingulate gyrus are associated with a profound intentional disorder termed akinetic mutism, suggesting that the cingulate gyrus provides motivational information to neocortical areas. Eidelberg and Galaburda (1984) demonstrated that the right cingulate gyrus had more input into the neocortex than did the left.

Intrahemispheric Networks

The intrahemispheric networks that are important in mediating intention have also not been fully elucidated. However, studies of patients with focal lesions as well as studies of monkeys suggest that the frontal lobes may play a critical role in intentional activity. For example, motor neglect of the limb has been reported in monkeys from dorsolateral frontal lesions (Watson et al., 1978) and while the ipsilesional limbs are not totally akinetic there is a hypokinesia as measured by reaction times. Medial frontal lesions are also associated with limb akinesia (Meador et al., 1986). An ocular directional akinesia can also be seen with dorsolateral frontal lesions and a directional limb hypokinesia may be seen with frontoparietal lesions (Heilman et al., 1985). In addition, motor impersistence is most frequently seen with dorsolateral frontal lesions (Kertesz et al., 1985), defective response inhibition of the eyes is seen with dorsolateral frontal lesions (Butter et al.,1989), and selective response inhibition of the limbs is associated with medial frontal lesions (Verfaellie and Heilman, 1987). Vilkki (1990) has demonstrated that motor perseveration may also be associated with frontal lesions.

The frontal cortex has strong projections to the striatum. While the dorso-lateral frontal lobe projects to the caudate, the supplementary motor area projects to the putamen, and the cingulate gyrus projects to the ventral striatum. The striatum projects to the internal portion of the globus pallidus or the pars reticularis of the substantia nigra, which in turn projects to thalamic nuclei [e.g., ventralis anterius (VA), ventralis lateralis (VL), medialis dorsalis (MD)]. These thalamic nuclei project back to the same area of the frontal cortex where this frontal, basal ganglia, and thalamic loop arises, including the dorsolateral frontal lobe, supplementary motor area, and cingulate gyrus.

In addition to the frontal lobes, intentional disorders may be associated with diseases that affect both the basal ganglia and the thalamus. The most common disorder that induces akinesia is Parkinson's disease. The akinesia associated with Parkinson's appears to be induced by a loss of the dopaminergic neurons that project to the striatum. Dopamine antagonists may also produce akinesia and dopamine agonists may reverse this akinesia. Thalamic lesions of VA/VL or the medial nuclei such as centromedian parafascicularis can also induce akinesia.

Not only do diseases that affect frontal lobe cortex, basal ganglia, and thalamus induce intentional disorders, but these disorders, especially akinesia, are also associated with diseases that affect the white matter that connects the frontal lobes with these subcortical structures. Therefore, akinesia is often associated with white matter diseases such as arteriosclerotic encephalopathy (Binswanger's disease or multiple lacunar infarcts), advanced multiple sclerosis, and hydrocephalus.

Lastly, akinesia has also been reported with temporoparietal lobe lesions (Valenstein et al., 1982). While the akinesia associated with basal ganglia diseases such as Parkinson's disease appears to be endo-evoked, the akinesias associated with frontal and parietal cortical dysfunction appear to be exo-evoked (Valenstein et al., 1982; Watson et al., 1978).

Based on the pathologic evidence cited one can postulate that the frontal lobes play a central role in an intentional network. The dorsolateral frontal lobes receive projections from both the parietal lobe, which is a polymodal association cortex, and from multimodal primary association cortices. The frontal lobe also has strong reciprocal connections to the cingulate gyrus, the medial thalamic nuclei, and nonreciprocal connections with the striatum, which project to the globus pallidus and substantia nigra and from there to the thalamus and back to the cortex as previously described.

The frontal lobe's connections with the inferior parietal lobe may provide the frontal lobe with stored knowledge (cognition) and the limbic connections may provide the frontal lobe with motivational information. Unimodal sensory and polymodal sensory association areas may provide information to the frontal lobe about external stimuli that may call the organism to action. Afferents from the mesencephalon as well as the reticular system, including the thalamus, may be important for modulating arousal and activation.

Physiologic studies have provided further support for the role of the frontal lobes in intention-motor activation. Suzuki and Azuma (1977) recorded from neurons in the dorsolateral frontal lobe of monkeys who were trained to make a rapid movement to a stimulus. When the animal was prepared to make a movement the cells were active. When the animal was not prepared to initiate a response as determined by a delay in response time these cells were less active. Stimulus parameters did not affect these cells' activity, suggesting that these cells were intentional neurons. Goldberg and Bushnell (1981) found that the dorsolateral frontal lobes contained neurons that discharge before purposeful saccades. Lesions of the frontal lobe destroy these intentional cells and in their absence there is defective activation of the motor neurons.

The manner in which these frontal lobe "intentional" neurons influence the motor neurons has not been definitely established. However, as discussed, the dorsolateral frontal lobe and the thalamic areas such as the ventrolateral, dorsomedial, and intralaminar nuclei share anatomic connections with each other and form a network with the basal ganglia, premotor, and motor cortex. Since lesions in these structures (dorsolateral frontal lobe, basal ganglia, ventrolateral thalamus, medial thalamus) and premotor areas (i.e., supplementary motor areas) induce akinesia, Watson and coworkers (1981) posited that this network mediates intentional activity.

We do not know if the four different forms of intentional activity we have discussed are mediated by the same network or if different systems or subsystems mediate different forms of intentional activity. Some of the intentional disorders we discussed may be related to the "release" of phylogenetically more primitive compensatory systems. For example, Goldberg and Bushnell demonstrated that neurons in the dorsolateral frontal lobes have a role in the preparation of saccadic eye movements. Based on Goldberg and Bushnell's work one would predict that a unilateral frontal lobe lesion would induce a directional akinesia of the eyes. However, Guitton and colleagues (1985) noted that patients with frontal lobe lesions could not saccade away from a stimulus before they made a saccade toward the stimulus (defective response inhibition). While a directional akinesia and defective response inhibition would appear to be mutually incompatible behaviors, Butter and associates (1989) repeatedly tested a patient who had a unilateral frontal lobe lesion using a crossed-response task. Initially the patient showed both contralesional unilateral sensory neglect and a directional contralesional akinesia. Subsequently the patient was able to detect contralesional stimuli and move his eyes in a contralesional direction. However, in the crossed-response task, when presented a contralesional stimulus that was a signal to move the eyes in an ipsilesional direction, the patient often incorrectly responded by first making a contralesional saccade before making an ipsilesional saccade. While Goldberg and Bushnell demonstrated that neurons in the dorsolateral frontal lobe have a role in preparing for a saccade, collicular neurons can perform the same type of preparatory functions, perhaps, after frontal lobe damage, recovery of the ability to initiate a contralesional saccade is mediated by the colliculus. However, activity of the colliculus, unlike the frontal lobes, cannot be altered by task instructions. Perhaps, normally, the dorsolateral frontal lobes exert an inhibitory influence on the colliculus that is absent after frontal lesions. This inhibitory effect cannot be direct, since no frontal lobe eye field cells have been reported that are tonically active except during saccades. However, the pars reticulata of the substantia nigra projects to the colliculus and has tonic activity. The frontal lobe may influence the substania nigra through its connections to the caudate. A similar release of inhibition may also be responsible for other nonocular defects where the brain damaged patients cannot either withhold or terminate a response.

REFERENCES

Benson DF. Aphasia. *In* Clinical Neuropsychology. KM Heilman and E Valenstein (eds), Oxford University Press, New York, 1985, p. 35.

Butter CM, Rapcsak SZ, Watson RT, Heilman KM. Changes in sensory in attention directional hypokinesia and release of the fixation reflex following a unilateral frontal lesion: a case report. Neuropsychologia 26:533–545, 1989.

Coslett HB, Heilman KM. Hemihypokinesia after right hemisphere strokes. Brain and Cognition 9:267–278, 1989.

Coslett HB, Bowers D, Fitzpatrick E, Haws B, Heilman KM. Directional hypokinesia and hemispatial inattention in neglect. Brain 113:475–486, 1990.

DeRenzi E, Faglioni P, Scotti G. Hemispheric contribution to the exploration of space through the visual and tactile modality. Cortex 6:191–203, 1970.

Eidelberg D, Galaburda AM. Inferior parietal lobule. Divergent architectonic asymmetries in the human brain. Archives of Neurology 41:843–852, 1984.

Goldberg ME, Bushnell MC. Behavioral enhancement of visual responses in monkey cerebral cortex, II. Modulation in frontal eye fields specifically related to saccades. Journal of Neurophysiology 46:773–787, 1981.

Guitton D, Buchtel HA, Douglas RM. Frontal lobe lesions in man cause difficulties in suppressing reflexive glances in an generating goal-directed saccades. Experimental Brain Research 58:455–472, 1985.

Heilman KM, Van den Abell T. Right hemisphere dominance for mediating cerebral activation. Neuropsychologia 17:315–321, 1979.

Heilman KM, Bowers D, Coslett B, Whelan H, Watson RT. Directional hypokinesia: Prolonged reaction times for leftward movements in patients with right hemisphere lesions and neglect. Neurology 35:855–868, 1985.

Heilman KM, Rothi LJG. Apraxia. *In* KM Heilman and E Valenstein (eds), Clinical Neuropsychology, 2nd Edition. Oxford University Press, New York, 1985.

Heilman KM, Watson RT, Rothi LJG. Limb apraxia. *In* S. Appel (ed), Current Neurology. Year Book Medical Publishers, Vol. 9, 1989, pp. 179–189.

Heilman KM, Bowers D, Watson RT. Performance on a hemispatial pointing task by patients with neglect syndrome. Neurology 33:661–664, 1983.

Howes D, Boller F. Simple reaction time: Evidence of focal impairment from a lesion of the right hemisphere. Brain 98:317–332, 1975.

Jones E. The precise diagnostic value of allochirea. Brain 30:490–532, 1907.

Kertesz A, Nicholson I, Cancelliere A, Kassa K, Black S. Motor impersistence. Neurology 35:662–666, 1985.

Luria AR. Two kinds of motor perseveration in massive injury to the frontal lobes. Brain 88:1–10, 1965.

Luria AR. Higher Cortical Functions in Man. Basic Books Inc., New York, pp. 324–340, 1966.

Meador K, Watson RT, Bowers D, Heilman KM. Hypometria with hemispatial and limb motor neglect. Brain 109:293–305, 1986.

Mishkin M, Ungerleider L, Macko KA. Object vision and spatial vision: Two cortical pathways. Trends in the Neurosciences 6:414–417, 1983.

Posner MI, Walker JA, Friedrich FF, Rafel RD. Effects of parietal injury on covert orienting of attention. Journal of Neuroscience 4:1863–74, 1984.

Rapcsak SZ, Cimino CR, Heilman KM. Attitudinal neglect. Neurology 38:277–281, 1988.

Roeltgen MG, Roeltgen DP, Heilman KM. Unilateral motor impersistence and hemispatial neglect from a striatal lesion. Neuropsychiatry, Neuropsychology and Behavioral Neurology 2:125–135, 1989.

Sandson J, Albert MC. Perseveration in behavioral neurology. Neurology 37:1736–1741, 1987.

Shelton, PA, Bowers D, Heilman KM. Peripersonal and vertical neglect. Brain 113:191–205, 1990.

Suzuki H, and Azuma M. Prefrontal neuronal activity during gazing at a light dot in the monkey. Brain Research 126:497–508, 1977.

Valenstein E, Heilman KM, Watson RT, Van den Abell T. Nonsensory neglect from parietotemporal lesions in monkeys. Neurology 32:1198–1201, 1982.

Verfaellie M, Bowers D, Heilman KM. Hemispheric asymmetries in mediating intention but not selection attention. Neuropsychologia 26:521–531, 1988.

Verfaellie M, Heilman KM. Response preparation and response inhibition following lesions of the medial frontal lobes. Archives of Neurology 44:1265–1275, 1987.

Vilkki J. Perseveration in memory for figures after frontal lobe lesions. Neuropsychologia 27:1101–1104, 1989.

Watson RT, Miller BD, Heilman KM. Non sensory neglect. Annals of Neurology 3:505–508, 1978.

Watson RT, Valenstein E, Heilman KM. Thalamic neglect: Possible role of the medial thalamus and nucleus reticularis in behavior. Archives of Neurology 38:501–506, 1981.

VI
Integration of Experimental Models with Studies of Patients

11

Somatic Markers and the Guidance of Behavior: Theory and Preliminary Testing

ANTONIO R. DAMASIO,
DANIEL TRANEL,
AND HANNA C. DAMASIO

The theory proposed here evolved as a response to the challenge posed by patient EVR. As has been discussed elsewhere in detail (Eslinger and Damasio, 1985), patient EVR developed profoundly abnormal personality characteristics following a bilateral ablation of ventromedial frontal cortices, which was required for the surgical treatment of a meningioma. Prior to the appearance of the tumor and to surgery (which took place when EVR was age 35), EVR was, from all possible perspectives, a normal individual. He was intelligent, hard-working, successful at securing a steady skilled job and at being promoted for his good performance. He was active in social affairs and was perceived as a leader and example by his siblings, and by others in his community. But the person that emerged after frontal surgery could hardly be more different. EVR has never again been able to maintain a job (he clearly remains skilled enough to hold one, but he cannot be counted on to report to work promptly or to execute all the intermediate steps of the tasks that are expected of him). His ability to plan his activities, both on a daily basis as well as into the future, is severely impaired. The planning may fail to include components that would obviously be advantageous for his future, and include instead peripheral business that is of no possible use. Often, on matters of relatively secondary import, e.g., what to wear, where to shop, what restaurant to go to, EVR is plunged into an endless debate. He is unable to make a rapid choice and, instead, pursues a course of interminable comparisons and successive deliberations among many possible options that become more and more difficult to distinguish. His final response selection, if it ever comes, may end up being random. An especially troubled area for his decision making has to do with social behaviors and, as a subset of those, with financial planning. It clearly is not easy for EVR to decide which persons are good and which ones are not, in terms of his future life course. A sense of what is socially appropriate, judging from the choices he makes in his "real-life" encounters, is clearly lacking, while it is obvious from his premorbid life and achievement that he once had a keen sense of social appropriateness. His relatives corroborate this, but the ecologic findings make it unequivocal.

In the end, EVR's decision making and planning are (1) qualitatively different from what they were before, and (2) clearly defective by reference to his own standards as well as those of his direct peers. In the long term, the defect leads to many punishing consequences for EVR. In general, these characteristics of behavior fit the criteria for sociopathy, as defined in the *Diagnostic and Statistical Manual of Mental Disorders* (DSM-III; American Psychiatric Association, 1980) (e.g., "inability to sustain consistent work behavior," "inability to maintain an enduring attachment to a sexual partner," "lack of ability to function as a responsible parent," "defective planning"). The key difference is that EVR's sociopathic personality manifestations appeared in adulthood, after his brain damage, rather than during the development of his personality. Thus, we have tentatively termed his condition "acquired sociopathy." It should be emphasized that there are other important differences between "acquired sociopathy" of the type manifest by EVR and similar patients, and the standard "developmental sociopathy" elaborated in DSM-III, e.g., the latter type of patient has far greater likelihood of being antisocial in a manner that is harmful to others, while the EVR-type is more likely to cause difficulties for the self; hence, parallels between the two conditions are, in part, strictly for heuristic purposes.

Against this background of ravage, we must describe the many aspects of his intellectual profile that remain not only intact but, indeed, outstanding. EVR is not just an intelligent man, but a superiorly intelligent one, a judgment supported by psychometric evidence (on the Wechsler Adult Intelligence Scale-Revised, EVR obtains IQ scores in the top 1–2 percentile [Verbal IQ = 132, Performance IQ = 135]), and by reflection on many hours of structured interviews ranging over varied topics. EVR can distinguish with great subtlety among highly ambiguous concepts, can use deduction and induction fluently, and can comment with charm and irony on myriad daily events. Numerous neuropsychologic tests make these judgments objective (e.g., Shipley-Hartford Vocabulary score = 37/40, Abstractions score = 40/40; Visual-Verbal Test score = 73/84). Naturally, EVR's language processing, at phonemic, lexical, syntactic, and discourse levels, is fully preserved.

Conventional learning and memory are also intact, as can be proven by EVR's perfect acquisition of all manner of events that occur in his daily life, by his perfect recollection of autobiographic details, and by formal neuropsychologic testing (e.g., Wechsler Memory Scale MQ = 145 [99th percentile]; Rey Auditory-Verbal Learning Test Trial 5 score = 14/15 [superior]; Benton Visual Retention Test score = 9/10 correct [superior]; Rey-Osterrieth Complex Figure recall score = 32/36 [99th percentile]). The partial exception to this lies with social knowledge. It might be argued that EVR has a selective memory defect for social knowledge; however, this would not be an accurate statement, because EVR can access social knowledge when he is questioned about it verbally, and even when a social problem is presented to him cast in verbal premises. It is perhaps more accurate to state that learning of social knowledge is impaired, since EVR clearly does not learn from his mistakes, and repeatedly selects response options that lead to negative consequences.

It is not possible to account for EVR's defects on the basis of general impairments of intelligence, memory, language, or perception. Furthermore, EVR and, along with him, other similar patients to whom we will refer as "EVR-like," also lack some subtle but supposedly characteristic signs of frontal lobe dysfunction, which tend to be highly correlated with defective decision making and planning. For instance, EVR produces perfect scores on the Wisconsin Card Sorting Test, the Category Test, and the Word Fluency Test, and his performances in paradigms requiring cognitive estimations (Shallice and Evans, 1978) and judgments of recency and frequency (Milner and Petrides, 1984) are flawless. He is not perseverative and he is not impulsive.

How, then, can we explain EVR's peculiar condition?

THE THEORY OF SOMATIC MARKERS

Background

We have proposed that although EVR is able to recognize the meaning of social situations, and to imagine possible responses to those situations, he is no longer able to select the most advantageous response, taking into account his autobiography and the contingencies of his environment. In brief, EVR not only possesses but still accesses knowledge about the *manifest* meaning of entities and events (the identity of a person or place), but also knowledge about their *implied* meaning (the positive or negative value of a person or action, possible response options to an event, and the imagined consequences that follow a given response immediately and later).

The distinction between manifest and implied meanings is critical to the understanding of EVR's problem, which we will attempt using as a framework our model for time-locked retroactivation (Damasio, 1989a,b). In this model, any level of meaning is seen as the result of the synchronous evocation of many separate cognitive components, whose ensemble defines entities and events based on their constituent features. The model posits that the co-evocations are the consequence of synchronously activating numerous anatomically separate regions in association cortices. The synchronous activations occur in early cortices that contain the neural inscriptions of component representations and are directed by feedback projections from convergence zones located over multiple cortical regions (interconnected both hierarchically and heterarchically). Because there is no single neuroanatomic region that holds the integrated "image" of a polysensory based set of events, meaning is critically dependent on timing. And because implied meanings require a far larger set of components for their definition than manifest meanings do, the problem of synchronization and subsequent attention looms larger. In short, from this perspective, the response selections required for appropriate decision making in social cognition and equivalent realms, necessitates the holding on-line, for long periods of time (in the order of several thousand milliseconds), highly heterogeneous sets of cognitive components that must be attended effectively, if a choice is to be made. Where we believe EVR fails is in the *selection of one among many response options,* displayed long after the triggering stimuli were first presented and often even after they are no longer perceivable. It should be noted that the defect in the operations we posit is related to frontal cortical dysfunction, and also, that the frontal cortices have long been presumed to be critical for neural operations in which responses to stimuli must be effected after a delay (Jacobsen, 1935; 1936). The latter notion has played a major role in the theoretic formulations of Fuster (1989) and Goldman-Rakic (1987) regarding frontal lobe function in primates.

The Proposed Mechanism for the Defect

We propose that the response selection impairment is due to a *defect in the activation of somatic markers* that must accompany the internal and automatic processing of possible response options. Deprived of a somatic marker to assist, both consciously and covertly, with response selection, EVR has a reduced chance of responding in the most advantageous manner, and a higher chance of generating responses that will lead to negative consequences. Let us explain with an example.

Imagine yourself confronted by the possibility of accompanying an acquaintance to a particular social event; or the possibility of entering a business partnership with yet another acquaintance. In either case, the premises of the situation (the identities of those involved, their previous relation to you, their social record) will be available to you from previous interactions, drawing on a variety of nonverbal and verbal parcellated knowledge (which, according to the model adduced previously, can be synchronously evoked in separate cortices). The implications of going or not going will also be available to you in all of their complexity, and in an equally distributed neural manner. In short, the premises of the situation, several response options, and several anticipated consequences, must be simultaneously available for your inspection, so that attention can bring them into consciousness.

Going to the social event may mean an immediate advantage, but it may be that the nature of the event implies that you will be criticized for attending it by your friends and relatives, resulting in a future net loss. And yet, you must decide on a course of action. This may be done either with deliberation, or automatically, or somewhere in between. What we are proposing is that normal individuals can be assisted in this complex decision-making process by *the appearance of a somatic signal that marks the ultimate consequences of the response option with a negative or positive somatic state.* In other words, response option "A," regardless of its predictable immediate reward, can evoke a future scenario that is potentially threatening to the individual, and is marked by a negative somatic state. The perceiver would then experience the reenactment of punishment (another way of putting it would be to say that a negative emotion would be felt).

The first effect of the somatic marker would then be to provide the subject with a conscious "gut feeling" on the merits of a given response, and force attention on the positive or negative nature of given response options based on their foreseeable consequences. But in addition, we also posit a second effect, which would be covert and which would modify the state of neural systems that propitiate appetitive or aversive behaviors, e.g., the dopamine and serotonin nonspecific systems that can alter processing in cerebral cortex. This effect would be activated by the somatic marker and would increase or reduce the chances of immediate response, e.g., a negative somatic state would inhibit appetitive behaviors and vice versa, even if the somatic state itself would not be attended to and would thus not be experienced consciously. This, in turn, could increase or reduce the chances of inhibiting a response or facilitating it.

The Plausibility of the Mechanism

At first glance, it might seem more efficient to have all sorts of decision making based on a fully rational computation of the merits and disadvantages of each response option. Why should one rely on a seemingly primitive "emotional" signal? The first answer is that, in all likelihood, such mechanisms were successfully developed in other species and have proven to be thoroughly effective in their ecologic niches. The second is that the sheer amount of possible response options makes it likely that an assistance device is required to sort out the responses that are more likely to be relevant for the overall goals of the organism in both the short and long term. In other words, an unassisted rational computation of many conflictual response options is probably quite inefficient, e.g., the organism might be paralyzed with indecision, as indeed EVR often is. The third answer has to do with the special value of somatic states in the acquisition of a large range of behaviors than one might call social and personal. This is because the acquisition of such behaviors is closely linked with punishment and reward, brought in by parenting, schooling, peer group influences, and other interactions during development, to ensure that certain key goals of the individual and the species are achieved according to the contingencies set by the social environment. Punishment and reward are perceived modifications of baseline somatic states, which induce perceptions along the range that includes pain and pleasure. It is reasonable to assume that in the same way that punishment and reward mark a given act as valuable or dangerous for the individual, during development, and are learned conjunctively, the reenactment of a state of pain or pleasure triggered by the internal representation of the consequence of a response option would mark that response option as positive or negative. The specific proposal is that the accompanying somatic state would ensure in most circumstances, and in a fairly automatic way, that responses whose consequences would be negative to the individual would be thoughtfully avoided or covertly suppressed.

If the preceding proposal does apply to EVR-type patients, it must be found that they (1) can access implied meanings to the situations in which they act defectively, and (2) fail to activate somatic states to those implied meanings. There is already considerable evidence to support the first requisite, but virtually none to support the second. In a study reported elsewhere (Damasio et al., 1990) and summarized in this chapter, we tested the hypothesis that EVR-type patients are no longer able to mount somatic states to complex stimuli charged with social significance.

TESTING THE PROPOSAL

We studied three subject groups. The first we called *bifrontal,* and comprised five subjects who had bilateral lesions in orbital and lower mesial frontal regions. The second was termed *brain-damaged controls,* and included six subjects who had lesions *outside* the ventromedial frontal cortices. The third consisted of *normal controls,* and included five subjects.

To assess somatic state activation, we utilized the electrodermal skin conductance response (SCR), because the SCR is a biologically and psychologically relevant index of autonomic neural activity (Boucsein, 1988; Edelberg, 1972; 1973; Fowles, 1986), and it reliably indexes the "signal value" of stimuli at both physiologic and psychologic levels (e.g., Bernstein, 1979; Raskin, 1973).

We utilized three categories of stimuli in the experiments: (1) *Elementary unconditioned* ("orienting") stimuli: These were basic "orienting" stimuli that reliably elicit SCRs from normal subjects (Fowles and Schneider, 1978; Raskin, 1973; Stern and Anschel, 1968), such as an unexpected loud hand-clap close to the subject's ears. (2) *Target pictures:* pictures depicting social disaster, mutilation, or nudity. Those pictures have strong "implied" meanings, i.e., they readily evoke emotional responses of pleasure or pain in normal subjects, and elicit high-amplitude, discriminatory SCRs (Greenwald et al., 1990; Lang and Greenwald, 1988). (3) *Nontarget pictures:* pictures depicting neutral material such as bland scenery and abstract patterns. These "nontargets" do not elicit large-amplitude SCRs from normal subjects (Lang and Greenwald, 1988), and they do not have strong "implied" meanings.

The set of 40 pictorial slides (10 targets and 30 nontargets) were randomly ordered and administered twice, consecutively. During the first administration (the PASSIVE response condition), the subject viewed the slides without making any verbal or motor response. During the second (ACTIVE response condition) the subject had to comment on the content of the slide and on the impact it made on the subject.

Following the ACTIVE condition, the subject participated in a short "debriefing" session to verify that the SCR data were not contaminated by inattentiveness or idiosyncratic mores and aesthetics. Questions were asked about the stimulus content and the feelings the subject had experienced while viewing the slides in the PASSIVE versus ACTIVE conditions.

Skin conductance was recorded from both hands, using equipment and techniques described elsewhere (Tranel and A. Damasio, 1988; Tranel and H. Damasio, 1989). The amplitude of the largest SCR that had onset within 1–5 seconds after stimulus onset was measured for both orienting stimuli and for the pictorial stimuli in both conditions.

For each subject we calculated a total of five scores: The average "orienting" SCR, and the average target and nontarget SCR for both response conditions. Averages were based on all available stimulus presentations (including nonres-

Table 11–1 Skin Conductance Magnitudes*

	Orienting response	Passive condition		Active condition	
		Target	Nontarget	Target	Nontarget
Normal controls	0.688	0.802	0.077	0.999	0.150
(n = 5)	(0.208)	(0.327)	(0.066)	(0.384)	(0.027)
Brain-damaged controls	0.520	0.594	0.137	0.949	0.289
(n = 6)	(0.503)	(0.565)	(0.234)	(0.901)	(0.313)
Bifrontals	0.950	0.125	0.049	0.323	0.074
(n = 5)	(0.347)	(0.145)	(0.088)	(0.294)	(0.153)

*In microSiemens (μS); S.D. in parentheses.

ponses counted as zero-amplitude SCRs), and are referred to as "magnitudes" (Venables and Christie, 1980). Nonparametric techniques were utilized for statistical analysis (Siegel and Castellan, 1988), since the data sets did not meet sufficiently the parametric assumptions of homogeneity of variance and normal distribution.

The results of the controls (normals and brain-damaged) and the bifrontals are shown in Table 11–1. Statistical analysis of these data indicated the following:

1. There were no differences between the orienting SCRs of the three subject groups (a Kruskal-Wallis one-way analysis of variance by ranks test was nonsignificant [$H = 2.08$, $p > .30$]).

2. Both the normal and brain-damaged controls showed sharp discrimination between the target and nontarget stimuli with a much larger SCR magnitude for the targets ($p > .05$, Sign Test), in both the Passive and Active conditions. This effect is in line with previous findings regarding the effects of highly charged visual stimuli on autonomic responses (e.g., Greenwald et al., 1990; Hare et al., 1970; Klorman et al., 1975).

3. The bifrontals failed to generate discriminatory SCRs to the target pictures in the PASSIVE condition ($p = .50$, Sign Test) but in the ACTIVE condition the target versus nontarget SCR magnitudes were significantly different ($p = 0.031$, Sign Test). This indicates that the bifrontals are substantially closer to normals in the ACTIVE condition.

As an example, the results from subject EVR are presented in detail in Table 11–2, together with some ancillary experiments that were used to follow-up and firmly document EVR's response patterns.

EVR's orienting SCRs were normal, and his orienting response magnitude was well within the range of the control groups. In the first experiment, however, he demonstrated a marked failure to generate normal SCRs to the target stimuli in the PASSIVE condition. There was no difference between his SCR magnitude for the targets versus the nontargets ($p > .33$, Mann-Whitney U test). In the ACTIVE condition, however, he showed normal discriminatory SCRs to the targets, with a target–nontarget difference that is significant and virtually identical to controls ($z = -3.87$, $p < .001$, Mann-Whitney U test).

Table 11-2 Skin Conductance Magnitudes for Subject EVR*

Condition	SCR magnitudes (in μS) (S.D.)	
Orienting response	0.650	
	Target	Nontarget
Initial experiment		
Passive	0.003	0.006
	(0.008)	(0.023)
Active	0.598	0.012
	(0.564)	(0.031)
A-B-A reversal experiment		
Passive	0.000	0.004
	(−)	(0.013)
Active	0.718	0.007
	(0.818)	(0.027)
Passive	0.008	0.031
	(0.018)	(0.092)
2-Year follow-up experiment		
Passive	0.002	0.004
	(0.005)	(0.012)
Active	0.576	0.020
	(0.356)	(0.042)

*In μS; S.D. in parentheses.

Several months after the initial study, EVR's SCRs were studied in an A-B-A reversal design with a new stimulus set. In this experiment, EVR was first exposed to a PASSIVE condition. An ACTIVE condition immediately followed, and then another PASSIVE condition. The stimulus set was the same across all three sections of this follow-up experiment, i.e., EVR viewed the same stimulus set three times consecutively. Once again, EVR showed normal SCRs to the target pictures only in the ACTIVE condition ($z = -6.28$, $p < .001$); in both PASSIVE situations, his responses remained severely impaired ($p > .50$ for target–nontarget comparisons in both PASSIVE conditions).

More than 2 years (27 months) after the initial experiment, we conducted a follow-up study of EVR, using still another set of stimuli but the same procedures as for the initial study. The outcome replicated previous findings, as EVR showed excellent SCR discrimination of the target pictures in the ACTIVE condition ($z = -5.76$, $p < .001$), but no discrimination in the PASSIVE condition ($p > .50$).

COMMENT

When our frontal lobe damaged subjects viewed complex and socially significant stimuli passively, their autonomic responses were abnormal and often were entirely absent. This remarkable and highly reproducible finding suggests that no somatic state was generated in response to the implied meanings that accompany the viewing of those stimuli. The finding cannot be explained by a primary autonomic dysfunction, because stimuli of a simpler and unconditioned nature still elicited normal autonomic responses in the same subjects. Furthermore, when the condition was modified to include an active, verbal commentary on the contents of each stimulus, the subjects did respond to the appropriate stimuli. This clearly reconfirms that the ability to generate autonomic responses has not been compromised, but rather, the mechanism for its triggering has been altered.

It has been shown previously that patients with frontal lobe lesions have defects in autonomic orienting responses (Luria, 1973; Luria and Homskaya, 1970), and a similar outcome has been reported for nonhuman primates with frontal ablations (Kimble et al., 1965). These studies, however, were aimed at measuring overall arousal. Our findings go well beyond this earlier work in demonstrating an autonomic defect that is specific to a certain stimulus type, response condition, and location of lesion.

Neural Basis: Description of Network

The core of damage in EVR-type patients is in the ventromedial sector of the frontal lobe. Both the medial orbital cortices and the lower mesial orbital cortices, along with subjacent white matter, are damaged bilaterally. These cortices, judging from what is known of nonhuman primate neuroanatomy, receive projections that hail from all sensory modalities, directly or indirectly (Chavis and Pandya, 1976; Jones and Powell, 1970; Pandya and Kuypers, 1969; Potter and Nauta, 1979). In turn, they are the only known source of projections from frontal regions toward central autonomic control structures (Nauta, 1971), and such projections have a demonstrated physiologic influence on visceral control (Hall et al., 1977). The ventromedial cortices have extensive bidirectional connections with the hippocampus and amygdala (Amaral and Price, 1984; Goldman-Rakic et al., 1984; Porrino et al., 1981; Van Hoesen et al., 1972; 1975).

This anatomic design is certainly compatible with the role we propose for the ventromedial cortices. We believe these cortices contain convergence zones that hold a record of temporal conjunctions of activity in varied neural units, e.g., sensory cortices, limbic structures. This would be a record of signals from regions that were active simultaneously and that, as a set, defined a given situation. A critical output of the ventromedial convergence zones would be to autonomic effectors such as the amygdala so that, when a given set of inputs to the ventromedial region would obtain, a pertinent output to amygdala would follow. Activation of the amygdala would in turn result in reenactment of a somatic state whose signal, intensity, and somatic distribution would be pertinent to the sensory set. Finally, the newly enacted somatic state would be perceived by somatosensory cortices in conjunction with the sensory set that had originated the entire cycle and that would have remained on-line.

The systems network necessary for these processes thus includes the following structures: (1) Ventromedial frontal cortices with convergence zones that record combinations of (a) the distributed representations of certain stimuli and the recalled representations they generate, (b) the somatic states that have been prevalently associated with the above; (2) central autonomic effectors, the amygdala in particular, which can activate somatic responses in viscera, vascular bed, endocrine system, and nonspecific neurotransmitter systems; and (3) somatosensory projection systems and cortices, especially those in the nondominant parietal region (see Tranel and H. Damasio, 1989, for preliminary evidence).

It is important to note that the evocation of a somatic marker for stimuli that are unconditioned and far more basic, for instance, a startling noise or a flash of light, requires a different and simpler network. It is possible that autonomic activation could be achieved by direct thalamic projections to amygdala or other autonomic effectors, long before signals about such stimuli would actually reach the cerebral cortex. The complex network outlined previously pertains only to those stimuli whose complexity, in terms of configurations and implications, requires processing in multiple sensory cortices and over longer delays.

Extension of the Theory to Nonsocial Decision-making Processes

Assuming that the brain has available a means to select good responses from bad in social situations, we suspect it is likely that the mechanism has been co-opted for behavioral guidance that is outside the realm of social cognition. The argument here is that nature would have evolved a highly successful mechanism of guidance to cope with problems whose answer might maximize survival or lead to danger. Although a large range of those problems pertains to the social realm directly, it is apparent that many other problems, albeit not social, are indirectly linked to precisely the same framework of survival versus danger, of ultimate advantage versus disadvantage, of ultimate gain and balance versus loss and disequilibrium. It is therefore plausible that a system geared to produce markers and signposts to guide "social" responses would have been adapted to assist with "intellectual" decision making. Naturally, the somatic markers would not be perceived in the form of "feelings." But they would still act covertly to highlight, in the form of an attentional mechanism, certain components over others, and to direct, in effect, the go, stop, and turn signals necessary for much decision making and planning on even the most abstract of topics.

A final comment is in order regarding the application of the theory and findings previously discussed to a population of psychiatric patients. First, it is possible that "developmental" sociopathy might be due to a developmental defect in the function of the neural system. The defect need not be in the same unit of the system, and need not be as profound. For instance, it might be sufficient to have a higher threshold of activation for somatic states such that most relevant stimuli would produce weak responses. Intriguingly, some evidence is already available in this regard. It has been shown, for example, that sociopaths show poor autonomic conditioning with aversive unconditioned stimuli (e.g., shock), defective autonomic responses in anticipation of aversive stimuli, and even impaired autonomic conditioning to appetitive stimuli (e.g., Hare and Quinn, 1971; Lykken, 1957; for review: Hare, 1978). But, in general, the mechanism would be the same. It is important to note that the differences between developmental and acquired sociopaths, namely, the greater benignity of the latter, do not invalidate this proposal. Acquired sociopaths, in spite of their profound defect, have lived a normal premorbid life during which they learned how to deal with social situations normally; developmental sociopaths never did. The previous normality of the system in the acquired sociopath is likely to compensate for the defect in numerous circumstances.

Another psychiatric condition that may be interpreted with the help of these findings is obsessive-compulsive disease. In short, we see it as the very opposite of sociopathy, i.e., a condition in which numerous trivial stimuli are allowed to generate somatic markers that force the attention of the perceiver and call for response implementation. The dysfunction would relate to the same network and, quite particularly, to ventromedial frontal cortices. For instance, it would be reasonable to discover that where ventromedial frontal cortices are damaged in acquired sociopaths, they should be underactive in developmental sociopaths, and probably overactive in obsessive-compulsive patients ("activity" being measured, for instance, by metabolic or cerebral blood flow rates). Along the same perspective, depressed and neurotic patients with a high degree of somatic suffering should reveal overactivity in ventromedial frontal cortices.

ACKNOWLEDGMENTS

This study was supported by NINDS Program Project Grant NS 19632.

REFERENCES

Amaral DG, Price JL. Amygdalo-cortical projections in the monkey (Macaca fascicularis). Journal of Comparative Neurology 230:465–496, 1984.

American Psychiatric Association. Diagnostic and Statistical Manual of Mental Disorders, 3rd Edition. Washington, DC, 1980.

Bernstein AS. The orienting response as novelty and significance detector: Reply to O'Gorman. Psychophysiology 16:263–273, 1979.

Boucsein W. Elektrodermale Aktivitat: Grundlagen, Methoden und Anwendungen. New York: Springer-Verlag, 1989.

Chavis DA, Pandya DN. Further observations on corticofrontal connections in the rhesus monkey. Brain Research 117:369–386, 1976.

Damasio AR. The brain binds entities and events by multiregional activation from convergence zones. Neural Computation 1:123–132, 1989a.

Damasio AR. Time-locked multiregional retroactivation: A systems-level proposal for the neural substrates of recall and recognition. Cognition 33:25–62, 1989b.

Damasio AR, Tranel D, Damasio H. Individuals with sociopathic behavior caused by frontal damage fail to respond autonomically to social stimuli. Behavioral Brain Research 41:81–94, 1990.

Damasio H, Damasio AR. Lesion Analysis in Neuropsychology. New York: Oxford University Press, 1989.

Edelberg R. The electrodermal system. In Greenfield, = NS, Sternbach RA (eds), Handbook of Psychophysiology. New York: Holt, Rinehart & Winston, 1972, pp. 367–418.

Edelberg R. Mechanisms of electrodermal adaptations for locomotion, manipulation, or defense. Progress in Physiological Psychology 5:155–209, 1973.

Eslinger PJ, Damasio AR. Severe disturbance of higher cognition after bilateral frontal lobe ablation: Patient EVR. Neurology 35:1731–1741, 1985.

Fowles DC. The eccrine system and electrodermal activity. *In* Coles MGH, Donchin E, Porges SW (eds), Psychophysiology: Systems, Processes, and Applications. New York: Guilford Press, 1986, pp. 51–96.

Fowles DC, Schneider RE. Electrolyte effects on measurements of palmar skin potential. Psychophysiology 15:474–482, 1978.

Fuster JM. The Prefrontal Cortex, 2nd Edition. New York: Raven Press, 1989.

Goldman-Rakic PS. Circuitry of primate prefrontal cortex and regulation of behavior by representational memory. *In* Plum, F (ed), Handbook of Physiology: The Nervous System, Vol 5. Bethesda, MD: American Physiological Society, 1987, pp. 373–417.

Goldman-Rakic PS, Selemon LD, Schwartz ML. Dual pathways connecting the dorsolateral prefrontal cortex with the hippocampal formation and parahippocampal cortex in the rhesus monkey. Neuroscience 12:719–743, 1984.

Greenwald MK, Cook EW, Lang PJ. Affective judgment and psychophysiological response: Dimensional covariation in the evaluation of pictorial stimuli. Journal of Psychophysiology (in press).

Hall RE, Livingston RB, Bloor CM. Orbital cortical influences on cardiovascular dynamics and myocardial structure in conscious monkeys. Journal of Neurosurgery 46:638–647, 1977.

Hare RD. Electrodermal and cardiovascular correlates of psychopathy. *In* Hare RD, Schalling D (eds), Psychopathic Behavior: Approaches to Research. New York: Wiley & Sons, 1978, pp. 107–143.

Hare RD, Wood K, Britain S, Shadman J. Autonomic responses to affective visual stimuli. Psychophysiology 7:408–417, 1970.

Hare RD, Quinn MJ. Psychopathy and autonomic conditioning. Journal of Abnormal Psychology 77:223–235, 1971.

Jacobsen CF. Functions of the frontal association area in primates. Archives of Neurology and Psychiatry 33:558–569, 1935.

Jacobsen CF. Studies of cerebral functions in primates: I. The functions of the frontal association areas in monkeys. Comparative Psychology Monographs 13:3–60, 1936.

Jones EG, Powell TPS. An anatomical study of converging sensory pathways within the cerebral cortex of the monkey. Brain 93:793–820, 1970.

Kimble DP, Bagshaw MH, Pribram KH. The GSR of monkeys during orienting and habituation after selective partial ablations of the cingulate and frontal cortex. Neuropsychologia 3:121–128, 1965.

Klorman R, Wiesenfeld A, Austin ML. Autonomic responses to affective visual stimuli. Psychophysiology 12:553–560, 1975.

Lang PJ, Greenwald MK. The international affective picture system standardization procedure and initial group results for affective judgments: Technical report 1A. Gainesville, FL: Center for Research in Psychophysiology, University of Florida, 1988.

Luria AR. The frontal lobes and the regulation of behavior. *In* Pribram KH, Luria AR (eds), Psychophysiology of the Frontal Lobes. New York: Academic Press, 1973, pp. 3–26.

Luria AR, Homskaya ED. Frontal lobes and the regulation of arousal processes. *In* Mostofsky, DI (ed), Attention: Contemporary Theory and Analysis. New York: Appleton-Century-Crofts, 1970, pp. 303–330.

Lykken DT. A study of anxiety in the sociopathic personality. Journal of Abnormal and Social Psychology 55:6–10, 1957.

Milner B, Petrides M. Behavioural effects of frontal-lobe lesions in man. Trends in Neurosciences 7:403–407,1984.

Nauta WJH. The problem of the frontal lobe: A reinterpretation. Journal of Psychiatric Research 8:167–187, 1971.

Pandya DN, Kuypers HGJM. Cortico-cortical connections in the rhesus monkey. Brain Research 13:13–36, 1969.

Porrino LJ, Crane AM, Goldman-Rakic PS. Direct and indirect pathways from the amygdala to the frontal lobe in rhesus monkeys. Journal of Comparative Neurology 198:121–136, 1981.

Potter H, Nauta WJH. A note on the problem of olfactory associations of the orbitofrontal cortex in the monkey. Neuroscience 4:316–367, 1979.

Raskin DC. Attention and arousal. In Prokasy WF, Raskin DC (eds), Electrodermal Activity in Psychological Research. New York: Academic Press. 1973, pp. 125–155.

Shallice T, Evans ME. The involvement of the frontal lobes in cognitive estimation. Cortex 14:294–303, 1978.

Siegel S, Castellan NJ. Non-parametric Statistics for the Behavioral Sciences, 2nd Edition. New York: McGraw-Hill, 1988.

Stern RM, Anschel C. Deep inspirations as stimuli for responses of the autonomic nervous system. Psychophysiology 6:132–141, 1968.

Tranel D, Damasio AR. Nonconscious face recognition in patients with face agnosia. Behavioural Brain Research 30:235–249, 1988.

Tranel D, Damasio H. Intact electrodermal skin conductance responses in a patient with bilateral amygdala damage. Neuropsychologia 27: 381–390, 1989.

Tranel D, Damasio H. Neuroanatomical correlates of skin conductance responses to "signal" stimuli. Psychophysiology 26:S61, 1989.

Van Hoesen GW, Pandya GN, Butters N. Cortical afferents to the entorhinal cortex of the rhesus monkey. Science 175:1471–1473, 1972.

Van Hoesen GW, Pandya GN, Butters N. Some connections of the entorhinal (area 28) and perirhinal (area 35) cortices of the rhesus monkey: II. Frontal lobe afferents. Brain Research 95:25–38, 1975.

Venables PH, Christie MJ. Electrodermal activity. In Martin I, Venables PH (eds), Techniques in Psychophysiology. New York: Wiley & Sons, 1980, pp. 3–67.

12

Delayed-Response Tasks: Parallels Between Experimental Ablation Studies and Findings in Patients with Frontal Lesions

MARLENE OSCAR-BERMAN,
PATRICK MCNAMARA,
AND MORRIS FREEDMAN

In this chapter we begin by defining a category of tasks usually referred to as delayed-response tasks. In particular, we describe the classic direct method delayed-response (DR) task, and the spatial delayed alternation (DA) task. Next, we briefly outline the neuroanatomic systems important for performing DR and DA tasks, and we review results of DR and DA testing in several human populations with neurologic dysfunction. One of our goals is to contribute toward an understanding of two basic issues: (1) The extent to which prefrontal cortex may be involved in DR and DA performance in humans, and (2) the nature of the neuropsychologic functions necessary for the successful performance of DR and DA tasks by humans. The ultimate aim is to clarify the behavioral manifestations of human brain disorders causing cognitive changes, and to help solve the enigma of the *frontal lobe syndrome.* We reasoned that initial evidence regarding these issues could be gleaned from careful examination of several patient groups with differing spared and impaired neuropsychologic abilities, but all with some degree of prefrontal pathology. In addition, we hoped to gain further insights into DR, DA, and prefrontal functions by applying knowledge about the neurochemical deficits in these same patient groups.

DEFINITIONS

Tasks known as delayed-response tasks (or delayed-reaction tasks, or spatial-delay tasks) refer generally to a class of time-based and response-based labora-

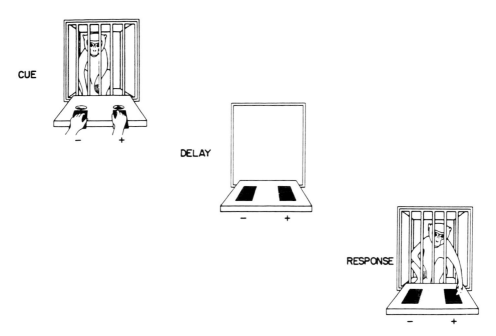

Figure 12-1 Three parts of a classic direct-method delayed-response trial. A reward is placed into a well under one of two identical stimuli differing only in spatial location. As soon as the wells are covered by the stimuli, a screen is lowered between the experimenter and the subject. After a delay (usually between 0 and 60 sec), the screen is raised with the tray containing the stimuli within the subject's reach. (From Goldman-Rakic, 1987, with permission from the author and publishers.)

tory procedures employed to measure mediation ability (or *cross-temporal bridging* ability; Fuster, 1989). Intact mediation ability is inferred from accurate choices made in the present, on the basis of information that was available in the immediate past. The first of this class of experimental paradigms to be introduced to psychology was the *direct-method* or *classic delayed-response* (DR) task (Hunter, 1913). In this simplest type of DR procedure, a piece of food (or some other reward) is placed by the experimenter into a reinforcement well under one of two identical stimuli differing only in their spatial location (Fig. 12–1). Baiting the well is accomplished out of reach, but in full view of a research participant (in this case, a hungry monkey). As soon as the wells are covered by the stimuli, a screen is lowered between the experimenter and the subject. After a variable delay (usually between 0 and 60 seconds), the screen is raised, with the tray containing the stimuli now within the subject's reach. The monkey displaces one of the stimuli and retrieves the food if the correct side is chosen; if the monkey chooses the incorrect side, no food is available. (Sometimes an indirect method is used, in which a cue such as a light signals the locus of the reinforcement.) The DR task is *time based* in that the subject must delay a choice until the opportunity to respond is made available. The task is not *response patterned,* because a regular sequence of responding, itself, is irrelevant to obtaining the reinforcements.

Another type of delayed-reaction task that is both time based and response patterned is *delayed alternation* (DA). DA tasks are usually given in an experimental apparatus identical to that used for measuring DR performance, and DA shares important features in common with DR: A delay between the stimulus and the opportunity to make a response, and a spatial cue as a salient stimulus dimension. However, the task requirements in DA and DR are quite different. In DA, stimulus–outcome relations regularly alternate across trials (French, 1964). The subjects must learn to alternate responding from left to right. On each trial, the side not previously chosen is rewarded, and a brief delay is interposed between trials (usually 5 seconds, with the screen lowered between the experimenter and the subject). (Sometimes the response sequence is doubled, LLRRLLRR . . . , and sometimes the response loci alternate nonspatially, e.g., between two distinctly different visual stimuli, but none of these variants will be considered here.) Thus, in the classic DR task, the subject utilizes spatial/attentional and mnemonic skills to notice and remember an external cue—the location of a reward placed there by the experimenter. In the DA task, the sources of cues are not conspicuous. Whether the cues about the locus of the reinforcement in the DA task originate inside the subject (e.g., where he or she last responded) and/or outside of the subject (whether or not a reward was available), the subject must learn to inhibit, on each trial, the previously rewarded response.

Several explanations have been offered regarding the nature of DR and DA deficits, but none has proved entirely satisfactory. These explanations generally include abnormalities in the following functions: Short-term memory (e.g., episodic memory and immediate memory), spatial information processing, response inhibition (and its corollary, perseveration), temporal chunking, kinesthetic feedback, and many others (for reviews: Arnold, 1984; Damasio, 1979; Freedman and Oscar-Berman, 1986a,c; Fuster, 1989; Goldman-Rakic, 1987; Pribram and Tubbs, 1967; Stamm, 1987; Stuss and Benson, 1986). Despite a lack of consensus regarding the precise nature of the functions being tapped by DR and DA tasks, it is universally assumed that they are sensitive measures of one or more cognitive functions linked to neuroanatomic systems of prefrontal cortex, and that successful performance on the tasks requires an ability to mediate cross-temporal contingencies.

NEUROANATOMIC SYSTEMS IN DR AND DA PERFORMANCE

Since the middle 1930s, when Jacobsen initially described selective DR deficits in monkeys with lesions of prefrontal cortex (Jacobsen, 1936), the impairment has been a hallmark of the damage. The inability of monkeys with bilateral prefrontal cortex lesions to perform DR tasks, even at the shortest delays, is striking. Likewise, these same animals have difficulty with DA tasks. For nearly a half a century, deficits on DR and DA tasks have been associated reliably with lesions of the prefrontal cortex in nonhuman animals (Warren and Akert, 1964). Because of its role in DR and DA tasks, prefrontal cortex has been labeled *mediator of cross-temporal contingencies* (Fuster, 1989), or *mediator of cross-temporal stimulus information* (Goldman-Rakic, 1989). Two large subdivisions of prefrontal cortex have been recognized to be important in normal DR and DA

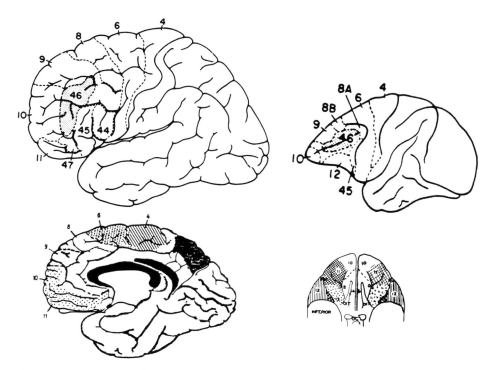

Figure 12-2   Cytoarchitectonic areas of a human brain (Brodmann, 1909) and the brain of a Rhesus monkey (Walker, 1940). (From Goldman-Rakic, 1987; Markowitsch, 1988; Walker, 1940, with permission.)

performance (Fig. 12–2): The dorsolateral and polar extent of the frontal lobes, and the ventral prefrontal region including the orbitofrontal surface and inferior convexity (Mishkin and Pribram, 1956; Numan, 1978; Oscar-Berman, 1975; Rosenkilde, 1979; Stuss and Benson, 1986; Warren and Akert, 1964). [The medial prefrontal sector, containing the anterior cingulate gyrus, is not included as a third subdivision because little evidence has linked that region directly with the tasks relevant to the present chapter (see Pribram, 1973).] The dorsolateral and ventral subdivisions of prefrontal cortex have correspondingly different cytoarchitectonic parcellations, neurochemical sensitivities, and connectional relationships with the rest of the brain. They are described in the following sections. Before proceeding, however, it must be emphasized that *the dichotomy is one of degree, and relies upon relative—not absolute—differences in the locations of neuroanatomic connections and in the contributions of neurotransmitter activity/innervation.*

Dorsolateral Prefrontal System

In monkeys and in humans, respectively, there are between six and ten cytoarchitectonically distinct areas within the dorsolateral prefrontal region (Walker, 1940; Brodmann, 1909). (The ventral prefrontal surface contains fewer distinct cell types.) In macaques, the dorsolateral region tied most directly to normal performance on spatial-delay tasks lies within the principal sulcus of the dorso-lateral surface [Walker's (1940) area 46. The corresponding cytoarchitectonic region in humans is Brodmann's (1909) area 46.]. In monkeys, lesions of the principal sulcus (area 46) produce deficits on DR and DA tasks as severe as those involving the entire dorsolateral prefrontal convexity. In fact, the cortex most critical for DR performance lies within the middle third sector of the principal sulcus (for reviews: Butters et al., 1972; Fuster, 1989; Goldman-Rakic, 1987; Pribram, 1987; Stamm, 1987; Stuss and Benson, 1986; Warren and Akert, 1964; Wilson, 1962).

Dorsolateral prefrontal cortex has reciprocal projections to and from other neocortical association cortices, limbic structures (via the cingulate cortex and ventral prefrontal cortex), and diencephalic regions (Fuster, 1989; Goldman-Rakic, 1987; Pandya and Barnes, 1987; Stuss and Benson, 1986). It has nonre-ciprocal efferent connections with basal ganglia sites, sending fibers to the ante-rior part of the head of the caudate nucleus (Johnson et al., 1968). Efferents also are sent to brain stem monoamine sites, suggesting that dorsolateral prefrontal cortex can control its own level of functional arousal (Arnsten and Goldman-Rakic, 1984; Weinberger et al., 1986). The dorsolateral prefrontal cortex itself is a primary neocortical target of ascending dopaminergic innervation (Bannon and Roth, 1983; Fuster, 1989; Javoy-Agid et al., 1989; Moore, 1982), although other monoaminergic innervation also is evident (Foote and Morrison, 1986; Goldman-Rakic, 1987; Javoy-Agid et al., 1989). An ascending catecholami-nergic pathway originates in anteromedial and ventral regions of the midbrain ventral tegmental area and then projects in a partially topographic manner onto dorsolateral prefrontal sites (Bannon and Roth, 1983; Dalsass et al., 1981; Fus-ter, 1989; Moore, 1982).

DR deficits can be produced by lesions of the head of the caudate (Battig et al., 1960), the dorsomedial nucleus of the thalamus (Isseroff et al., 1982; Schul-man, 1964), and the subthalamus (Adey et al., 1962). Mild DA deficits can be produced by lesions of the same subcortical sites important for DR performance, but in addition, DA performance is mildly sensitive to damage of the hippocam-pus with and without the amygdala (Mahut, 1971; Rosvold and Szwarcbart, 1964), inferotemporal cortex (Mahut and Cordeau, 1963), cingulate cortex (Pri-bram et al., 1962), and the hypothalamus (Rosvold, 1972). Brozoski and col-leagues (1979) demonstrated that a significant deficit in performance on a DA task, induced by depletion of dopamine stores from dorsolateral cortex, could be reversed selectively with a dopaminergic agonist.

In summary, dorsolateral prefrontal cortex is predominantly and recipro-cally interconnected with other neocortical association areas (directly, or via the diencephalon), and nonreciprocally connected with striatal and brain stem sites. Catecholaminergic (especially dopaminergic) innervation of dorsolateral pre-frontal cortex is important in normal performance on delayed reaction tasks.

Ventral Prefrontal System

The orbitofrontal sector of ventral prefrontal cortex has been associated more often with deficits on DA tasks than on DR tasks (Fuster, 1989; Goldman-Rakic,

1987; Warren and Akert, 1964). Orbitofrontal cortex displays a pattern of connections paralleling that of dorsolateral cortex, but the two systems are clearly and distinctly different. Primary orbitofrontal connections are with the medial thalamus (the magnocellular region of the dorsomedial nucleus), the hypothalamus, the ventrolateral portion of the head of the caudate, and the amygdala. [Dorsolateral cortex connects with a more lateral region of the dorsomedial nucleus of the thalamus (as well as to ventral and anterior thalamic areas), the anterolateral portion of the head of the caudate, the hippocampus, and many neocortical regions (Fuster, 1989).] In general, compared with dorsolateral cortex, orbital cortex is (1) more densely interconnected with limbic sites (Mishkin, 1964; Nauta and Domesick, 1981) and with the basal forebrain (e.g., the medial septal area, the diagonal band of Broca, and the nucleus basalis of Meynert; Mesulam et al., 1983), and (2) less interconnected with other neocortical association areas (Eslinger and Damasio, 1985; Pribram, 1987).

Orbitofrontal cortex is host to a variety of neurochemical influences because of its intimate connectivity with hypothalamic and limbic sites (Martinez, 1983). In addition, neurons of the nucleus basalis of Meynert in the basal forebrain provide the major source of cholinergic innervation to the entire neocortex, including the ventral prefrontal sector (Mesulam et al., 1983; Mesulam et al., 1986). However, these basal forebrain cholinergic neurons *receive* cortical inputs from only a few areas; the orbitofrontal (but not dorsolateral) prefrontal region is one source of these cortical inputs to the basal forebrain (Mesulam and Mufson, 1984). Thus, while orbitofrontal cortex sends efferents into cholinergic basal forebrain sites, dorsolateral prefrontal cortex sends efferents to brain stem monoamine sites. Consequently, orbital prefrontal cortex may have the ability to control its own level of functional arousal (as does dorsolateral prefrontal cortex via a different neurotransmitter system). Interestingly, Richardson and DeLong (1986) reported that neurons in the basal forebrain tended to fire selectively at, or immediately before, reward delivery in a spatial-delay task. In summary, then, orbitofrontal cortex appears to be linked predominantly with limbic and basal forebrain sites and thereby linked more with forebrain cholinergic than with catecholaminergic systems (see also Javoy-Agid et al., 1989). In this regard, however, it must be noted that while a growing body of neurochemical evidence (including distributions of neurotransmitter markers) generally respects these large regional divisions (Javoy-Agid et al., 1989), measures of the cholinergic marker enzyme, cholineacetyltransferase, have demonstrated equal levels of intrinsic cholinergic activity in 10 distinct frontal areas (including areas 46, 11, and 12) of normal postmortem human brains (Kish et al., 1989). These studies suggest that while intrinsic cholinergic activity appears to be uniform across prefrontal cortical regions, cholinergic innervation is not.

It is important to point out that although deficits on DR occur in monkeys after lesions within either the dorsolateral or the ventral frontal system, impairments are most striking following dorsolateral frontal damage (Oscar-Berman, 1975; Warren and Akert, 1964). We know of only one direct comparison of the effects of lesions of the two frontal systems on spatial DA performance (Passingham, 1975). In that study, two groups of monkeys with lesions of the different prefrontal systems were tested on a DA task that did not eliminate visual cues (hence contained aspects of the DR task); both groups performed poorly. However, we will assume that since the more typical DA task is primarily response patterned, and response inhibition is closely associated with orbitofrontal cortex, lesions there would likely lead to DA deficits at least as severe as dorsolateral lesions. Another task used more typically than DA to display orbitofrontal-based deficits is object alternation (requiring subjects to alternate choosing one of two visually distinct objects whose left-right positions vary randomly from trial to trial).

Summary

Whatever the important distinguishing features between DR and DA tasks, it is clear that accurate performance on them relies upon relatively different underlying neuroanatomic, neurochemical, and neuropsychologic mechanisms linked with the frontal lobes. Prefrontal cortex is host to at least two subsystems: Dorsolateral and ventral. Thus, while the dorsolateral system contains intimate connections with other neocortical sites, its connections with limbic sites are less striking than the orbitofrontal system's. The dorsolateral system is more closely linked with the catecholaminergic network than with cholinergic transmitters, and, although it is important for successful performance on both DR and DA, it is especially important for DR performance. Visuospatial mnemonic and attentional functions have been linked to the principal sulcus within the dorsolateral prefrontal cortex. By contrast, functions involved (somehow) in response inhibition have been linked to the orbitofrontal cortex. The ventral system, of which the orbitofrontal cortex is a part, is intimately connected with basal forebrain and limbic structures; its connections with other neocortical regions are not as extensive as the dorsolateral system's. The ventral system is more closely linked with the cholinergic network than with catecholaminergic transmitters. Like the dorsolateral system, the ventral system supports successful performance on both DA and DR, but it is especially important for DA performance.

Human Prefrontal Systems

The original work on neuroanatomic systems involved in DR and DA performance was based on nonhuman models. In humans, however, evidence regarding a prefrontal functional separation along dorsolateral and ventral dimensions is less clear than with nonhuman primates. One important reason for this obfuscation in humans is the heterogeneity of patient samples being studied: Human brain lesions usually occur in diverse prefrontal sites; are of variable size; may be unilateral or asymmetrically bilateral; are a result of different etiologic influences; occur at different time periods in a lifespan; and so on. Another reason for the confusion is the heterogeneity of procedures by which functional changes are assessed. In our own attempts to clarify the functional significance of human prefrontal cortex, we have tried to deal with both of these enormous problems by keeping our patient samples as homogeneous as possible, and by supplementing results of clinical neuropsychologic evaluations with information about the patients' abilities to perform DR and DA tasks. Based on the assumption of significant functional, anatomic, and neurochemical homologies between monkey and human brain systems, including those of prefrontal cortex (Mitchell and Erwin, 1987; Pandya and Barnes, 1987; Steklis and Erwin, 1988), we chose to test our patient groups on DR and DA tasks. We chose DR and DA specifically because of their special sensitivity to frontal dysfunction in nonhuman primates. The assumption of homology among primate species permits the use of a potentially rich source of insight into the cognitive functions of the frontal lobes in humans, namely, numerous behavioral testing paradigms originally designed to measure the effects of circumscribed brain lesions in monkeys.

HUMAN NEUROLOGIC PATIENTS WITH PREFRONTAL PATHOLOGY

Recall that two important goals of the present chapter are (1) to determine the extent to which prefrontal cortex may be involved in DR and DA performance in humans, and (2) to clarify the nature of the neuropsychologic functions necessary for the successful performance of DR and DA tasks by humans. To those ends, we now review results of DR and DA testing in nine groups of patients with neurologic symptoms suggesting prefrontal pathology. Our review is augmented, when possible, by information about neurochemical deficits in the patient groups, in order to supplement neuroanatomic and functional facts about their disorders.

The groups we have studied include patients with the following neurologic conditions: (1) Bilateral prefrontal lesions from tumor or trauma (Freedman and Oscar-Berman, 1986a); (2) alcoholic Korsakoff's syndrome (Oscar-Berman et al., 1982); (3) anterior communicating artery disease (Freedman and Oscar-Berman, 1986a); (4) Parkinson's disease with dementia, and (5) Parkinson's disease without dementia (Freedman and Oscar-Berman, 1986b); (6) Alzheimer's disease (Freedman and Oscar-Berman, 1986b); (7) olivopontocerebellar atrophy (El-Awar et al., 1989); (8) Broca's aphasia (Oscar-Berman et al., 1982); and (9) Huntington's disease (Oscar-Berman et al., 1982). Deficits on DR and DA were inferred when performance of any of the patient groups was significantly different from that of normal and/or non-Korsakoff alcoholic controls (Freedman and Oscar-Berman, 1986a,b; Oscar-Berman et al., 1982). Information about age, intelligence, and DR/DA performance of the groups is displayed in Table 12–1. The groups all were tested on DR (with delays of 0, 10, 30, and 60 seconds) and DA (5 seconds) under similar laboratory conditions, including similar apparatuses, procedures, and reinforcements.

Evidence from Clinical Neuropsychology

In numerous independent studies, patients suffering from any of the neurologic conditions just listed have demonstrated neuropsychologic changes consistent with frontal dysfunction (Damasio, 1979; Damasio et al., 1985; Kish et al., 1988; Moscovitch et al., 1986; Stuss and Benson, 1986; Taylor et al., 1986). Neuropsychologic tests that depend on intact frontal functions for successful performance include the Wisconsin Card Sorting Test (Heaton, 1981; Milner, 1963;

Table 12–1 Mean Ages, IQs (Wechsler Adult Intelligence Scale), and Performance Levels on DR and DA Tasks of the Groups of Patients Tested.

	N	Age	FSIQ	VIQ	PIQ	DR	DA
Normal controls	22	65	101*	. .	. .	− −	− −
Non-Korsakoff alcoholics	2–13	40	111	113	104	− −	− −
Broca's aphasics	8–11	51	. .	. .	91	− −	− −
Parkinsonians without dementia	13	62	100*	. .	. .	− −	− −
Parkinsonians with dementia	15	72	84*	. .	. .	+ +	− −
ACoA patients	5	46	109	. .	. .	− −	(−/+)
Huntington patients	8–15	46	81	84	80	− −	+ +
OPCA patients	10–11	33	. .	89	. .	− −	+ +
Korsakoff patients	12	54	104	105	103	(−/+)	+ +
Alzheimer patients	14	68	81*	. .	. .	+ +	+ +
Bifrontal trauma or tumor	6	49	90	. .	. .	+ +	+ +

Asterisks indicate that IQ was estimated from scores on the Dementia Rating Scale (Coblentz et al., 1973). Absence of deficit on DR or DA is indicated by − −; presence of deficit is indicated by + +; some question of deficit is indicated by (−/+). (The smaller N for group indicates the number of patients with IQ measures.)
OPCA = olivopontocerebellar atrophy.

1964), tests of verbal fluency (Butters et al., 1987), Luria's response inhibition go–no-go test (Luria, 1980), and the Stroop color-word interference test (in which subjects must respond to color words written in assorted colors; Stroop, 1935). Although the Wisconsin Card Sorting Test is considered to be among the best markers of frontal lobe disease in humans (Damasio, 1979; Kolb and Whishaw, 1985; Lezak, 1983; Weinberger et al., 1986), poor performance on any of these tests usually reflects abnormal perseverative responding (Lezak, 1983). Unless otherwise detailed, it can be assumed that all of the groups to be discussed have demonstrated clinical evidence of frontal pathology, including poor performance on some or all of the aforementioned tests.

Patients with Bilateral Frontal Lobe Lesions

For over a century, and despite an ever increasing literature on neuropsychologic changes of frontal patients, the *frontal lobe syndrome* has remained somewhat of an enigma. In 1868, the famous case of Phineas Gage was described, and it remains, today, a good example of the salient characteristics of the human prefrontal syndrome. Gage was a reliable foreman of mild temperament who became irresponsible, profane, and easily provoked subsequent to an accident in which an iron bar passed though his frontal lobes; however, his cognitive capacities remained relatively intact. In subsequent reports of human frontal damage, a highly diverse spectrum of *personality* changes has been described, yet only one facet of *cognitive* change has clearly stood out, i.e., abnormal perseverative responding (Lezak, 1983; Lhermitte et al., 1986; Stuss and Benson, 1986; Teuber, 1955; Valenstein, 1980). The abnormality is one of response inhibition, especially marked on tests of problem solving, abstract reasoning, attention, imitation, motor control, and sequencing. It also has been described as an impairment in *executive functioning* (Lezak, 1983; Lhermitte et al., 1986; Stuss and

Benson, 1986). At present, we know of no studies in which neurotransmitter assays have been performed on frontal patients, but based upon results of neurochemical studies of monkey brains, and of normal postmortem human brains, it is likely that at least two transmitter systems will prove to be important: One with special relevance in dorsolateral prefrontal functioning, and one with special relevance in orbitofrontal functioning.

In our work with DR and DA paradigms, performance of patients with bilateral damage to prefrontal cortex served as the prototype for comparisons with all of the other patient groups we studied. They all had intelligence quotients (IQs) within normal range and showed a clinical profile of abnormal perseveration on neuropsychologic testing. Of the six frontal patients we examined, computerized tomography (CT) scans demonstrated predominantly orbitofrontal involvement in four, and two patients had predominantly dorsolateral frontal damage (Freedman and Oscar-Berman, 1986a).

Patients with Alcoholic Korsakoff's Syndrome

Profound anterograde amnésia is the most obvious characteristic of patients with alcoholic Korsakoff's syndrome. In addition, Korsakoff patients exhibit clinical signs associated with bifrontal pathology, including perseverative responding (for reviews: Butters et al., 1987; Moscovitch et al., 1986; and Oscar-Berman, 1980; 1984). Neuropathologic and neuroradiographic evidence reveals cortical atrophy in these patients, with notable prefrontal involvement (N. Butters and T. Jernigan, personal communication; Cala et al., 1978). Atrophy also has been reported in midline diencephalic structures, especially the dorsomedial nucleus of the thalamus, and the mammillary bodies of the hypothalamus (Talland and Waugh, 1969; Victor et al., 1971). The thalamic sites have strong connections with large regions of prefrontal cortex (Warren and Akert, 1964); the hypothalamic connections are primarily from the ventral prefrontal sector (Nauta and Domesick, 1981).

There is a growing body of evidence for cholinergic dysfunction in Korsakoff patients. Cell loss has been reported in the basal forebrain area, particularly the nucleus basalis of Meynert (Arendt et al., 1983), along with reduction in brain cholinergic activity. [The basal forebrain receives projections from various neocortical sites including orbitofrontal—but not dorsolateral prefrontal—cortex (Mesulam et al., 1983).] Also, performance on memory tests has been shown to decline with ingestion of an anticholinergic agent such as scopolamine (Drachman, 1977). In addition to the findings of cholinergic dysfunction in Korsakoff's syndrome, there is evidence implicating catecholaminergic dysfunction in these patients as well (for review: Joyce, 1987). First, the neuropathology associated with Korsakoff's disease frequently involves the site of origin of ascending noradrenergic pathways (Victor et al., 1971). Second, behavioral deficits have been related to reduced brain norepinephrine and dopamine activity in Korsakoff patients (McEntee and Mair, 1978; Mair et al., 1982; 1985). And third, although catecholamine levels in cerebrospinal fluid (CSF) samples from Korsakoff patients are not reduced, memory deficits can be reversed transiently with clonidine (a noradrenergic agonist), and memory can be improved during withdrawal from clonidine therapy (i.e., at the time when noradrenergic activity would be elevated; Martin et al., 1987; McEntee and Mair, 1980). However, improved performance might have been the result of generalized arousal associated with the withdrawal state.

Patients with Anterior Communicating Artery Disease (ACoA)

Anterograde amnesia usually is associated with ACoA (Talland et al., 1967). However, depending upon the extent of damage from a ruptured anterior communicating artery, and the surgical procedure by which it is treated, ACoA patients can have variable degrees of short-term memory loss (Alexander and Freedman, 1984; Gade, 1982; Gade and Mortenson, 1989). Perseverative responding, as measured by performance on the Wisconsin Card Sorting Test, has been found to be as severe in ACoA as it is in patients with bilateral frontal lesions (Freedman and Oscar-Berman, 1986a). The major brain regions implicated in the pathology of this group are the nuclei of the basal forebrain, including the nucleus basalis of Meynert and medial septal sites (Damasio et al., 1985; Gade, 1982; Philips et al., 1987). The nucleus basalis of Meynert projects to various regions including paralimbic and hippocampal sites, while receiving projections directly from orbitofrontal cortex; medial septal sites tend to project to the hippocampus (Mesulam et al., 1983; Mesulam and Mufson, 1984; Olton and Wenk, 1987). At this time, we know of no studies of neurochemical dysfunction in patients with ACoA. Because the lesion involves the basal forebrain, however, cholinergic dysfunction has been suggested (Damasio et al., 1985; Gade and Mortenson, 1989).

Patients with Parkinson's Disease

Movement disturbances accompany Parkinson's disease, whether or not dementia is present. In addition, Parkinson patients frequently exhibit difficulty in initiating tasks and often perform at a slowed rate (Bachman and Albert, 1985). They evidence frontal-like abstract reasoning and perseverative behaviors (for reviews: Agnoli et al., 1984; Bachman and Albert, 1985; Mayeux and Stern, 1982; Ruberg and Agid, 1988; Taylor et al., 1986). Although the primary pathology in Parkinson's disease involves degeneration of neurons in the basal ganglia and substantia nigra, numerous neuropathologic and radiologic studies implicate frontal damage as well (see reviews cited above). Thus, the brains of patients with Parkinson's disease show cortical atrophy with moderate to severe neuronal loss in frontal cortex (Ruberg and Agid, 1988). Interestingly, although prefrontal cortex sends efferent neuronal fibers onto sites in the basal ganglia, there appear to be no corresponding afferent inputs from basal ganglia to prefrontal cortex (Divac and Oberg, 1979).

Catecholaminergic deficits are well documented in Parkinson's disease (Agid et al., 1987; Bachman and Albert, 1985; Brown and Marsden, 1984; Mann and Yates, 1986; Ruberg and Agid, 1988). Striatal dopamine is particularly reduced, and CSF dopamine metabolite levels positively correlate with severity of the disease (Agid et al., 1987). The striatal dopaminergic lesions can result in behavioral changes similar to those observed with prefrontal lesions (see Bachman and Albert, 1985, and Fuster, 1989). Moreover, lesions of mesocortico-limbic dopamine neurons, and noradrenergic lesions of the locus coeruleus may contribute to attentional and memory deficits in Parkinson patients (Ruberg and Agid, 1988). Other neurotransmitters are affected as well, including the cholinergic system. While cholinergic innervation of the striatum is preserved, it is deficient in the hippocampus and cerebral cortex (Ruberg and Agid, 1988). There is controversy about the role of cholinergic dysfunction in the dementia of Parkinson's disease. It has been postulated that cholinergic lesions denervating the hippocampus and cerebral cortex affect memory in a more direct way than the catecholaminergic lesions, or affect a "different mnemonic mechanism" (Ruberg and Agid, 1988, p. 192). However, it is difficult to assess the impact of cholinergic deficits in the dementia of Parkinson's disease for the following reasons: (1) The neurochemical deficits in all brain regions are mild when compared to the striatal dopaminergic deficits; (2) cholinergic innervation of hippocampus is compromised whether or not dementia is present (Ruberg and Agid, 1988); (3) the dementia may not be related to lesions of the cholinergic nucleus basalis of Meynert (Ball, 1984); and (4) although Parkinsonian dementia seems to be a direct function of degree of neocortical cholinergic loss (Agid et al., 1987; Ruberg and Agid, 1988), in olivopontocerebellar atrophy (OPCA) (not associated with severe dementia), cortical cholinergic deficiencies are as profound as those of Alzheimer's disease (Kish et al., 1989). Nonetheless, it may be that at least two subtypes of cognitive impairments exist in Parkinson's disease, one primarily a result of the dopaminergic deafferentation, and one primarily a result of a combination of dopaminergic plus cholinergic deficiencies.

Patients with Alzheimer's Disease

Patients with Alzheimer's disease perform poorly on the standard clinical neuropsychologic tests sensitive to frontal dysfunction (Butters et al., 1987). Numerous studies of neuropathologic changes and neurotransmitter deficiencies in Alzheimer patients have documented extensive cell loss and cholinergic deficits throughout the cerebral cortex, including prefrontal regions (e.g., Hansen et al., 1988). In addition, reviews of the literature on cholinergic changes in Alzheimer's disease have called attention to loss of neurons within the basal forebrain, and its projections to the limbic system (Ball, 1984; Mann and Yates, 1986). As mentioned earlier, basal forebrain nuclei receive projections from orbitofrontal cortex, and thus, degeneration of neurons within the nucleus basalis of Meynert will have an impact especially on orbitofrontal functioning. Finally, there is evidence that some Alzheimer patients have catecholaminergic (dopamine) deficits as well (Mann and Yates, 1986); they are less profound than the cholinergic deficits.

Patients with Olivopontocerebellar Atrophy (OPCA)

The salient characteristic of patients with OPCA is their severe cerebellar ataxia (Schut, 1950). Although cognitive deterioration appears mild by comparison to

the movement disturbance, deficits by OPCA patients on tests of frontal functioning have been reported (El-Awar et al., 1989; Kish et al., 1988). Loss of neurons in the substantia inominata, as well as reduced activity of choline acetyltransferase and acetylcholinesterase, have been documented in this disease (see
Kish et al., 1988; 1989). The reduction in cortical cholinergic activity in OPCA
is as severe as in Alzheimer's disease, but unlike Alzheimer's disease, cholinergic
activity in the amygdala and hippocampus has been found to be either normal
or only mildly reduced (Kish et al., 1988; 1989).

Patients with Huntington's Disease

Huntington's disease is associated with profound atrophy of the caudate nuclei
and putamen, causing uncontrollable choreiform movements. Both of these
basal ganglion structures receive projections from prefrontal sites, and cortical
atrophy accompanies the subcortical degeneration—especially in the frontal and
temporal lobes (Divac and Oberg, 1979; Mann and Yates, 1986; Goldman-
Rakic, 1987). In the late stages of their disease, Huntington patients demonstrate
many of the disinhibited personality changes characteristic of patients with bilateral prefrontal damage, and they also have been shown to perform poorly on
numerous neuropsychologic tests of frontal (and temporal) functioning (Butters
et al., 1987; Fisher et al., 1983; Oscar-Berman, 1984). In addition, although
GABA-ergic deficits are certainly more prominent than cholinergic or catecholaminergic deficits in Huntington's disease, significant losses of choline acetyltransferase activity have been observed in the nucleus accumbens, septal nuclei,
and hippocampus, as well as in striatal sites (Spokes, 1980). Cholinergic deficits
intensify as the disease progresses.

Patients with Broca's Aphasia

The outstanding deficit in Broca's aphasia is a reduction in language production
(e.g., telegraphic speech), although mild comprehension deficits have been
reported as well (Goodglass and Kaplan, 1972; Stuss and Benson, 1986). Historically, the lesion classically associated with Broca's aphasia has been localized
at the foot of the third frontal convolution, unilaterally on the left dorsolateral
surface (Goodglass and Kaplan, 1972). However, there is evidence that the lesion
usually includes insular sites deep to opercular cortex (Mohr et al., 1978). Therefore, both orbitofrontal and dorsolateral regions may be involved in Broca's
aphasia, depending on the degree to which the lesion extends below the classic
Broca's area. Patients with Broca's aphasia typically do not show personality
changes usually associated with bilateral prefrontal pathology, but many do
show cognitive changes characterized by abnormal perseveration (Allison and
Hurwitz, 1967; Sandson and Albert, 1984). In our work with these patients, we
were especially interested in their ability to perform DR and DA tasks, because
their prefrontal lesions are unilateral (and hence, their deficits on DR and DA
were expected to be mild, if at all), and because they do not have normal verbal
mediation ability to help them bridge the gap across delays.
    Although we know of no empirical evidence about neurotransmitter deficits

in patients with circumscribed frontal lesions, including those with Broca's aphasia, the studies reviewed earlier would suggest that abnormalities would be more prominent in the catecholaminergic system than in the cholinergic system in patients with Broca's aphasia (if the lesions are restricted to dorsolateral sites); cholinergic mechanisms (more so than catecholaminergic) would be disrupted in patients with unilateral or bifrontal lesions in the orbitofrontal region. [This assertion is made despite the fact that (1) neurons throughout the cerebral cortex normally and primarily are GABA-ergic and glutaminergic, and (2) cytoarchitectonically distinct frontal areas have relatively uniform, low levels of cholinergic activity (Kish et al., 1989).]

Summary

In summary, neuropsychologic, neuroanatomic, and neurochemical evidence indicate that all of the preceding patient groups share some prefrontal dysfunction. There is overlapping pathology of dorsolateral and ventral systems in the disorders we have reviewed, with the exception of rare patients having bilateral focal prefrontal lesions. Nonetheless, the groups appear to be divided along lines that respect the two prefrontal subdivisions, with some groups more heavily influenced by dorsolateral than by orbitofrontal dysfunction, and other groups more heavily influenced by orbitofrontal than by dorsolateral dysfunction. However, it is important to stress the following caveat: *The dichotomy is one of emphasis, and relies upon quantitatively different degrees of dysfunction, damage, and neurotransmitter deficiencies.* Ventral prefrontal damage and cholinergic dysfunction (where evidence is available) are more prominent in patients with Alzheimer's disease, OPCA, ACoA, Korsakoff's syndrome, and late stage Huntington's disease than the other neurologic conditions we considered. By contrast, dorsolateral damage and catecholaminergic dysfunction (again, where evidence is available) are more prominent in patients with Parkinson's disease, Broca's aphasia (and variably, in patients with Korsakoff's syndrome). Interestingly, in the patient groups we have studied, performance on DR and DA tasks also respects the two prefrontal systems: Relative to other groups, patients with predominantly (but not exclusively) ventral system pathology perform poorly on DA; patients with predominantly (but not exclusively) dorsolateral system pathology perform poorly on DR; and patients with severe damage to both systems perform poorly on both DR and DA (see Table 12–1). Evidence on results of DR and DA testing in the groups now will be considered.

DR AND DA PERFORMANCE BY HUMAN NEUROLOGIC PATIENTS

To review, we have reasoned that if DR performance is closely coupled to the dorsolateral prefrontal cortex in humans, as it seems to be in monkeys, patients with predominantly dorsolateral pathology should evidence deficits on DR tasks. That is, Parkinson patients and, to a lesser extent, patients with Korsakoff's syndrome and, perhaps, Broca's aphasia would be expected to perform poorly on DR. Furthermore, if DA is closely tied to the ventral prefrontal system, patients with predominantly orbitofrontal pathology would be expected to perform poorly on DA problems compared to the other groups. Patients in this category would include those with ACoA, Alzheimer's disease, OPCA, late stage Huntington's disease, and (a subgroup of) Korsakoff's patients. Finally, patients with cortical damage that overspreads the entire prefrontal region would be expected to perform poorly on both tasks. Such patients would include those with Alzheimer's disease and, of course, large bifrontal damage of any etiology.

DR

Results of DR and DA testing on nine neurologic patient groups and two control groups are summarized in Table 12–1. Relative to control subjects, three neurologic groups were significantly impaired on DR problems: Alzheimer patients with dementia (Freedman and Oscar-Berman, 1986b), equally demented Parkinson patients (Freedman and Oscar-Berman, 1986b), and patients with bilateral prefrontal lesions (Freedman and Oscar-Berman, 1986a). Although the patients with frontal lesions and those with Alzheimer's disease did poorly on both DA and DR, it is important to note that Parkinson patients with dementia evidenced no deficit on DA. Interestingly, a group of Parkinson patients without clinical or psychometric evidence of dementia, showed no DR nor DA deficits.

Catecholamine Dysfunction?

Patients with Parkinson's disease suffer profound dopaminergic dysfunction (Hornykiewicz and Kish, 1984). In addition to cell loss in the substantia nigra pars compacta, degeneration of the dopaminergic neurons in the ventral tegmental area has been documented (Ruberg and Agid, 1988). The latter nuclei project directly onto dorsolateral prefrontal cortex, while the former project to the head of the caudate (Carpenter, 1976). The anterodorsal sector of the head of the caudate, in turn, receives direct projections from dorsolateral prefrontal cortex (Johnson et al., 1968). It is noteworthy that within the caudate nucleus in Parkinson patients, it is the anterior portion of the caudate head that undergoes the most severe loss of dopamine concentration (Kish et al., 1986). Thus, a catecholaminergic deficiency resulting from damage to a major part of the dorsolateral prefrontal system appears to be intimately tied to DR deficits in the dementia of Parkinson's disease. In Alzheimer's disease, since prefrontal damage is not restricted to the ventral (cholinergic) system, and since some patients evidence significant dopaminergic deficits (Mann and Yates, 1986), their DR deficits also may be linked to dorsolateral damage. Finally, two of our six patients with bifrontal lesions had predominantly dorsolateral lesions, and therefore dopaminergic dysfunction cannot be ruled out as a factor in the frontals' DR deficits.

    In summary, since deficits on DR are prominent following dorsolateral prefrontal damage, and since catecholaminergic (especially dopaminergic) innervation of dorsolateral prefrontal cortex (Bannon and Roth, 1983; Goldman-Rakic, 1987; Weinberger et al., 1986) appears to be involved in normal performance on delayed reaction tasks (Goldman-Rakic, 1989), we suggest that catecholaminergic dysfunction may be an important underlying component of poor DR performance. Animal studies have shown that deficits on DR occur after lesions within the dorsolateral and the ventral prefrontal systems, but are more prominent after dorsolateral damage (Oscar-Berman, 1975; 1978). Lesions in the head of the caudate (Divac, 1972), the dorsomedial thalamus (Schulman, 1964), and subthalamus (Adey et al., 1962) also are associated with DR deficits. The first two of these structures receive direct projections from dorsolateral prefrontal cortex and dopaminergic projections from midbrain sites (Goldman-Rakic, 1987; Moore, 1982); the subthalamus is intimately connected with the dopaminergic substantia nigra and globus pallidus (Bradford, 1986).

DA

As can be seen in Table 12–1, relative to control subjects, five neurologic groups were significantly impaired on delayed alternation problems: Korsakoff patients (Freedman and Oscar-Berman, 1986a; Oscar-Berman et al., 1982); Alzheimer patients (Freedman and Oscar-Berman, 1986b); patients with OPCA (El-Awar et al., 1989); Huntington patients (Oscar-Berman et al., 1982); and patients with bilateral prefrontal lesions (Freedman and Oscar-Berman, 1986a). In addition, although the impairment demonstrated by ACoA patients was not statistically significant, there was considerable variability in their performance, suggesting that it should not be considered entirely normal. By contrast, patients with Parkinson's disease or Broca's aphasia did not evidence significant deficits on DA relative to controls.

Cholinergic Dysfunction?

Since orbitofrontal cortex is intimately linked to cholinergic basal forebrain nuclei (Javoy-Agid et al., 1989 Mesulam et al., 1983; Olton, 1989), we suggest that cholinergic dysfunction may be an important underlying component of the DA-related cognitive deficits in the patient populations we have tested. Cholinergic dysfunction has been noted in Alzheimer's disease (Price et al., 1982), in Korsakoff's syndrome (Arendt et al., 1983), in OPCA (Kish et al., 1988), and in Huntington's disease (Spokes, 1980). Although to our knowledge cholinergic dysfunction has not yet been reported in patients with ACoA, nor in patients with circumscribed bifrontal lesions, such findings would seem likely for reasons stated earlier. In summary, each of the patient groups with a significant DA deficit also has—or likely has—a clinically significant cholinergic disturbance. Are there parallel findings in nonhuman primates with lesions in cholinergic systems?

As noted in the section, "Neuroanatomical Systems in DA and DR," animal studies have shown that lesions of any of the following brain regions can impair DA performance: Dorsolateral or orbitofrontal cortex, hippocampus (with and without the amygdala), the head of the caudate nucleus, and the hypothalamus. Orbitofrontal cortex and the hippocampus in nonhumans (and humans) have been implicated in other tests requiring spatial skills and normal response inhibition (Damasio, 1979; Goldman-Rakic, 1987; Javoy-Agid et al.,

1989; Kolb and Whishaw, 1985; O'Keefe and Nadel, 1978). Likewise, cholinergic circuits have been implicated in mnemonic spatial processing and response inhibition (Beatty and Troster, 1988; Kopelman, 1986; Olton and Wenk, 1987; Pandya and Yeterian, 1984). The frontal cortex and the hippocampus are densely innervated by cholinergic fibers (Mesulam et al., 1983; Olton and Wenk, 1987). The cholinergic substantia inominata (especially medial septal sites) innervates hippocampus and is interconnected with most limbic regions (Mesulam and Mufson, 1984). In addition, the hippocampal CA fields and fornical efferents are cholinergic (Mesulam, 1988). Although the anterior portion of the head of the caudate receives dopaminergic innervation, there is evidence that its ventrolateral aspect receives cholinergic innervation (Haber, 1986). Cholinergic innervation and activity have been reported for hypothalamic and amygdala sites (Bjorklund et al., 1987; Bradford, 1986). Based on the majority of findings, therefore, it appears that cholinergic forebrain systems may play a role in DA-related functions in nonhuman primates.

Neuropsychologic Functions in DR and DA

We have reviewed considerable evidence to support the view that some aspect(s) of performance on DR tasks is mediated by different neuroanatomic and neurochemical systems than performance on DA tasks. At this point, it appears that the functional differences (derived originally from work with nonhuman primates) have something to do, on the one hand, with visuospatial mnemonic and attentional functions (disrupted by damage in dorsolateral-prefrontal and catecholaminergic systems), and, on the other hand, functions involved in response inhibition (disrupted by damage in orbitofrontal and cholinergic systems). Do clinical neuropsychologic findings in the patient groups we have tested support this view? In other words, do the patient groups with DR impairments also show severe deficits in visuospatial mnemonic and attentional functions, and do the patient groups with DA impairments show abnormal response perseveration? Available evidence suggests that short-term memory is not critical to successful DR performance, but that visuospatial and attentional factors may be. Further, intact inhibitory response mechanisms do appear to be needed for successful DA performance.

DR: Visuospatial, Memory, and Attentional Functions?

The patient groups who performed poorly on DR were those with bilateral prefrontal damage, Alzheimer's or Parkinson's disease, and (to some extent) Korsakoff's syndrome. Parkinson patients with dementia—the group with the most severe DR deficit—are characterized as having frontal-like "coloration (nothing is implied about the severity of the symptoms)" (Ruberg and Agid, 1988, p. 181); they have some visuospatial deficits, but do not show severe anterograde amnesia (Freedman and Albert, 1985; Freedman and Oscar-Berman, 1986c; 1987; Mayeux and Stern, 1982; Ruberg and Agid, 1988). Alzheimer and Korsakoff groups have well-documented visuospatial, memory, and attentional deficits, with short-term memory impairments being most salient (Butters et al., 1987;

Cummings and Benson, 1983; Ellis and Oscar-Berman, 1989; Freedman and Oscar-Berman, 1986c; 1987; Khan, 1986). Patients with bifrontal damage also have visuospatial, memory, and attentional deficits, but these are mild by contrast to Alzheimer and Korsakoff patients (Butters et al., 1987; Ellis and Oscar-Berman, 1989; Khan, 1986; Oscar-Berman, 1980; 1984). Severe anterograde amnesia, however, is characteristic of most ACoA patients (Damasio et al., 1985; Gade, 1982; Moscovitch et al., 1986), who evidence no DR deficit (and variable performance levels on DA). Short-term memory impairments in patients with OPCA or Huntington's disease (who performed poorly on DA only), as well as non-Korsakoff alcoholics (who were unimpaired on DR and DA), have been described, but are not as severe as in Korsakoff's syndrome, ACoA, and Alzheimer's disease (e.g., Butters et al., 1987; Lezak, 1983). Additionally, among the bifrontal patients, we found no relationship between Wechsler Memory Scale scores and impairment on DR (or DA; Freedman and Oscar-Berman, 1986a).

It appears, then, that while the presence of anterograde amnesia does not in itself present a major obstacle to successful performance on DR, the influence of visuospatial abnormalities is possible. Likewise, attentional deficits cannot be ruled out, since they have been demonstrated in Alzheimer, Korsakoff, Huntington, and OPCA patients (see preceding references), and have not been adequately assessed in the other groups. Further, the idea of attentional factors being important in DR is congruent with the neurochemistry of the forebrain: Catecholaminergic systems—most seriously compromised in Parkinson's disease— have been implicated in attentional functions (Clark et al., 1987).

DA: Abnormal Perseverative Responding?

The patient groups with significant DA deficits were those with bifrontal damage, and Alzheimer's, Korsakoff's, OPCA, and Huntington's diseases; several ACoA patients also showed DA deficits. Abnormal perseverative responding is a notable characteristic of patients with bifrontal lesions (Damasio, 1979), Korsakoff's syndrome (Oscar-Berman, 1973; 1980), and Alzheimer's disease (Terry and Katzman, 1983). Kish and his colleagues (Kish et al., 1988; 1989) have reported strong perseverative responding by OPCA patients on several neurobehavioral measures, and several investigators have noted abnormal perseveration in Huntington patients (Butters et al., 1987; Fisher et al., 1983). We found that perseveration on the Wisconsin Card Sorting Test correlated significantly with number of errors on DA and DR by the patients with bifrontal lesions and by those with Korsakoff's syndrome or ACoA (Freedman and Oscar-Berman, 1986a); of the frontal patients, perseveration was especially marked in those with predominantly orbitofrontal lesions (Eslinger and Damasio, 1985; Freedman and Oscar-Berman, 1986a). Stuss and associates (1982) reported a relationship between bilateral orbitofrontal lesions in humans and sensitivity to proactive interference. Further, the idea that the ability to inhibit perseverative responding is important to DA performance is supported by the neurochemistry of the forebrain: Cholinergic systems have been postulated to support response programming and memory functions (Kopelman, 1986; Numan, 1978; Richardson and DeLong, 1986).

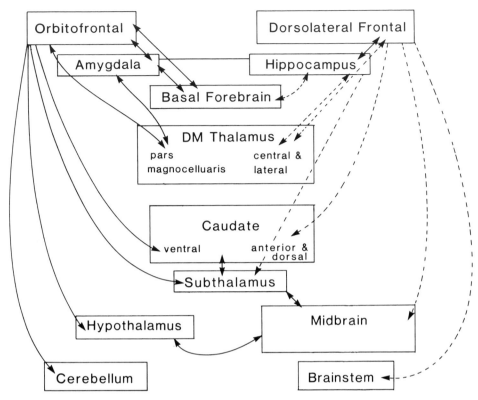

Figure 12-3   Schematic representation of two major prefrontal neuroanatomic systems.

Other Neuropsychologic Functions

In human DR and DA performance, cross-temporal bridging can be mediated by language. The use of language-related strategies, however, is not essential to successful performance on the tasks. This assertion is based mainly upon results with the Broca's aphasics, whose expressive language capacity is minimal, but whose DR and DA performance levels were intact. In addition, DR performance was deficient in Parkinson patients, whose language function is mildly impaired (showing anomia; Cummings and Benson, 1983), but their DA performance was intact.

CONCLUSIONS

We have shown that DR and DA studies in humans can complement those of the nonhuman animal literature. Much can be learned about the nature of the neurologic disturbance in a studied population, and conversely, constraints can be imposed on theories that seek to explain the nature of the brain functions tapped by DR and DA tasks.

The prefrontal cortex in humans and monkeys contains at least two parallel systems: One on the dorsolateral surface, and one located ventrally (Fig. 12-3).

Remarkably, the neurobehavioral, neuroanatomic and neurochemical organization of the prefrontal cortex respects this division. Patients who typically demonstrate predominantly catecholaminergic dysfunction tend to have difficulty with DR tasks; patients who typically demonstrate cholinergic deficits tend to have difficulty with DA tasks; and patients with significant involvement of catecholaminergic as well as cholinergic neurotransmitter systems perform poorly on both DR and DA. Again, it is essential to emphasize that this dichotomy is intended only as a useful way of organizing a vast amount of data derived from an extremely diverse and rapidly growing literature. In describing parallels between human and nonhuman frontal function and structure, we have not considered many alternative tasks sensitive to frontal pathology. We chose DR and DA tasks because of their consistency in eliciting deficits in monkeys and people with bilateral prefrontal lesions. For future studies, we suggest using a simple object reversal procedure (e.g., object alternation) in addition to DR and DA, because object alternation is more selectively sensitive to orbitofrontal dysfunction than DA (Butter, 1969; Freedman, 1990). We also have not considered the role of other neurotransmitter systems important in neurologic disease. Nor have we described interaction effects, interactions among neurotransmitters, and interactions of brain structures/pathways involved with the two major prefrontal systems. We chose to concentrate on catecholaminergic and cholinergic systems because they both preferentially innervate the prefrontal neuroanatomic systems involved in DR and DA; they both have been demonstrated to have relevance for human cognition; and they both have been determined to be directly implicated in the pathology of the diseases we have studied.

ACKNOWLEDGMENTS

Dr. Berman's research was supported by grants from the U.S. Department of Health and Human Services (NIAAA #AA07112, and NINCDS #NS06209), and by funds from the U.S. Department of Veterans Affairs. Dr. Freedman's support came from the Medical Research Council of Canada, the Physicians' Services Incorporated Foundation, the Ontario Mental Health Foundation, and the Gerontology Research Council of Canada. The authors acknowledge the helpful comments of Dr. Stephen J. Kish, Dr. David Gansler, Ms. Susan Lanzoni, and Ms. Jennifer Rautine.

REFERENCES

Adey WR, Walter DO, Lindsley DF. Subthalamic lesions: Effects on learned behavior and correlated hippocampal and subcortical slow-wave activity. Arch Neurol 6:194–207, 1962.

Agid Y, Javoy-Agid F, Ruberg M. Biochemistry of neurotransmitters in Parkinson's disease. *In* Marsden CD, Fahn S (eds), Movement Disorders, Vol 2. New York: Butterworths, 1987, pp. 166–230.

Agnoli A, Ruggieri S, Meco G, Casacchia M, Denaro A, Conti L, Bedini L, Stocchi F, Fioravanti M, Franzese A, Lazzari R. An appraisal of the problem of dementia in Parkinson's disease. *In* Hassler RG, Christ JF (eds), Advances in Neurology, Vol 40: Parkinson-Specific Motor and Mental Disorders. New York: Raven Press, 1984, pp. 299–306.

Alexander M, Freedman M. Amnesia after anterior communicating artery rupture. Neurology 34:752–757, 1984.

Allison RS, Hurwitz LJ. On perseveration in aphasics. Brain 90:429–448, 1967.

Arendt T, Bigl V, Arendt A, Tennestedt A. Loss of neurons in the nucleus basalis of Meynert in Alzheimer's disease, paralysis agitans, and Korsakoff's disease. Acta Neuropathol 61:101–108, 1983.

Arnold MB. Memory and the Brain. London: Lawrence Erlbaum, 1984.

Arnsten AFT, Goldman-Rakic PS. Selective prefrontal cortical projections to the region of the locus coeruleus and raphe nuclei in the Rhesus monkey. Brain Res 306:9–18, 1984.

Bachman DL, Albert ML. The dopaminergic syndromes of dementia. In Pilleri G, Tagliavini F (eds), Cerebral Aging and Degenerative Dementias. Waldau-Bern, Switzerland: Institute of Neuroanatomy, University of Berne, 1985, pp. 91–119.

Ball MJ. The morphological basis of dementia in Parkinson's disease. Can J Neurol Sci 11:180–184, 1984.

Bannon MJ, Roth RH. Pharmacology of mesocortical dopamine neurons. Pharmacol Rev 35:53–68, 1983.

Battig K, Rosvold HE, Mishkin M. Comparison of the effects of frontal and caudate lesions on delayed-response and alternation in monkeys. J Comp Physiol Psychol 53:400–404, 1960.

Beatty WW, Troster AI. Neuropsychology of spatial memory. In Whitaker HA (ed), Contemporary Reviews in Neuropsychology. New York: Springer-Verlag, 1988, pp. 77–108.

Bjorklund A, Hokfelt T, Swanson LW (eds), Handbook of Chemical Neuroanatomy. Vol 5: Integrated Systems of the CNS, Part I. Hypothalamus, Hippocampus, Amygdala, Retina. New York: Elsevier, 1987.

Bradford, HE. Chemical Neurobiology. New York: WH Freeman and Co., 1986.

Brodmann K. Vergleichen Histologische Lokalisation der Grosshirnrinde in Ihren Prinzipien Dargestellt auf Grund des Zellenbaues. Leipzig: Barth, 1909.

Brown RG, Marsden CD. How common is dementia in Parkinson's disease? Lancet 1:1262–1265, 1984.

Brozoski T, Brown RM, Rosvold HE, Goldman PS. Cognitive deficit caused by depletion of dopamine in prefrontal cortex of Rhesus monkey. Science 205:929–931, 1979.

Butter, CM. Perseveration in extinction and in discrimination reversal tasks following selective frontal ablations in Macaca mulatta. Physiol Behav 4:163–171, 1969.

Butters N, Granholm E, Salmon DP, Grant I. Episodic and semantic memory: A comparison of amnesic and demented patients. J Clin Exp Neuropsychol 9:479–497, 1987.

Butters N, Pandya DN, Stein D, Rosen J. A search for the spatial engram within the frontal lobes of monkeys. Acta Neurobiol Experimentalis Warsaw 32:305–329, 1972.

Cala LA, Jones B, Mastaglia FL, Wiley B. Brain atrophy and intellectual impairment in heavy drinkers-a clinical, psychometric and computerized tomography study. Aust NZ J Med 8:147–153, 1978.

Carpenter M. Human Neuroanatomy. Baltimore: William & Wilkins, 1976.

Clark CR, Geffen GM, Geffen LB. Catecholamines and attention I: Animal and clinical studies. Neurosci Biobehav Reviews 11:341–352, 1987.

Coblentz JM, Mattis S, Zingesser LH, Kasoff SS, Wisniewski HM, Katzman R. Presenile dementia: Clinical aspects and evaluation of cerebrospinal fluid dynamics. Arch Neurol 29:299–308, 1973.

Cummings JL, Benson DF. Dementia: A Clinical Approach. Boston: Butterworths, 1983.

Dalsass M, Kiser S, Mendershausen M, German DC. Medial prefrontal cortical projections to the region of the dorsal periventricular catecholamine system. Neuroscience 6:657–65, 1981.

Damasio AR. The frontal lobes. In Heilman KM, Valenstein E (eds), Clinical Neuropsychology. New York: Oxford University Press, 1979, pp. 360–412.

Damasio AR, Graff-Radford NR, Eslinger PJ, Damasio H, Kassell N. Amnesia following basal forebrain lesions. Arch Neurol 3:263–271, 1985.

Divac I. Neostriatum and functions of the frontal cortex. Acta Neurobiol Experimentalis Warsaw 32:461–478, 1972.

Divac I, Oberg RGE. Current conceptions of neostriatal functions: History, and an evaluation. In Divac I, Oberg RGE (eds), The Neostriatum. New York: Pergamon Press, 1979, pp. 215–230.

Drachman DA. Memory and cognitive function in man: Does the cholinergic system have a specific role? Neurology 27:783–790, 1977.

El-Awar M, Kish S, Oscar-Berman M, Robitaille Y, Schut L, Freedman M. Selective delayed alternation deficits in dominantly-inherited olivopontocerebellar atrophy. Brain and Cognition, 1991.

Ellis RJ, Oscar-Berman, M. Alcoholism, aging, and functional hemispheric asymmetries. Psychol Bull 106:128–147, 1989.

Eslinger PJ, Damasio AR. Severe disturbance of higher cognition after bilateral frontal lobe ablation: Patient EVR. Neurology 35:1731–1741, 1985.

Fisher JM, Kennedy JL, Caine ED, Shoulson I. Dementia in Huntington's disease: A cross sectional analysis of intellectual decline. Advances in Neurology. Vol 38: The Dementias. New York: Raven, 1983, pp. 229–238.

Foote SL, Morrison JH. Extrathalamic modulation of cortical function. Ann Rev Neurosci 10:67–95, 1986.

Freedman M. Object alternation and orbitofrontal system dysfunction in Alzheimer's and Parkinson's disease. Brain and Cognition 14:134–143, 1990..

Freedman M, Albert ML. Subcortical dementia. In Frederiks JAM (ed), The Handbook of Clinical Neurology, Vol 2, 46: Neurobehavioral Disorders. New York: Elsevier Science, 1985, pp. 311–316.

Freedman M, Oscar-Berman M. Bilateral frontal lobe disease and selective delayed-response deficits in humans. Behav Neurosci 100:337–342, 1986a.

Freedman M, Oscar-Berman M. Selective delayed response deficits in Parkinson's and Alzheimer's disease. Arch Neurol 43:886–890, 1986b.

Freedman M, Oscar-Berman M. Comparative neuropsychology of cortical and subcortical dementia. Can J Neurol Sci 13:410–414, 1986c.

Freedman M, Oscar-Berman M. Tactile discrimination learning deficits in Alzheimer's and Parkinson's diseases. Arch Neurol 44:394–398, 1987.

French GM. The frontal lobes and association. In Warren JM, Akert, K (eds), The Frontal Granular Cortex and Behavior. New York: McGraw-Hill, 1964, pp. 56–73.

Fuster JM. The Prefrontal Cortex. New York: Raven Press, 1989.

Gade A. Amnesia after operations on aneurysms of the anterior communicating artery. Surg Neurol 18:46–49, 1982.

Gade A, Mortenson EL. Temporal gradient in the remote memory impairment of amnesic patients with lesions in the basal forebrain. Unpublished manuscript, 1989.

Goldman-Rakic PS. Circuitry of primate prefrontal cortex and regulation of behavior by representational memory. In Plum F (ed), Handbook of Physiology: The Nervous System. Vol 5. Bethesda: American Physiological Society, 1987, pp. 373–417.

Goldman-Rakic PS. Memory functions of prefrontal cortex and their relevance to dementia. Paper presented at the first annual meeting of the Memory Disorders Research Society, Boston, MA, October, 1989.

Goodglass H, Kaplan E. The Assessment of Aphasia and Related Disorders. Philadelphia: Lea & Febiger, 1972.

Haber SN. Neurotransmitters in the human and nonhuman primate basal ganglia. Hum Neurobiol 5:159–68, 1986.

Hansen LA, DeTeresa R, Davies P, Terry RD. Neocortical morphometry, lesion counts and choline acetyltransferase levels in the age spectrum of Alzheimer's disease. Neurology 38:48–54, 1988.

Heaton RK. Wisconsin Card Sorting Test Manual. Odessa, FL: Psychological Assessment Resources, 1981.

Hornykiewicz O, Kish SJ. Neurochemical basis of dementia in Parkinson's disease. Can J Neurol Sci 11:185–190, 1984.

Hunter WS. The delayed reaction in animals and children. Behav Monogr 2:1–86, 1913.

Isseroff A, Rosvold HE, Galkin TW, Goldman-Rakic P. Spatial memory impairments following damage to the mediodorsal nucleus of the thalamus in Rhesus monkeys. Brain Res 232:97–113, 1982.

Jacobsen CF. Studies of cerebral function in primates. Comp Psychol Monogr 13:1–68, 1936.

Javoy-Agid F, Scatton B, Ruberg M, L'Heureux R, Cervera P, Raisman R, Matloteaux J-M, Beck H, Agid Y. Distribution of monoaminergic, cholinergic, and GABAergic markers in the human cerebral cortex. Neuroscience 39:251–259, 1989.

Johnson TN, Rosvold HE, Mishkin M. Projections of behaviorally defined sectors of the prefrontal cortex to the basal ganglia, septum and diencephalon of the monkey. Exp Neurol 21:20–34, 1968.

Joyce EM. The neurochemistry of Korsakoff's syndrome. *In* Stahl SM, Iversen SD, Goodman EC (eds), Cognitive Neurochemistry. Oxford: Oxford University Press, 1987, pp. 327–345.

Khan AU. Clinical Disorders of Memory. New York: Plenum Medical Book Co, 1986.

Kish SJ, El-Awar M, Schut L, Leach L, Oscar-Berman M, Freedman M. Cognitive deficits in olivopontocerebellar atrophy: Implications for the cholinergic hypothesis of Alzheimer's dementia. Ann Neurol 24:200–206, 1988.

Kish SJ, Rajput A, Gilbert J, Rozdilsky B, Chang LY, Shannak K, Hornykiewicz O. Elevated α-aminobutyric acid level in striatal but not extrastriatal brain regions in Parkinson's disease: Correlation with striatal dopamine loss. Ann Neurol 20:26–31, 1986.

Kish SJ, Robitaille Y, El-Awar M, Deck JHN, Simmons J, Schut L, Chang LY, DiStephano L, Freedman M. Non-Alzheimer type pattern of brain choline acetyltransferase reduction in dominantly inherited olivopontocerebellar atrophy. Ann Neurol 22:362–367, 1989.

Kolb B, Whishaw IQ. Fundamentals of Human Neuropsychology, 2nd Edition. New York: WH Freeman, 1985.

Kopelman MD. The cholinergic neurotransmitter system in human memory and dementia: A review. Q J Exp Psychol 38A:535–573, 1986.

Lezak MD. Neuropsychological Assessment, 2nd Edition. New York: Oxford University Press, 1983.

Lhermitte F, Pillon B, Serdaru M. Human autonomy and the frontal lobes. I: Imitation and utilization behavior: A neuropsychological study of 75 patients. Ann Neurol 19:326–334, 1986.

Luria AR. Higher Cortical Functions in Man, 2nd Edition. New York: Basic Books, 1980.

Mahut H. Spatial and object reversal learning in monkeys with partial temporal lobe ablations. Neuropsychologia 9:409–424, 1971.

Mahut H, Cordeau JP. Spatial reversal deficit in monkeys with amygdalo-hippocampal ablations. Exp Neurol 7:426–434, 1963.

Mair RG, McEntee WJ, Zatorre RJ. Brain norepinephrine and dopamine activity: Correlation with specific behavioral deficits in Korsakoff's psychosis. Neurology 32:66–67, 1982.

Mair RG, McEntee WJ, Zatorre RJ. Monoamine activity correlates with psychometric deficits in Korsakoff's disease. Behav Brain Res 15:247–254, 1985.

Mann DMN, Yates PO. Neurotransmitter deficits in Alzheimer's disease and in other dementing disorders. Hum Neurobiol 5:147–158, 1986.

Markowitsch HJ. Anatomical and functional organization of the primate prefrontal cortical system. In Steklis HD, Erwin J (eds), Comparative Primate Biology, Vol 4: Neurosciences. New York: Alan R Liss, 1988, pp. 99–153.

Martin PR, Weingartner H, Gordon EK, Burns RS, Linnoila M, Kopin IJ, Ebert MH. Central nervous system catecholamine metabolsim in Korsakoff's psychosis. Ann Neurol 15:184–187, 1987.

Martinez JL. Endogenous modulators of learning and memory. In Cooper ST (ed), Theory in Psychopharmacology, Vol 2. New York: Academic Press, 1983, pp. 48–74.

Mayeux R, Stern Y. Intellectual dysfunction and dementia in Parkinson's disease. In Mayeux R, Rosen WG (eds), The Dementias. New York: Raven Press, 1982, pp 211–227.

McEntee WJ, Mair RG. Memory impairment in Korsakoff's psychosis: A correlation with brain noradrenergic activity. Science 202:905–907, 1978.

McEntee WJ, Mair RG. Memory enhancement in Korsakoff's psychosis by clonidine: Further evidence for a noradrenergic deficit. Ann Neurol 7:466–470, 1980.

Mesulam M-M. Central cholinergic pathways: Neuroanatomy and some behavioral implications. In Avoli M, Reader TA, Dykes RW, Gloor P (eds), Neurotransmitters and Cortical Function, From Molecules to Mind. New York: Plenum, 1988, pp. 237–260.

Mesulam M-M, Mufson EJ. Neural inputs into the nucleus basalis of the substantia innominata (CH4) in the Rhesus monkey. Brain 107:253–274, 1984.

Mesulam M-M, Mufson EJ, Levey AI, Wainer BH. Cholinergic innervation of cortex by the basal forebrain: Cytochemistry and cortical connections of the septal area, diagonal band nuclei, nucleus basalis (substantia innominata) and hypothalamus in the Rhesus monkey. J Comp Neurol 214:170–197, 1983.

Mesulam M-M, Volicer L, Marquis JK, Mufson EJ, Green C. Systematic regional differences in the cholinergic innervation of the primate cerebral cortex: Distribution of enzyme activities and some behavioral implications. Ann Neurol 19:144–151, 1986.

Milner B. Effects of different brain lesions on card sorting: The role of the frontal lobes. Arch Neurol 9:90–100, 1963.

Milner B. Some effects of frontal lobectomy in man. In Warren JM, Akert K (eds), The Frontal Granular Cortex and Behavior. New York: McGraw-Hill, 1964, pp. 313–334.

Mishkin M. Perseveration of central sets after frontal lesions in monkeys. In Warren JM, Akert K (eds), The Frontal Granular Cortex and Behavior. New York: McGraw-Hill, 1964, pp. 219–241.

Mishkin M, Pribram KH. Analyses of the effects of frontal lesions in monkey: II. Variations of delayed response. J Comp Physiol Psychol 49:36–40, 1956.

Mitchell G, Erwin J (eds). Comparative Primate Biology. Vol 2, Part B, Behavior, Cognition, and Motivation. New York: Alan R Liss, 1987.

Mohr JP, Pessin MS, Finkelstein S, Funkenstein HH, Duncan GW, Davis KR. Broca: aphasia, pathologic and clinical. Neurology 28:311–324, 1978.

Moore RY. Catecholamine neuron systems in brain. Ann Neurol 12:321–327, 1982.

Moscovitch M, Winocur G, McLachlan D. Memory as assessed by recognition and reading time in normal and memory-impaired people with Alzheimer's disease and other neurological disorders. J Exp Psychol [Gen] 115:331–347, 1986.

Nauta WJH, Domesick VB. Neural associations of the limbic system. *In* Beckman AL (ed), The Neural Basis of Behavior. Jamaica, NY: Spectrum, 1981.

Numan R. Cortical-limbic mechanisms and response control: A theoretical review. Physiol Psychol 6:445–470, 1978.

O'Keefe J, Nadel L. The Hippocampus as a Cognitive Map. New York: Clarendon Press, 1978.

Olton DS. Frontal cortex timing and memory. Neuropsychologia 27:121–130, 1989.

Olton DS, Wenk GL. Dementia: Animal models of the cognitive impairments produced by degeneration of the basal forebrain cholinergic system. *In* Meltzer HY (ed), Psychopharmacology: The Third Generation of Progress. New York: Raven Press, 1987, pp. 941–953.

Oscar-Berman M. Hypothesis testing and focusing behavior during concept formation by amnesic Korsakoff patients. Neuropsychologia 11:191–198, 1973.

Oscar-Berman M. The effects of dorsolateral-frontal and ventrolateral-orbitofrontal lesions on spatial discrimination learning and delayed response in two modalities. Neuropsychologia 13:237–246, 1975.

Oscar-Berman M. The effects of dorsolateral-frontal and ventrolateral-orbitofrontal lesions on nonspatial test performance. Neuropsychologia 16:259–267, 1978.

Oscar-Berman M. Neuropsychological consequences of long-term chronic alcoholism. Am Sci 68:410–419, 1980.

Oscar-Berman M. Comparative neuropsychology and alcoholic Korsakoff's disease. *In* Squire L, Butters N (eds), Neuropsychology of Memory. New York: Guilford Press, 1984, pp. 194–202.

Oscar-Berman M, Zola-Morgan SM, Oberg RGE, Bonner RT, Comparative neuropsychology and Korsakoff's syndrome III: Delayed response, delayed alternation and DRL performance. Neuropsychologia 20:187–202, 1982.

Pandya DN, Barnes CL. Architecture and connections of the frontal lobe. *In* Perecman E (ed), The Frontal Lobes Revisited. New York: IRBN Press, 1987, pp. 41–72.

Pandya DN, Yeterian EH. Proposed neural circuitry for spatial memory in the primate brain. Neuropsychologia 22:109–122, 1984.

Passingham R. Delayed matching after selective prefrontal lesions in monkeys (Macaca mulatta). Brain Res 92:89–102, 1975.

Philips S, Sangalang V, Stearns G. Basal forebrain infarction. A clinicopathologic correlation. Arch Neurol 44:1134–1138, 1987.

Pribram KH. The primate frontal cortex: Executive of the brain. *In* Pribram KH, Luria AR (eds), Psychophysiology of the Frontal Lobes. New York: Academic Press, 1973, pp. 293–314.

Pribram KH. The subdivisions of the frontal cortex revisited. *In* Perecman E (ed), The Frontal Lobes Revisited. New York: IRBN Press, 1987, pp 11–40.

Pribram KH, Tubbs WE. Short-term memory, parsing and the primate frontal cortex. Science 156:1765–1767, 1967.

Pribram KH, Wilson WA, Connors J. Effects of lesions of the medial forebrain on alternation behavior of Rhesus monkeys. Exp Neurol 6:36–47, 1962.

Price DL, Whitehouse PJ, Struble RG, Clark AW, Coyle JT, DeLong MR, Hedreen JC. Basal forebrain cholinergic systems in Alzheimer's disease and related dementias. Neurosci Commentaries 1:84–92, 1982.

Richardson RT, DeLong MR. Nucleus basalis of Meynert neuronal activity during a delayed response task in monkey. Brain Res 399:364–368, 1986.

Rosenkilde CE. Functional heterogeneity of the prefrontal cortex in the monkey. A review. Behav Neural Biol 25:301–345, 1979.

Rosvold HE. The frontal lobe system: Cortical-subcortical interrelationships. Acta Neurobiol Exp Warsaw 32:439–460, 1972.

Rosvold HE, Szwarcbart MK. Neural structures involved in delayed-response performance. *In* Warren JM, Akert K (eds), The Frontal Granular Cortex and Behavior. New York: McGraw-Hill, 1964, pp. 1–15.

Ruberg M, Agid Y. Dementia in Parkinson's disease. *In* Iversen LL, Iversen SD, Snyder SH (eds), Handbook of Psychopharmacology. Vol 20. Psychopharmacology of the Aging Nervous System. New York: Plenum, 1988, pp. 157–206.

Sandson J, Albert ML. Varieties of perseveration. Neuropsychologia 22:715–732, 1984.

Schulman S. Impaired delayed response from thalamic lesions. Arch Neurol 11:477–499, 1964.

Schut JW. Hereditary ataxia: Clinical study through six generations. Arch Neurol Psychiatry 168:75–95, 1950.

Spokes EGS. Neurochemical alterations in Huntington's chorea: A study of post mortem brain tissue. Brain 103:179–210, 1980.

Stamm JF. The riddle of the monkey's delayed-response deficit has been solved. *In* Perecman E (ed), The Frontal Lobes Revisited. New York: IRBN Press, 1987, pp. 73–89.

Steklis HD, Erwin J (eds), Comparative Primate Biology. Vol 4: Neurosciences. New York: Alan R Liss Inc, 1988.

Stroop JR. Studies of interference in serial verbal reactions. J Exp Psychol 18:643–662, 1935.

Stuss DT, Benson DF. The Frontal Lobes. New York: Raven Press, 1986.

Stuss DT, Kaplan E, Benson DF, Weir WS, Chiulli S, Sarazin FF. Evidence for the involvement of orbitalfrontal cortex in memory functions: An interference effect. J Comp Physiol Psychol 96:913–925, 1982.

Talland GA, Sweet W, Ballantine T. Amnesic syndrome with anterior communicating artery aneurysm. J Nerv Ment Dis 145:179–192, 1967.

Talland GA, Waugh NC (eds). The Pathology of Memory. New York: Academic Press, 1969.

Taylor AE, Saint-Cyr JA, Lang AE. Frontal lobe dysfunction in Parkinson's disease: The cortical focus of neostriatal outflow. Brain 109:845–883, 1986.

Terry RD, Katzman R. Senile dementia of the Alzheimer type. Ann Neurol 14:497–506, 1983.

Teuber HL. Physiological psychology. Annual Review of Psychology. Palo Alto: Annual Reviews Inc, 1955, pp. 267–296.

Valenstein ES (ed). The Psychosurgery Debate. Scientific, Legal, and Ethical Perspectives. San Francisco: WH Freeman & Co, 1980.

Victor M, Adams RD, Collins GH. The Wernicke-Korsakoff Syndrome. Philadelphia: Davis, 1971.

Walker AE. A cytoarchitectural study of the prefrontal area of the macaque monkey. J Comp Neurol 73:59–86, 1940.

Warren JM, Akert K (eds). The Frontal Granular Cortex and Behavior. New York: McGraw-Hill, 1964.

Weinberger DR, Berman KF, Zec RF. Physiological dysfunction of dorsolateral prefrontal cortex in schizophrenia. I: Regional cerebral blood flow (rCBF) evidence. Arch Gen Psychiatry 43:114–125, 1986.

Wilson WA Jr. Alternation in normal and frontal monkeys as a function of response and outcome of the previous trial. J Comp Physiol Psychol 55:701–704, 1962.

13

Learning Impairments Following Excisions of the Primate Frontal Cortex

MICHAEL PETRIDES

This chapter will review a series of studies demonstrating that the human frontal cortex plays a major role in the learning of conditional associative tasks (Petrides, 1985a; 1990). In such tasks, the subjects are faced with a situation in which there are various possible responses that can be performed on any given trial, but each one of these responses is correct only when it is performed in the presence of the appropriate sensory signal. The signals and the responses bear no relationship to one another, and, thus, to master such a task, the subjects have to learn the particular responses that must be performed in the presence of the different cues.

In the studies described here, the performance of patients with frontal lobe excisions on conditional tasks was compared with that of patients with unilateral temporal lobectomies, as well as that of unoperated normal control subjects. As can be seen in Figures 13–1 and 13–2, the extent and precise locus of the frontal excisions varied from case to case. In all cases, however, the motor cortex on the precentral gyrus was spared, and when the operation was carried out in the left hemisphere, the speech area of Broca was never removed. The temporal lobectomies always included the anterior temporal neocortex and the amygdaloid nucleus and, in some cases, extended posteriorly along the mesial temporal lobe to involve an extensive part of the hippocampus or parahippocampal gyrus (Fig. 13–3).

Excisions of the frontal cortex, such as those illustrated in Figures 13–1 and 13–2, do not cause any obvious motor or sensory defects and they do not impair performance on conventional intelligence tests and various perceptual, linguistic, and memory tasks that have proven to be sensitive indicators of posterior cortical or mesial temporal lobe lesions (Milner, 1971; 1975). Many of these patients, however, show poor adjustment to everyday life, often exhibiting poor regulation of behavior by various environmental signals. It is conceivable that at least one aspect of their poor social adjustment may originate from a more fundamental impairment in their ability to retrieve, in a situation where there are

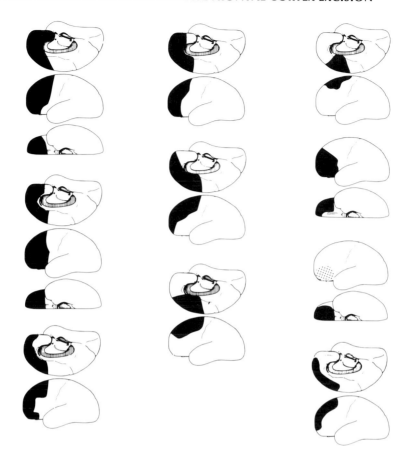

Figure 13–1 Representative cases with cortical excisions from the left frontal lobe. These diagrams are based on the surgeon's drawing at the time of operation.

many competing responses, the particular ones being signaled by different sensory cues. A number of conditional tasks were developed and used to investigate performance of patients with frontal cortical lesions in situations requiring selection between alternative responses on the basis of arbitrary sensory signals. Some of these studies will be described below.

SPATIAL CONDITIONAL RESPONSES

In one of the early conditional tasks that were developed for work with patients, the subjects were required to point to different spatial locations in response to the presentation of visual stimuli (Petrides, 1985a, Experiment 1). In this task, the subjects were seated in front of a table on which there were six white cards forming a horizontal row, and six blue lamps placed behind the response cards in an irregular but constant arrangement (Fig. 13–4).

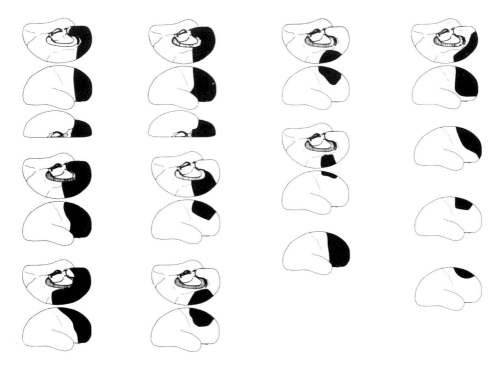

Figure 13–2 Representative cases with cortical excisions from the right frontal lobe.

Figure 13–3 Diagrams showing the lateral extent of cortical excisions in three left and three right temporal lobe cases.

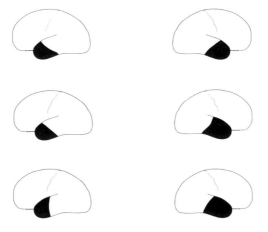

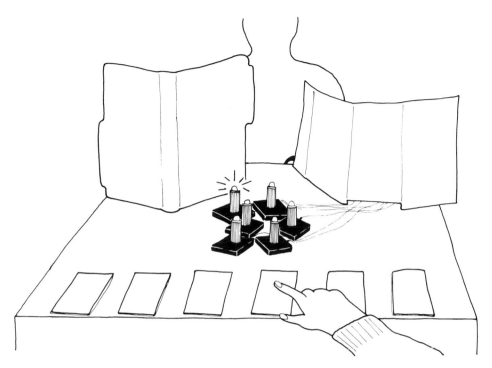

Figure 13-4 Schematic drawing of the experimental arrangement in the spatial conditional task.

The subjects were told that each card was correct for one, and only one, of the six blue lamps and that they would have to learn to point to the correct card when a given blue lamp was lit. On each testing trial, one of the lamps was lit and the subjects had to respond by touching one of the cards. If they touched the correct card, they were told that their response was correct and the lamp was turned off. If they touched an incorrect card, they were told that their response was wrong, and had to point to other cards until they discovered the correct one. After a correct response, the lamp was turned off and the next trial was initiated by turning on another lamp. Testing was terminated when the subjects reached the learning criterion, which was defined as 18 consecutive correct responses, or when a maximum of 180 trials were administered.

Patients with either left or right frontal cortical excisions were severely impaired in learning this task, many of these patients failed to reach criterion within the limits of testing (Fig. 13–5). By contrast, patients with left temporal lobe excisions and patients with right temporal lobe excisions *without* extensive damage to the hippocampus performed as well as the normal control subjects on this task. However, when the right temporal lobe excisions included additional extensive damage to the hippocampal system, impairments on this task emerged.

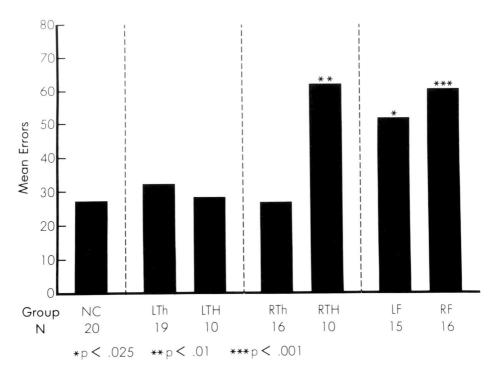

Figure 13-5 Mean error scores for the various groups on the spatial conditional task. NC, normal control group; LTh, left temporal lobe group with little hippocampal involvement; LTH, left temporal lobe group with extensive hippocampal involvement; RTh, right temporal lobe group with little hippocampal involvement; RTH, right temporal lobe group with extensive hippocampal involvement; LF, left frontal lobe group; RF, right frontal lobe group.

These findings demonstrated a striking impairment in the learning of a conditional task in patients with unilateral frontal cortical damage. In addition, the fact that patients with right temporal lobe excisions with extensive damage of the hippocampus were also impaired points to the importance of the functional interaction between the frontal neocortex and the limbic regions within the right temporal lobe for the learning of this task. There is considerable evidence that limbic areas within the mesial temporal lobe are critical for learning and memory (Milner, 1972; Mishkin, 1982) and that, in the human brain, the right hippocampal system is particularly involved in spatial learning and memory (Corkin, 1965; Smith and Milner, 1981).

NONSPATIAL CONDITIONAL RESPONSES: HAND POSTURES

The study just described raised the question of whether the severe impairment that was observed after frontal lobe lesions on the spatial conditional task was a reflection of a more general impairment in this type of learning involving other

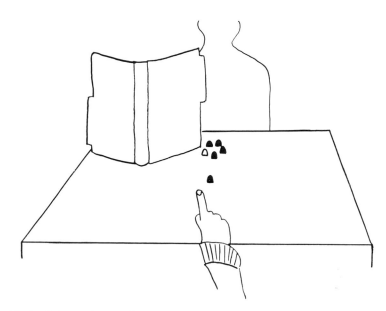

Figure 13–6   Schematic drawing of the experimental arrangement in the conditional task involving hand postures.

kinds of responses. This question was addressed in another study in which the patients had to master a conditional task requiring the performance of different hand postures (Petrides, 1985a, Experiment 2). In this task, the subjects were first taught six hand postures and, when they had learned these postures, testing on the conditional task was initiated. Six different colored stimuli were placed on the table in front of the subjects, who were told that each one of these stimuli would be the cue for the performance of a specific hand posture (Fig. 13–6). Testing proceeded as follows. On each trial, one of the colored stimuli was placed in front of the others and the subjects had to respond by producing the hand posture that they thought was correct for that stimulus. After each response, the experimenter told the subjects whether they were correct or not. If an incorrect response was made, the subjects had to try one of the other hand postures until they found the correct one. When the correct response was produced, the trial was terminated by replacing that stimulus among the others. The relative position of the stimuli was then changed, and the next trial was administered. As can be seen in Figure 13–7, patients with either left or right frontal lobe excisions were again severely impaired, whereas patients with temporal lobe excisions were not, except for the patients with left temporal lobe lesions including extensive damage to the hippocampal region.

These findings clearly demonstrated that the frontal neocortex is critical for conditional learning and that its contribution appears to be a general one involving the learning of different types of conditional responses. It must be emphasized at this point that the impairment observed in the patients with frontal lobe lesions was *not* secondary to difficulties in discriminating between the stimuli or

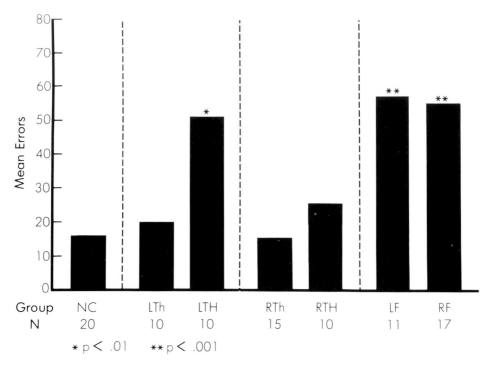

Figure 13-7   Mean error scores for the various groups on the conditional task involving hand postures. The abbreviations are the same as those used in Figure 13-5.

in performing the different responses. For instance, these patients had learned the six hand postures before testing began and could readily name the color of each stimulus. In addition, on each trial if the subject had made an error by producing an incorrect response to the particular stimulus presented, he had to make the other postures until he found the correct one before going on to the next trial. Thus, throughout the testing session it was evident that the subject knew and could perform from memory the various responses but was not able to learn the correct postures for the different stimuli.

As was the case for the spatial conditional task, learning of the present task also required significant functional interaction between the frontal neocortex and the limbic regions within the mesial temporal lobe. In this case, however, the left hippocampal region was the critical one. This region is known to play a major role in verbal learning and memory (Milner, 1971), and its involvement in the present conditional task may have resulted from the tendency of many subjects to verbalize the associations between the hand postures and the colored stimuli. It may, on the other hand, reflect a more primary contribution of the left hippocampal region in the learning of certain motor tasks, in agreement with the notion that certain aspects of motor control may depend more on the left hemisphere (see DeRenzi et al., 1980; Geschwind, 1967; Kimura and Archibald, 1974).

NONSPATIAL CONDITIONAL LEARNING: ABSTRACT DESIGNS

In the two tasks already described, the responses that the subjects had been required to perform were distinct movements, i.e., making different hand postures or pointing to various positions. Work with nonhuman primates, however, demonstrated that excisions of posterior dorsolateral frontal cortex can impair performance on a conditional task that requires selection between responses that need not be distinct movements. Monkeys with such lesions were shown to be markedly impaired on a conditional task in which they had to respond by choosing the appropriate one of two visually distinct boxes that varied randomly in position from trial to trial (Petrides, 1985b). Since the boxes did not occupy a constant position, the required responses were to select the appropriate visual stimulus rather than to point to a distinct location.

To explore the possibility that just as in nonhuman primates the impairment on conditional tasks in patients with frontal lobe lesions is a more general one and not restricted to tasks involving the performance of distinct movements, a new task was developed and administered to the patients. When particular colored stimuli were presented, the subjects had to respond by selecting, from a set of six abstract designs, the correct one for the stimulus shown. The subjects sat at a table on which there was a stack of cards, each one having the same six designs printed on it but with the position of these designs varying randomly from card to card. On the table, there also were six different colored stimuli, and a trial was initiated when the experimenter placed one of these in front of the others (Fig. 13–8). The subjects responded by pointing to one of the designs that were printed on the top card. After their response, they were told whether they had pointed to the correct design or not. If an incorrect response was made, the subjects had to point to other designs until they found the correct one. The colored stimulus for that trial was then placed among the others, the subjects turned over to the next card and a new trial was initiated when another stimulus was presented by the experimenter. As in the other conditional tasks with patients, testing continued until the subjects reached criterion or 180 trials had been administered.

As can be seen in Figure 13–9, patients with either left or right frontal lobe excisions were significantly impaired in learning this task in contrast to patients with left or right temporal lobe excisions who performed as well as the normal control subjects. These findings extend the earlier work with patients by demonstrating that the role of the human frontal cortex in conditional learning is not limited to situations requiring distinct movements but is a more general one involving the control of a variety of responses. Since the position of the designs that the subjects had to select in the present task varied randomly on different trials, the correct responses were neither directed toward particular points in space nor were they distinct hand postures, but rather responses that could be defined only in terms of the goal that had to be achieved, (e.g., select design X).

The deficit observed on the present task in patients with excisions from the frontal cortex cannot be due to difficulties in discriminating between the colored stimuli and the different abstract designs or in scanning the display of six designs

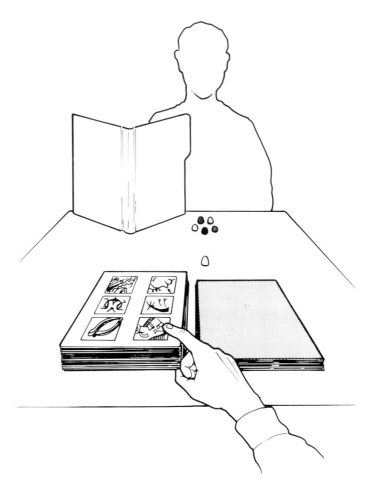

Figure 13-8 Schematic drawing of the experimental arrangement in the conditional task involving abstract designs.

in order to locate a particular one. Before testing on the conditional task had begun, the experimenter helped the subjects familiarize themselves with the designs by pointing to one of the designs on the top card and the subjects had to turn over to the next card and locate, within the new arrangement, the design that the experimenter had touched. Patients with frontal lesions could readily name the different colored stimuli and could identify any design from among the set of six designs. Thus, on the conditional task these patients exhibited a specific impairment in learning to select designs conditional upon the presentation of different visual cues.

Patients with temporal lobe excisions with or without extensive damage to the hippocampal complex were not impaired. By contrast, on the earlier tasks, patients with temporal lobectomies including removal of extensive parts of the hippocampal complex exhibited impairments that varied with the side of the excision. Extensive damage of the right hippocampal region impaired acquisi-

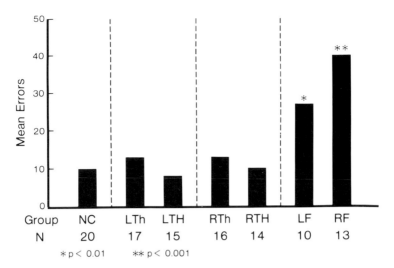

Figure 13-9   Mean error scores for the various groups on the conditional task involving abstract designs. The abbreviations are the same as those used in Figure 13-5.

tion of the conditional task with spatial responses, whereas left hippocampal damage resulted in a deficit on the task involving different hand postures. The lack of impairment on the present conditional task emphasizes the importance of the material to be learned for demonstrating impairments after unilateral hippocampal damage. The abstract designs used in this task had previously been used in the context of another memory task. The results of that study indicated that this material is processed primarily by neural mechanisms within the right hemisphere (Petrides and Milner, 1982).In the present study, the use of colored stimuli, which the subjects could readily encode in verbal terms, in combination with the abstract designs, may have resulted in a task that did not depend *primarily* on either the left or right mesial temporal lobe structures for its processing. Thus, *unilateral* excisions of mesial temporal lobe structures may not have been sufficient to impair performance on this task.

Studies with Nonhuman Primates

The frontal cortex constitutes a very large and structurally heterogeneous region of the primate cerebral cortex. It encompasses many different cytoarchitectonic areas that have their own unique connections with other cortical areas, as well as with a great number of subcortical neural structures (Barbas and Mesulam, 1981; 1985; Barbas and Pandya, 1989; Pandya and Yeterian, 1985; Petrides and Pandya, 1984; 1988). The anatomic evidence, therefore, suggests the existence of a number of relatively distinct functional subsystems within the frontal cortex, a hypothesis that is also supported by investigations of the behavioral effects of excisions restricted to specific parts of the frontal cortex (see Fuster, 1980).

In investigations with patients, it is extremely difficult to identify the critical areas of the frontal cortex that are involved in particular cognitive processes,

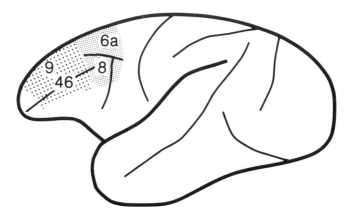

Figure 13-10 Schematic diagram of the lateral surface of the brain of the monkey, showing the posterior region of the dorsolateral frontal cortex, i.e., the periarcuate cortex (area 8 and rostral area 6) and the midlateral frontal cortex within and dorsal to the sulcus principalis (area 46 and area 9).

because the therapeutic excisions are rarely confined to distinct cytoarchitectonic areas. To overcome this problem, a series of studies with nonhuman primates were conducted, to establish the critical region within the dorsolateral frontal cortex for the learning and performance of conditional tasks. This work demonstrated that the periarcuate region of the dorsolateral frontal cortex (i.e., cytoarchitectonic area 8 and rostral area 6) constitutes a major component of a neural circuit necessary for the learning and performance of conditional tasks (Petrides, 1982; 1985b; 1986; 1987).

Two of the experiments with nonhuman primates will be presented here by way of illustration. In one experiment, monkeys with lesions restricted within the periarcuate cortex or the principalis cortex (Fig. 13-10) were compared with normal control animals on a motor conditional task modeled on the human task requiring the performance of different movements of the hand. In this task, the monkeys faced a box with two manipulanda attached to it. One of the manipulanda was a short stick that the animals could grip and the other was a button that they could touch with the palm of their hand (Fig. 13-11). This box could be pushed back by the animal to collect a reward (a peanut), which was delivered through a flexible tube joined to the box. The animals were first trained to perform these movements to receive rewards and were then tested on the conditional task. They now had to learn to perform one or the other movement conditional upon the presentation of one of two visual stimuli. In particular, they had to grip the stick when a green circular bottle-cover was presented, but to place their hand on the button when a blue and yellow toy truck was shown. As can be seen in Figure 13-12, the animals that had lesions restricted to the periarcuate cortex were not able to learn the task within the limits of testing (i.e., 1,020 trials), whereas those that had lesions of the periprincipalis region were only slightly slower than the normal animals in learning the task. It is important to emphasize that the deficit exhibited by the monkeys with periarcuate lesions

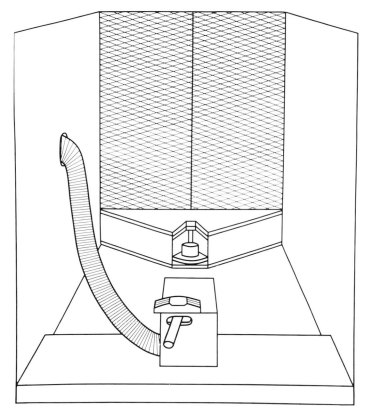

Figure 13–11 Schematic drawing of the experimental arrangement in the motor conditional task used with monkeys.

Figure 13–12 Trials to criterion on the motor conditional task. The monkeys with periarcuate lesions failed to reach criterion within the limits of testing (1,020 trials).

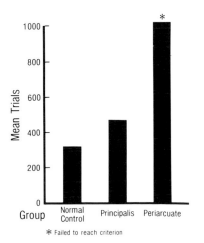

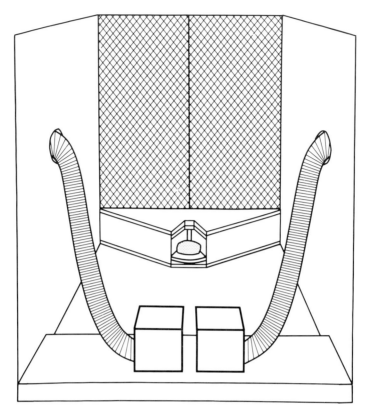

Figure 13–13 Schematic drawing of the experimental arrangement in the conditional task in which the monkey had to select between the lit and the unlit box.

on this task could not be attributed to a difficulty with the motor aspects of the task, because these animals had no obvious motor defects and had learned without difficulty to make both movements before testing began. It is particularly noteworthy that, during testing, the periarcuate animals quickly learned to wait for the presentation of a stimulus and to respond by performing one or the other of the two movements. Clearly, these animals knew that they had to perform one or the other response to obtain the reward but were not able to learn to perform the correct response for the particular stimulus presented. For other experiments that strengthen this conclusion, see Petrides, 1982; 1986 and Halsband and Passingham, 1982.

In another experiment, monkeys with periarcuate lesions were tested on a conditional task in which the required responses were to select between two visually distinct boxes whose positions varied randomly from trial to trial (Fig. 13–13). These boxes were constructed out of white opaque perspex, and, inside each one of them, there was a small light bulb that could be turned on or off by the experimenter. On any given trial, one of the boxes, chosen according to a random sequence, was lit and the other remained unlit. These boxes could be pushed back by the animal to receive a reward that was delivered through a flex-

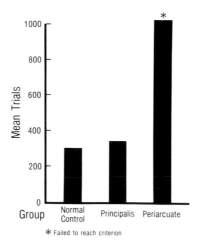

Figure 13-14   Trials to criterion on the conditional task requiring selection between the lit and unlit boxes. The monkeys with periarcuate lesions failed to reach criterion within the limits of testing (1,020 trials).

ible tube attached to each box. Behind the two test boxes, there was an apparatus with an opening at the front through which a stimulus could be presented. In the conditional task, the monkeys had to learn to open the lit box to receive a reward when stimulus A (a toy clown) was shown, but to open the unlit box when stimulus B (a yellow disc) was presented. The animals with periarcuate lesions were severely impaired in learning this task (Fig. 13-14). These same animals, however, were able to acquire at a normal rate two control tasks that had been administered to them before the conditional task. In one of these control tasks, the monkeys had to learn to open *only* the lit box when a cue was presented. When the animals had mastered this task, they were tested on another control task in which they had to break the previous habit by responding now to the unlit box. The results of these control experiments demonstrated that monkeys with periarcuate lesions could learn to respond by opening one of two visually distinct boxes when a signal to do so was presented and could reverse their response habit at a normal rate. It is clear from these experiments that the periarcuate animals could perceive the difference between the lit and the unlit boxes, could learn to wait until the cue was presented, and, then, having identified the lit box (or the unlit one, in the reversal task), to open it to receive their reward. These animals, however, could not master the task when the requirements were to select between the lit and the unlit box depending on the particular cue presented on any given trial.

CONCLUDING COMMENTS

The investigations described here have demonstrated that patients with frontal cortical excisions exhibit severe impairments in the performance of conditional associative tasks. These patients can learn and perform without any difficulty the various responses and can readily discriminate between the different stimuli that are used as cues for the production of these responses. They are, however, severely impaired when they have to retrieve from the set of alternative responses those that must be performed in the presence of the various cues.

The work with nonhuman primates has demonstrated that the posterior dorsolateral frontal cortex, i.e., the cortex within and around the arcuate sulcus, is a critical region for the acquisition and performance of such tasks. Animals with lesions restricted to this region of the frontal cortex perform poorly on conditional tasks. These animals, just as is the case with the patients, fail in selecting the correct response on different trials, even though they know the set of alternative responses, can produce them, and can discriminate normally between the various signals.

The animal work has further shown that within the posterior dorsolateral frontal cortex (periarcuate cortex), there is further specialization according to the type of responses that are required in the conditonal tasks. We now know, for instance, that lesions restricted to rostral area 6 impair performance on conditional tasks in which the animals have to select between different movements, whereas lesions restricted to the anterior arcuate region (area 8) impair performance on tasks requiring selection between visually distinct objects (Petrides, 1987). These findings are consistent with neuroanatomic work showing that rostral area 6 is predominantly linked to the somatosensory "association" cortex and the motor cortex, whereas area 8 is closely related to visual "association" cortex (see Pandya and Yeterian, 1985).

Electrophysiologic investigations have shown that single cells within the periarcuate region of the frontal cortex respond to visual (Gentilucci et al., 1983; Godschalk et al., 1981; Kubota and Hamada, 1978; Mohler et al., 1973; Rizzolatti et al., 1981a) and somaesthetic (Rizzolatti et al., 1981b) stimuli and that many cells in this region exhibit modulations of their response patterns according to the "instructional" significance of the stimuli rather than to their physical characteristics (Weinrich and Wise, 1982; Weinrich et al., 1984; Wise and Mauritz, 1985). These findings are consistent with the hypothesis that the periarcuate region of the frontal cortex plays a critical role in neural circuits for the selection of responses on the basis of different sensory signals.

REFERENCES

Barbas H, Mesulam M-M. Organization of afferent input to subdivisions of area 8 in the rhesus monkey. J Comp Neurol 200:407–431, 1981.

Barbas H, Mesulam M-M. Cortical afferent input to the principalis region of the rhesus monkey. Neuroscience 15:619–637, 1985.

Barbas H, Pandya DN. Architecture and intrinsic connections of the prefrontal cortex in the rhesus monkey. J Comp Neurol 286:353–375, 1989.

Corkin S. Tactually-guided maze learning in man: Effects of unilateral cortical excisions and bilateral hippocampal lesions. Neuropsychologia 3:339–351, 1965.

De Renzi E, Motti R, Nichelli P. Imitating gestures: A quantitative approach to ideomotor apraxia. Arch Neurol 37:6–10, 1980.

Fuster JM. The Prefrontal Cortex: Anatomy, Physiology, and Neuropsychology of the Frontal Lobe. New York: Raven Press, 1980.

Gentilucci M, Scandolara C, Pigarev IN, Rizzolatti G. Visual responses in the postarcuate cortex (area 6) of the monkey that are independent of eye position. Exp Brain Res 50:464–468, 1983.

Geschwind N. The apraxias. In Straus EW, Griffith RM (ed), Phenomenology of Will and Action. Philadelphia: Duquesne University Press, 1967, pp. 91–102.

Godschalk M, Lemon RN, Nijs HGT, Kuypers HGJM. Behaviour of neurons in monkey peri-arcuate cortex and precentral cortex before and during visually guided arm and hand movements. Exp Brain Res 44:113–116, 1981.

Halsband U, Passingham R. The role of premotor and parietal cortex in the direction of action. Brain Res 240:368–372, 1982.

Kimura D, Archibald Y. Motor functions of the left hemisphere. Brain 97:337–350, 1974.

Kubota K, Hamada I. Visual tracking and neuron activity in the post-arcuate area in monkeys. J Physiol (Paris) 74:297–312, 1978.

Milner B. Interhemispheric differences in the localization of psychological processes in man. Br Med Bull 27:272–277, 1971.

Milner B. Disorders of learning and memory after temporal lobe lesions in man. Clin Neurosurg 19:421–446, 1972.

Milner B. Psychological aspects of focal epilepsy and its neurosurgical management. In Purpura DO, Penry JK, Walter RD (eds), Advances in Neurology. Vol 8. New York: Raven Press, 1975, pp. 299–321.

Mishkin M. A memory system in the monkey. Phil Trans R Soc Lond B 298:85–95, 1982.

Mohler CW, Goldberg ME, Wurtz RH. Visual receptive fields of frontal eye field neurons. Brain Res 61:385–389, 1973.

Pandya DN, Yeterian EII. Architecture and connections of cortical association areas. In Peters A, Jones EG (eds), Cerebral Cortex. Vol. 4. New York: Plenum Press, 1985, pp. 3–60.

Petrides M. Motor conditional associative-learning after selective prefrontal lesions in the monkey. Behav Brain Res 5:407–413, 1982.

Petrides M. Deficits on conditional associative-learning tasks after frontal- and temporal-lobe lesions in man. Neuropsychologia 23:601–614, 1985a.

Petrides M. Deficits in non-spatial conditional associative learning after periarcuate lesions in the monkey. Behav Brain Res 16:95–101, 1985b.

Petrides M. The effect of periarcuate lesions in the monkey on the performance of symmetrically and asymmetrically reinforced visual and auditory go, no-go tasks. J Neurosci 6:2054–2063, 1986.

Petrides M. Conditional learning and the primate frontal cortex. In Perecman E (ed), The Frontal Lobes Revisited. New York: The IRBN Press, 1987, Ch 5, pp. 91–108.

Petrides M. Nonspatial conditional learning impaired in patients with unilateral frontal- but not unilateral temporal-lobe excisions. Neuropsychologia 28:137–49, 1990.

Petrides M, Milner, B. Deficits on subject-ordered tasks after frontal- and temporal-lobe lesions in man. Neuropsychologia 20:249–262, 1982.

Petrides M, Pandya DN. Projections to the frontal cortex from the posterior parietal region in the rhesus monkey. J Comp Neurol 228:105–116, 1984.

Petrides M, Pandya DN. Association fiber pathways to the frontal cortex from the superior temporal region in the rhesus monkey. J Comp Neurol 273:52–66, 1988.

Rizzolatti G, Scandolara C, Matelli M, Gentilucci M. Afferent properties of periarcuate neurons in macaque monkeys. II. Visual responses. Behav Brain Res 2:147–163, 1981a.

Rizzolatti G, Scandolara C, Matelli M, Gentilucci M. Afferent properties of periarcuate neurons in macaque monkeys. I. Somatosensory responses. Behav Brain Res 2:125–146, 1981b.

Smith ML, Milner B. The role of the right hippocampus in the recall of spatial location. Neuropsychologia 19:781–793, 1981.

Weinrich M, Wise SP. The premotor cortex of the monkey. J Neurosci 2:1329–1345, 1982.

Weinrich M, Wise SP, Mauritz K-H. A neurophysiological study of the premotor cortex in the rhesus monkey. Brain 107:385–414, 1984.

Wise SP, Mauritz K-H. Set-related neuronal activity in the premotor cortex of rhesus monkeys: Effects of changes in motor set. Proc R Soc Lond [Biol] 223:331–354, 1985.

VII
Neuropsychiatric and Developmental Effects of Frontal Lobe Damage

14
Prefrontal Cortex Dysfunction in Schizophrenia

DANIEL R. WEINBERGER,
KAREN FAITH BERMAN,
AND DAVID G. DANIEL

The notion that schizophrenia involves dysfunction of the frontal lobes dates back at least to Emil Kraepelin. In his view, the primary behavioral deficit in this disorder was a "destruction of the mainsprings of volition" secondary to anatomic pathology of the frontal cortex (Kraepelin, 1907). While consistent evidence of neuropathologic changes in the frontal lobe has not as yet emerged from research in schizophrenia, Kraepelin's emphasis on symptoms suggestive of frontal dysfunction has been echoed throughout this century in phenomenologic studies of this illness. In addition to diminished will and impaired judgment, a variety of other clinical features often seen in patients with schizophrenia have been considered as possibly secondary to frontal lobe, especially prefrontal cortex, dysfunction. These include blunted affect, poor insight, social withdrawal, reduced motivation, distractibility, attentional deficits, and impairments in smooth pursuit and in anticipatory saccadic eye movements (Weinberger, 1988).

Although Kraepelin believed that fundamental cognitive processes such as orientation and memory were usually preserved in patients with this illness, recent data have increasingly cast this shibboleth in doubt. As neuropsychologic studies have explored cognitive function in this disorder in greater detail, it has become clear that many patients manifest profound cognitive impairment. The impairment involves a number of functions, including sustained attention and vigilance, recall memory, and problem solving (Goldberg and Weinberger, 1986; 1988). Verbal and visuospatial skills are relatively preserved. Since this pattern of neuropsychologic deficits is also seen in patients with prefrontal injury, it has been interpreted as further suggestion of prefrontal dysfunction in patients with schizophrenia.

In the case of problem-solving tasks, the difficulties exhibited by some patients with schizophrenia are striking, in terms of both their extent and their similarity to the difficulties of patients with prefrontal injury. For example, Goldberg and colleagues (1987) administered the Wisconsin Card Sorting Test (WCS), a problem-solving abstract reasoning task sensitive to prefrontal injury, to several groups of patients with chronic schizophrenia and attempted to teach them how to do the task. In general, patients with schizophrenia do poorly on this test. After several trials during which patients performed in the impaired range, Goldberg and colleagues administered card by card instructions, which enabled patients to perform at the normal level. However, 15 minutes later, when they took the same test without explicit instruction, they performed at the same level of impairment as the first time they performed the task. This failure to use past experience to modify their behavior, to appear, in Teuber's words, "impervious to error information" (Teuber, 1972) is a characteristic of patients with prefrontal dysfunction.

While the phenomenologic similarity between some features of patients with schizophrenia and of patients with prefrontal injury is circumstantial evidence of prefrontal dysfunction in the former case, it is not direct and certainly not conclusive evidence. Direct evidence of prefrontal physiologic dysfunction has emerged from some brain imaging studies of regional cerebral blood flow (rCBF) and regional brain glucose utilization. In this chapter, we will review data from a series of studies performed in our rCBF laboratory at the National Institute of Mental Health that implicate prefrontal physiologic dysfunction as an important pathophysiologic correlate of schizophrenia. This work was originally inspired by the pioneering studies of David Ingvar and colleagues in Lund, Sweden, who reported in 1973 that compared with normal controls, patients with schizophrenia had less prefrontal rCBF relative to posterior rCBF, a finding that they referred to as "hypofrontality" (Ingvar and Franzen, 1974a,b). They observed that the more withdrawn, mute, and affectively blunted the patient, the more hypofrontal the rCBF pattern. This finding suggested a clinical-pathophysiologic correlation for certain symptoms of schizophrenia and prompted Ingvar to propose that schizophrenia involved a physiologic deficit in neural mechanisms that normally activate prefrontal cortex (Ingvar, 1981).

The finding of physiologic hypofrontality in schizophrenia has been replicated in several rCBF and glucose utilization studies (for review: Weinberger and Berman, 1988). However, negative reports have also appeared. In our view, and as the studies reviewed in this chapter illustrate, the finding of hypofrontality appears to be dependent on the behavioral state of the patients during the brain imaging experiment. To the extent that physiologic data in general are dynamic and defined by the conditions under which they are acquired, it is not surprising that the results of such experiments will vary depending on these conditions. In every rCBF and glucose utilization study of patients with schizophrenia performed while patients were engaged in a task that demanded prefrontal activation, they have been found to be "hypofrontal" (for review: Berman and Weinberger, 1986; Weinberger and Berman, 1986; Weinberger and Kleinman, 1986). These studies suggest that certain neural mechanisms involved in behavior specific activation of prefrontal cortex are dysfunctional in this disorder.

rCBF DURING THE WISCONSIN CARD SORTING TEST

We have performed four studies of rCBF in patients with schizophrenia and in normal control subjects while they were engaged in the WCS. This test was chosen because of its relative specificity and sensitivity to prefrontal dysfunction and because we hypothesized that it would be associated with physiologic activation of this brain region in normal individuals. The test was automated so that it could be administered to subjects seated in a dental chair with their head immobilized in a helmetlike apparatus that contained 32 gamma ray detectors. Patients inhaled radioactive 133-xenon gas that served as a tracer of rCBF. The xenon washout method developed by Obrist (1975) was used to quantify rCBF. Although this method has relatively limited resolution compared with current tomographic techniques such as positron emission tomography (PET) and single photon emission computerized tomography (SPECT), and provides information only about the cortex, it is noninvasive, quantitative, and involves no discomfort. The simplicity and the comfort of the procedure may be important factors in reducing physiologic "noise." Moreover, the xenon rCBF method remains the only available valid, quantitative method for the in vivo determination of rCBF.

Our initial study compared 24 normal individuals with 20 patients with chronic schizophrenia (mean age 29) who had been withdrawn from all medications and maintained medication-free for a minimum of 4 weeks (Weinberger et al., 1986). rCBF was determined during three states: Resting with eyes closed, and in two cognitive activation states presented in counterbalanced order. One was the WCS, and the other was a simple number matching (NM) test. This latter condition was conceived as a control for the physiologic correlates of the nonspecific mental activity that occur during the WCS task. These include the correlates of visual activation, motor responses, individual psychologic experiences of undergoing an rCBF procedure, etc. Since these nonspecific physiologic signals are liable to obscure the specific physiologic signals related to the higher-order cognitive processing involved in doing the WCS, subtracting the rCBF data during the NM from the data acquired during the WCS would, at least in theory, enhance our appreciation of the specific signal related to the WCS.

There were no significant differences in absolute rCBF between patients and controls during either the resting or the NM conditions. During the WCS, however, the difference between the patients and controls was highly significant. rCBF to the dorsolateral prefrontal cortex (DLPFC) of the patients was significantly lower. When rCBF during the NM was compared with rCBF during the WCS within individuals, we found that while normals increased prefrontal activity during the WCS compared with their own cerebral activity during the NM, patients did not. A between group comparison of change in rCBF from NM to WCS was also significant for the DLPFC.

To address the question of whether the findings would vary with clinical and medication state, we also studied using the identical activation protocol, a sample of 24 similar patients after 6 weeks of a fixed standard dose of haloperidol (Berman et al., 1986). Despite the fact that most of the patients were clinically less symptomatic, the rCBF results were the same.

Similar results have been found in two additional independent samples of patients, including another cohort of medication-free patients (N = 16) (Weinberger et al., 1988c) and a sample of monozygotic twins who were discordant for the illness (10 pairs). In the former study, the patients again showed reduced DLPFC activity during the WCS but not during the other conditions, and the degree of activation during the DLPFC task compared with the control task significantly differentiated the groups (Berman et al., 1989).

One problem with the data in this study and in the earlier studies is that there is a large degree of interindividual variation, and while the group means differ, there is considerable overlap in the individual data values from one group to another. Thus, it is difficult to determine whether the mean differences characterize the majority of patients or only a subgroup. This question illustrates how drawing conclusions about "normality" and "abnormality" from physiologic data such as rCBF is problematic without controlling for the numerous sources of interindividual variation that affect these data. The problem is analogous to estimating normality and abnormality from data about pulse rate without knowing about age, sex, physical activity, level of physical conditioning, etc.

The primary rationale for the twin study was to control for many of these sources of variation. Discordant monozygotic twins should be uniquely well matched for the factors that affect rCBF during these studies except for those related to the illness. The results of this study demonstrated that not only did the affected twins have significantly reduced DLPFC rCBF during the WCS when compared with their unaffected co-twins, but in every pair the affected twin had less prefrontal activity than did their healthy co-twin (Berman et al., 1989). This degree of discrimination has never been appreciated in studies of independent, i.e., unmatched, groups. The results suggest that when "ideal" controls are available, evidence of relative prefrontal hypoactivity may be a consistent pathophysiologic characteristic of the brains of patients with schizophrenia. The twin data also provided further information about the role of prior neuroleptic treatment. Although we had previously shown that DLPFC rCBF was not affected by acute medication status, we could not rule out that prior treatment had not produced irreversible changes in the capacity to activate the prefrontal cortex. In the twin study, reliable histories of exposure to antipsychotic drugs were attained, and the data indicated that the patients who had received the greatest quantities of these agents during their life tended to have, in fact, the highest DLPFC rCBF.

PREFRONTAL HYPOACTIVITY: EPIPHENOMENON OR PRIMARY PATHOPHYSIOLOGY?

The results of these rCBF studies indicate that prefrontal hypoactivity is a replicable physiologic finding in patients with schizophrenia examined during this prefrontally linked cognitive task. They suggest that this disorder is associated with dysfunction of neural mechanisms involved in behaviorally specific activation of DLPFC. There are, however, other possible interpretations of the data. For example, prefrontal hypoactivity in these patients may be a correlate of inattentiveness, uncooperativeness, or lack of mental effort, having nothing to do with regionally and behaviorally specific neural systems. It is also possible that simply doing poorly on a test, as patients with schizophrenia do on the WCS, is responsible for prefrontal hypoactivity. To address these possible explanations for the rCBF data, a series of studies was undertaken that involved other activation procedures that were at least as demanding as the WCS in terms of attention, motivation, and mental effort, but that did not appear to require activation of the DLPFC over baseline in normal individuals. In other words, these tests shared the nonspecific aspects of mental effort, motivation, attention, etc., with the WCS but were not "prefrontal tasks" and did not appear to involve the task-specific neural mechanisms that are enlisted during the WCS to physiologically activate the DLPFC. In theory, if the results of the WCS rCBF data were secondary to the nonspecific demands of the test that were shared by the nonprefrontal tasks, then patients should appear hypofrontal on these tasks as well. If patients were not hypofrontal during these additional tasks, then it is not likely to be the nonspecific aspects of the WCS condition that underlie prefrontal hypoactivity seen during this condition.

The first of the nonfrontal studies utilized a visual continuous performance task (CPT) that consisted of two conditions: A simple reaction time test, where subjects pressed a button every time they saw an "X" appear on a screen; and a more complicated task where subjects were required to press a button only when an "X" was preceded by an "A." This latter condition was dynamically paced, so that each subject would be certain to reach his or her own point of maximum performance. Despite the fact that this test involves considerable effort and concentration and that the patients' performances were much worse than the controls', rCBF did not differ between the groups during either of these conditions (Berman et al., 1986). Comparing the simple with the complex task in the normal group revealed that DLPFC was not activated during the more demanding condition any more than it was during the simple condition, suggesting that it was not a DLPFC-mediated task.

We also studied a group of medication-free patients on a version of the Speech Sounds Perception Test (SSPT) (Berman et al., 1987). This involved having patients discriminate differences and similarities in fragments of speech that they heard through earphones. The control task consisted of similar sounds without the performance of the discrimination exercise. While patients appeared globally less activated, i.e., had slightly less global increase in rCBF in the discrimination as compared with the baseline task, they were not relatively hypofrontal. As with the CPT conditions, this task required considerable effort, attention, cooperation, etc., but did not appear to be in normals a DLPFC selective behavior.

Since neither the CPT nor the SSPT involves abstract thinking, the comparison of these tasks with the WCS is still problematic. Perhaps the most appropriate counterpoint to the WCS study is an rCBF study of Ravens Progressive Matrices (RPM). This abstract reasoning, problem-solving test shares many features with the WCS, the CPT, and the SSPT, including the nonspecific attention and effort characteristics, but unlike the CPT and SSPT, it is also a reasoning task (as is the WCS). We administered the RPM to 24 normal individuals and determined rCBF during performance of this test and during performance of a control task that consisted of matching abstract forms similar to those appearing in the matrices of the RPM test (Berman et al., 1988a). The RPM task was associated with activation of posterior temporal and inferior parietal cortex, and not with activation (over baseline) of the DLPFC. Medication-free patients with schizophrenia were not hypoactive in DLPFC when compared with the normals during this condition.

Taken together, these studies strongly suggest that prefrontal hypoactivity during the WCS in patients with schizophrenia is not because of nonspecific factors such as test difficulty, poor performance, demands for concentration, attention, effort, and motivation, or even for abstract thinking and problem solving, but rather because of the demand for specific physiologic activation of the DLPFC. The results point to failure of the function of regionally specific neural mechanisms that subserve this activation process. Not surprisingly, this failure is most apparent during behaviors that require enhanced or focused output from DLPFC.

rCBF DURING THE WCS IN OTHER NEUROPSYCHIATRIC DISORDERS

In order to explore the specificity of this pathophysiologic finding to schizophrenia, we have examined several groups of patients with other disorders that have been associated with impairment of prefrontal cognitive functions, including patients with depression, Huntington's disease, Down's syndrome, and Parkinson's disease (PD). In a study of 10 patients with severe depression, several of whom had been psychotic and had received neuroleptic medications, we did not find prefrontal hypoactivity during the WCS task (Berman et al., unpublished). In patients with Huntington's disease (HD), who perform quite poorly on the WCS, rCBF was not only not reduced, it tended to be slightly increased (Weinberger et al., 1988b). Moreover, the degree to which prefrontal rCBF was increased correlated with the degree of caudate atrophy on computerized tomography (CT) scan. This result suggested that the mechanisms of prefrontal activation were intact in at least early HD and that the mechanism of prefrontal cognitive failure in this disorder was not related to a failure of activating systems. The correlation of prefrontal rCBF activation with caudate atrophy implicated failure on the output side, consistent with the location of the primary pathology in the head of the caudate nucleus, the major corticofugal projection of DLPFC. This study also highlights how physiologic imaging data can be used to characterize different pathophysiologic mechanisms for the same behavioral deficit.

The study of young adult patients with Down's syndrome, a population who perform very poorly on the WCS, found that this group also activated DLPFC normally during the WCS task (Berman et al., 1988b). In Down's syndrome, as in HD, the mechanisms that activate DLPFC in response to behavioral conditions that demand such activation appear to be intact. This also illustrates once again that physiologic activation per se does not necessarily mean normal cognitive function.

CLUES TO THE MECHANISM OF PREFRONTAL HYPOFUNCTION IN SCHIZOPHRENIA

The studies of patients with Huntington's disease and Down's syndrome suggest that neither pathology that is intrinsic to prefrontal cortex (i.e., cytoarchitectural maldevelopment as in Down's syndrome) nor pathology that is downstream from prefrontal cortex (i.e., as in HD) necessarily impair physiologic activation. Animal studies suggest that activation of prefrontal cortex is likely subserved by ascending afferentation systems from the thalamus (Nauta and Domesick, 1982), basal forebrain (i.e., cholinergic) and brain stem (i.e., dopaminergic, noradrenergic, and serotonergic), none of which are consistently pathologic in young adult patients with Down's syndrome or in early HD.

In our work, an initial clue that the brain stem afferentation system might be involved in schizophrenia came from a study of patients with PD (Weinberger et al., 1988a). Ten patients with primarily mild to moderately severe illness (clinical stages I and II in most cases) underwent the WCS rCBF protocol. Despite normal performance on the test, there was a significant correlation ($r = -.73$, $p = .01$) between prefrontal rCBF during the WCS and percentage perseverative errors committed on the task. This consistent relationship between physiology and performance was seen previously only in patients with schizophrenia (Weinberger et al., 1986). None of the other patient populations and none of our normal control populations demonstrated this relationship. Moreover, in the patients with PD, the same parameter that predicted performance on the WCS (i.e., prefrontal rCBF) also correlated with clinical measures linked to nigral dopaminergic activity, i.e., stage of illness ($r = -.86$, $p < .01$), rigidity ($r = -.66$, $p < .05$), and bradykinesia ($r = -.65$, $p < .06$). The results suggest that in this nondemented patient population, prefrontal dopaminergic function is compromised, perhaps not enough to impair cognitive function, but enough so that it has become a critical and predictive factor in prefrontal activation. It is reasonable to assume that patients with more advanced disease, many of whom manifest prefrontal cognitive deficits (Lees and Smith, 1983; Taylor et al., 1986), probably have even less prefrontal dopaminergic activity as suggested by rCBF studies that have reported reduced prefrontal rCBF in such patients (Bes et al., 1983). The results of recent postmortem studies of brains of patients with PD support this conjecture by demonstrating a link between cognitive deficits and loss of ventral tegmental dopaminergic neurons that project to the cortex (Rinne et al., 1989).

Further evidence for a possible role of prefrontal dopaminergic projections in patients with schizophrenia came from cerebrospinal fluid (CSF) monoaminergic metabolite data. The concentrations in CSF of homovanillic acid (HVA), the primary human dopamine metabolite, strongly predicted ($r = .81$, $p < .003$) prefrontal rCBF during the WCS in 10 of the unmedicated schizophrenic patients in whom both of these measures were available (Weinberger et al., 1988c). A similar relationship between CSF HVA and rCBF did not exist during other cognitive conditions, including the RPM. This relationship between CSF HVA concentrations and behavior-specific rCBF is not easy to interpret. The origin of CSF HVA is complex, with contributions from the basal ganglia, spinal cord, as well as the cortex. In monkeys, recent data suggest that prefrontal HVA concentrations may correlate with CSF HVA concentrations more strongly than do HVA concentrations in other brain regions, implying that CSF HVA levels may reflect activity in cortical dopaminergic projections (Ellsworth et al., 1987). Another difficulty in interpreting the correlation in the patients with schizophrenia is that the CSF collection was not done during the rCBF procedure. In spite of these uncertainties, the fact that this correlation was found only with prefrontal rCBF, and that it existed only with rCBF acquired during the specific prefrontal behavior, suggests that dopaminergic projections to the prefrontal cortex participate in the mechanism of physiologic activation of this region when there is a behavioral imperative for this activation. It should be noted that a similar though slightly less robust correlation was also found for the CSF metabolite of serotonin, i.e., 5'-HIAA, suggesting a possible role for serotonergic afferentation of the prefrontal cortex, as well.

PREFRONTAL HYPOACTIVITY IN SCHIZOPHRENIA: IS IT REVERSIBLE?

If hypometabolism in schizophrenia is related to subcortical dopaminergic afferent neuronal activity, it should be possible to pharmacologically augment this activity with dopamimetic agents and reverse this pathophysiologic condition. If diminished dopaminergic activity is the primary factor responsible for diminished prefrontal function, then the behavioral correlates of this hypofunctional state should also be reversible in the same manner. Geraud and associates (1987) reported evidence to support the first possibility. They administered piribidil, a mixed catecholaminergic receptor agonist, to a group of patients with chronic schizophrenia who were "hypofrontal" during the "resting state" by xenon inhalation rCBF examination. The drug normalized the rCBF pattern. The authors did not report the behavioral correlates of this effect.

We studied the effect of apomorphine, a dopamine receptor agonist, on rCBF in eight chronically psychotic patients, six of whom had chronic schizophrenia (Daniel et al., 1989). Our standard WCS/NM paradigm was used in a placebo-controlled, crossover, and counterbalanced design. We administered apomorphine/placebo before the subjects began the WCS task. In every patient with schizophrenia, prefrontal rCBF relative to nonfrontal rCBF increased after apomorphine. The prefrontal index, a measure of relative prefrontal rCBF, during the WCS was significantly greater after apomorphine than after placebo, suggesting that enhanced prefrontal dopaminergic afferent activity may increase prefrontal physiologic activity. Unfortunately, the results of this study are open to several other interpretations. For instance, we could not rule out that the rCBF change was a primary vascular phenomenon, not related to increased cortical neuronal activity. We also did not find a significant change in performance on the WCS test, a change that would have suggested that the physiologic effect translated into cognitive function.

In order to obviate some of these uncertainties, we have studied another sample of similar patients, using amphetamine as the dopamimetic agent (Daniel et al., in press). Though amphetamine is a mixed biogenic aminergic agonist, it has a longer biologic half-life and could be given before either of the cognitive activation rCBF procedures were performed. This made it possible to look at the effect of amphetamine on activation, i.e., the difference between rCBF during the WCS and rCBF during the NM task. This approach probably controls for primary vascular effects that should not be behaviorally specific. In this study rCBF was measured with a dynamic single photon emission computerized tomography (SPECT) method for monitoring xenon-133 saturation and desaturation. Two effects of amphetamine were observed. First, it produced a regionally nonselective and behaviorally nonspecific reduction in brain rCBF. Compared with placebo, rCBF after amphetamine was reduced globally during both the NM and the WCS conditions. This is consistent with several other in vivo brain metabolism studies in humans (Abreu, 1949; Kahn et al., 1989; Mathew and Wilson, 1985; Volkow et al., 1987). The striking finding was that the degree of activation, i.e., the change in rCBF during the WCS as compared with the NM, increased significantly especially in the left DLPFC. Moreover, there was a slight but significant improvement in performance on the WCS, and WCS performance and DLPFC rCBF correlated positively only after amphetamine. These results are consistent with the hypothesis that dopaminergic function at the cortical level is involved in the behavior-specific deficit in prefrontal activation seen in patients with schizophrenia. They also suggest that, as in animals (Sawaguchi, 1987), enhanced catecholaminergic input to the human prefrontal cortex improves physiologic "signal to noise."

PREFRONTAL HYPOACTIVITY AND LIMBIC NEUROPATHOLOGY IN SCHIZOPHRENIA

During the past decade, there has been a resurgence of interest in anatomic neuropathologic studies of schizophrenia, spurred primarily by the availability of in vivo anatomic techniques such as CT and magnetic resonance imaging (MRI). Recent studies using these techniques have reliably demonstrated that patients with this diagnosis have larger lateral and third ventricles and more prominent cortical sulci than do normal individuals of the same age (for review: Jaskiw et al., 1988; Kelsoe et al., 1988; Shelton and Weinberger, 1986). Moreover, MRI studies and postmortem histopathologic studies have reported that subtle deviations of the size and cytoarchitecture of medial temporal lobe structures such as the hippocampus and parahippocampal gyrus are consistent findings in the brains of patients with this disorder and may underlie the finding of ventricular enlargement (Bogerts et al., 1985; Brown et al., 1986; Suddath et al., 1988; Suddath et al., 1990). Evidence of anatomic pathology of the prefrontal cortex has been limited (Weinberger et al., 1979; Shelton et al., 1988) and is certainly less robust a finding than is pathology of the anterior-medial temporal lobe. However, the question of prefrontal anatomic pathology should remain open at this time considering the greater difficulty in appreciating subtle architectural deviations in neocortex as compared with archicortex.

Two studies have suggested that prefrontal physiologic hypoactivity may be linked to subcortical anatomic pathology in patients with schizophrenia. In the first, we observed a correlation (r = −.50, p < .01) between prefrontal rCBF during the WCS and ventricular size on CT in a sample of 30 patients with schizophrenia. This significant correlation was not observed during the NM task. The results suggest that to the degree that ventricular enlargement in schizophrenia reflects the extent of limbic pathology, to which it has been linked in at least one MRI study (Suddath et al., 1988), this pathology has an impact on prefrontal function during the WCS but not during nonprefrontal tasks. Since the WCS is a working memory task, in the sense that information from the recent past must be kept in mind in order to act appropriately, it is logical to assume that this task involves communication between prefrontal cortex and anterior-medial temporal lobe structures. Activation of this system (i.e., prefrontal cortex, hippocampus, and one of the midstations that link them—the thalamus) has been demonstrated in vivo in monkeys performing working memory tasks (Friedman et al., 1990). If the pathologic condition of the anterior-medial temporal lobe in schizophrenia affects communication across this network during such tasks, the existence of this condition may have its greatest impact on prefrontal activity and function when communication through prefrontal–anterior-medial temporal connectivity is needed. This might explain why prefrontal hypoactivity is seen during the working memory task but not during other tasks.

Support for this assumption has emerged from our study of monozygotic twins who are discordant for the illness. An interesting correlation between structural and functional pathology was found in this sample. The most consistent anatomic finding on MRI was reduced size of the anterior hippocampus, which was smaller in the affected member of 14 of 15 twin pairs (Suddath et al., 1990). The difference within a twin pair in hippocampal size in the left hemisphere, a putative measure of the degree of pathologic involvement of this region, correlated strongly with the difference in prefrontal activation during the WCS as compared with the NM tasks, a putative measure of behavior-specific prefrontal hypofunction (unpublished data).

CONCLUSIONS

It has been suspected throughout this century that patients with schizophrenia have disease of the frontal lobe. Until relatively recently, this suspicion was based on the phenomenologic similarity between many of the clinical features of schizophrenia and those of patients with injury to the prefrontal cortex. While replicable scientific evidence for neuropathologic changes in the frontal lobe of patients with schizophrenia has not been a consistent finding, evidence for physiologic dysfunction of this part of the brain has been frequently observed in studies of rCBF and glucose metabolism using brain imaging technologies. The data indicate that the conditions under which the studies of rCBF and metabolism are performed are important if not critical for the demonstration of prefrontal hypofunction. To date, every study that examined patients with schizophrenia during a cognitive task that activates prefrontal cortex in normal individuals has found that patients with schizophrenia, as a group, have reduced prefrontal function. In studies of monozygotic twins who are discordant for the illness, the affected twin has consistently had less prefrontal activity during a prefrontally activating cognitive task than their unaffected co-twin, suggesting that subtle prefrontal hypofunction may be a fairly consistent pathophysiologic correlate of schizophrenia.

The mechanism of prefrontal hypofunction in this disorder is obscure. It appears to be different from that of some other disorders that involve prefrontal-type cognitive deficits, such as HD and Down's syndrome. The similarity of the rCBF data in schizophrenia to that of patients with PD suggests a common pathophysiologic mechanism, perhaps reduced function in ascending catecholaminergic projections to the cortex. A link between prefrontal hypofunction in patients with schizophrenia and putative pathology of the anterior-medial temporal lobe suggests an additional mechanism, one of altered communication through pathways that subserve working memory. The relationship of prefrontal hypofunction with the classic psychotic symptoms of schizophrenia, those symptoms that are thought to be related to excessive limbic dopaminergic activity, is also obscure. However, the possibility that they may be related has opened new areas of investigation into the role of cortical modulation of subcortical dopaminergic activity (Jaskiw et al., 1988; Pycock et al., 1980). Preliminary animal studies suggest that prefrontal hypofunction may result in excessive subcortical dopaminergic activity that is especially prominent under stressful conditions.

REFERENCES

Abreu BE, Liddle GW, Burks AL, Sutherland V, Elliot HW, Simon A, Margolis L: Influence of amphetamine sulfate on cerebral metabolism and blood flow in man. J Am Pharmacol Assoc 38:186–188, 1949.

Berman KF, Doran AR, Pickar D, Weinberger DR: Cortical function during cognitive activation in depression: A comparison with normal subjects and patients with schizophrenia (unpublished).

Berman KF, Rosenbaum SCW, Brasher CA, et al: Cortical physiology during auditory discrimination in schizophrenia: A regional cerebral blood flow study. Soc Neurosci Abst p. 651, 1987.

Berman KF, Illowsky BP, Weinberger DR: Physiologic dysfunction of dorsolateral prefrontal cortex in schizophrenia. IV: Further evidence for regional and behavioral specificity. Arch Gen Psychiatry 45:616–623, 1988a.

Berman KF, Schapiro MB, Friedland RP, et al: Regional cortical blood flow during cognitive activation in Down's syndrome. Soc Neurosci Abst p. 1012, 1988b.

Berman KF, Torrey EF, Daniel DG, Weinberger DR: Prefrontal cortical blood flow in monozygotic twins concordant and discordant for schizophrenia. Schizophr Res 2:129, 1989.

Berman KF, Weinberger DR: Cerebral blood flow studies in schizophrenia. In Nasrallah HA, Weinberger DR (eds), The Neurology of Schizophrenia. Elsevier Science Publishers, 1986, pp. 277–308.

Berman KF, Zec RF, Weinberger DR: Physiologic dysfunction of dorsolateral prefrontal cortex in schizophrenia. II: Role of neuroleptic treatment, attention, and mental effort. Arch Gen Psychiatry 43:126–135, 1986.

Bes A, Guell A, Fabre N, Dupui Ph, Victor G, Geraud G: Cerebral blood flow studied by Xenon-133 inhalation technique in Parkinsonism: Loss of hyperfrontal pattern. J Cereb Blood Flow Metabol 3:33–37, 1983.

Bogerts B, Meerz E, Schonfeldt-Bausch R: Basal ganglia and limbic system pathology in schizophrenia: A morphometric study of brain volume and shrinkage. Arch Gen Psychiatry 42:784–791, 1985.

Brown RM, Colter N, Corsellis Jan, et al: Post mortem evidence of structural brain changes in schizophrenia: Differences in brain weight, temporal horn area, anterior parahippocampal gyrus compared with affective disorder. Arch Gen Psychiatry 43:36–42, 1986.

Daniel DG, Berman KF, Weinberger DR: The effect of apomorphine on regional cerebral blood flow in schizophrenia. J Neuropsychiatry Clin Neurosci 1:377–384, 1989.

Daniel DG, Weinberger DR, Jones D, Zigun J, Coppola R, Kleinman J, Bigelow L, Goldberg TE: Effect of amphetamine on regional cerebral blood flow during cognitive activation in schizophrenia (unpublished).

Ellsworth JD, Leahy DJ, Roth RJ Jr, Rudman D Jr: Homovanillic acid concentration in brain, CSF, and plasma as indicators of central dopamine function in primates. J Neural Transm 68:51–62, 1987.

Friedman HR, Janas JD, Goldman-Rakic PS: Enhancement of metabolic activity in the diencephalon of monkeys performing working memory tasks: A 2-deoxyglucose study in behaving Rhesus monkeys. J Cogn Neurosci 2(1):18–31, 1990.

Geraud G, Arne-Bes MC, Guell A, et al: Reversibility of hemodynamic hypofrontality in schizophrenia. J Cereb Blood Flow Metab 7:9–12, 1987.

Goldberg TE, Weinberger DR: Methodological issues in the neuropsychological approach to schizophrenia. In Nasrallah HA, Weinberger DR (eds), The Neurology of Schizophrenia. Elsevier N Holland, Amsterdam, 1986, pp. 141–156.

Goldberg TE, Weinberger DR: Neuropsychological studies of schizophrenia. Schizophr Bull 14:179–184, 1988.

Goldberg TE, Weinberger DR, Berman KF, Pliskin NH, Hyde N: Further evidence for dementia of the prefrontal type in schizophrenia. Arch Gen Psychiatry 44:1008–1014, 1987.

Ingvar DH: Measurements of regional cerebral blood flow and metabolism in psychopathological states. Eur Neurol 20(3):294–296, 1981.

Ingvar DH, Franzen G: Abnormalities of cerebral blood flow distribution in patients with chronic schizophrenia. Acta Psychiatr Scand 50:425–462, 1974a.

Ingvar DH, Franzen G: Distribution of cerebral activity in chronic schizophrenia. Lancet 2:1484–1486, 1974b.

Jaskiw JE, Christison G, Freed WJ, Weinberger DR: Behavioral effects of dopaminergic agonists and antagonists in the prefrontal cortex. Soc Neurosci Abst 663, 1988.

Kahn DA, Prohovnik I, Lucas LR, Sackeim HA: The associated effects of amphetamines on arousal and cortical blood flow in humans. Biol Psychiatry 25:755–767, 1989.

Kelsoe JR, Cadet JL, Pickar D, Weinberger DR: Quantitative neuroanatomy in schizophrenia: A controlled MRI study. Arch Gen Psychiatry 45:533–541, 1988.

Kraepelin E: Dementia Praecox in Paraphrenia. Barclay RM, Robertson GN (Trans.), Robert E. Krieger Publishing, New York, 1971.

Lees AJ, Smith E: Cognitive deficits in the early stages of Parkinson's disease. Brain 106:257–270, 1983.

Mathew RJ, Wilson WH: Dextroamphetamine induced changes in regional cerebral blood flow. Psychopharmacology 87:298–302, 1985.

Nauta WJH, Domesick VB: Neural associations of the limbic system. Neural Basis of Behavior 10:175–206, 1982.

Obrist WD, Thompson HK, Wang HS, Wilkinson WE: Regional cerebral blood flow estimated by 133 xenon inhalation. Stroke 6:245–256, 1975.

Pycock CJ, Kerwin RW, Carter CJ: Effect of lesion of cortical dopamine terminals on subcortical dopamine in rats. Nature 286:74–77, 1980.

Rinne JO, Rummukainen J, Paljarvi L, Rinne UK: Dementia in Parkinson's Disease is related to neuronal loss in the medical substantia nigra. Ann Neurol 26:47–50, 1989.

Sawaguchi T: Catecholamine sensitivities of neurons related to a visual reaction task in the monkey prefrontal cortex. J Neurophysiol 58(5):110–122, 1987.

Shelton RC, Karson CN, Doran AN, Pickar D, Bigelow LB, Weinberger DR: Cerebral structural pathology in schizophrenia: Evidence for a selective prefrontal cortical defect. Am J Psychiatry 145:154–163, 1988.

Shelton RC, Weinberger DR: X-ray computerized tomography studies in schizophrenia: A review and synthesis. In Nasrallah HA, Weinberger DR (eds), The Neurology of Schizophrenia. Elsevier N Holland Amsterdam, 1986, pp. 207–215.

Suddath RL, Casanova MF, Goldberg TE, Daniel DG, Kelsoe JR, Weinberger DR: Temporal lobe pathology in schizophrenia: A quantitative magnetic resonance imaging study. Am J Psychiatry 146:464–472, 1988.

Suddath RL, Christison GW, Torrey EF, Casanova MF, Weinberger DR: Anatomical abnormalities in the brains of monozygotic twins discordant for schizophrenia. N Engl J Med 322:789–94, 1990.

Taylor AE, Saint-Cyr A, Lang AE: Parkinson's disease and depression: A critical re-evaluation. Brain 109(2):279–292, 1986.

Teuber HL: Neuropsychology: Effects of focal brain lesions. Neurosci Res Prog Bull 10:383–384, 1972.

Volkow N, Angrist B, Wolf A, et al: Effects of amphetamine on local cerebral metabolism in normal and schizophrenic subjects as determined by positron emission tomography. Psychopharmacology 92:241–246, 1987.

Weinberger DR: Schizophrenia and the frontal lobes. Trends in Neuroscience 11:367–370, 1988.

Weinberger DR, Berman KF: Speculation on the meaning of cerebral metabolic hypofrontality in schizophrenia. Schizophr Bull 14(2):157–168, 1988.

Weinberger DR, Berman KF, Chase TN: Cortical dopamine and human cognition. Ann NY Acad Sci 537:330–338, 1988a.

Weinberger DR, Berman KF, Iadarola M, et al: Prefrontal cortical blood flow and cognitive function in Huntington's disease. J Neurol Neurosurg Psychiatry 51:94–104, 1988b.

Weinberger DR, Berman KF, Illowsky BP: Physiologic dysfunction of dorsolateral prefrontal cortex in schizophrenia. III: A new cohort and evidence for a monoaminergic mechanism. Arch Gen Psychiatry 45:609–615, 1988c.

Weinberger DR, Berman KF, Zec RF: Physiologic dysfunction of dorsolateral prefrontal cortex in schizophrenia. I: regional cerebral blood flow evidence (rCBF). Arch Gen Psychiatry 43:114–125, 1986.

Weinberger DR, Kleinman JE: Observations of the brain in schizophrenia. In Hales RE, Frances AJ (eds), Psychiatric Update, American Psychiatry Association Annual Review, APA Press, Washington, DC, 42–67, 1986.

Weinberger DR, Torrey EF, Neophytides AN, Wyatt RJ: Structural abnormalities in the cerebral cortex of chronic schizophrenic patients. Arch Gen Psychiatry 36:935–939, 1979.

15

The Role of the Frontal Lobes in Affective Disorder Following Stroke

SERGIO E. STARKSTEIN
AND ROBERT G. ROBINSON

In spite of the large amount of experimental and clinical evidence indicating that the frontal lobes play an important role in behavior and emotion, the frontal lobes remain one of the most enigmatic areas of the brain. Using laboratory animals, the initial investigations of the role of the frontal lobes in behavior conducted in the early 1900s generally produced negative findings. Compared with the clear motor or sensory deficits produced by lesions around the central sulcus, more anterior lesions in the frontal cortex produced no obvious behavioral changes. In 1948, however, Ward reported that after cingulotomy, their animals appeared tamer toward both cagemates and human handlers. Monkeys showed "no grooming behavior, no acts of affection towards companions, and seemed as if they had lost their social conscience . . . and the ability to forecast the social repercussions of their own actions."

Based on these laboratory observations as well as human data such as the Phineas T. Gage case and others (Harlow, 1868), the era of psychosurgery started. Psychosurgery involved the production of surgical lesions within white matter of the frontal lobes. Follow-up studies of patients with leukotomies, however, shed additional light on the association between lesions in specific frontal lobe areas and mood changes. Orbitofrontal leukotomies, for instance, were frequently reported to produce euphoria and emotional disinhibition. This procedure was therefore utilized in patients with depression and catatonic stupor (Reitman, 1946). On the other hand, lesions of the frontal convexity were noted to produce quieting effects and emotional flattening and therefore were most useful in manic patients (McLardy and Meyer, 1949).

After the psychosurgery era, the interest in the relationship between behavior and frontal lobes subsided. By the early seventies, however, the interest in the role of the frontal lobe in behavior and emotion reemerged. Blumer and coworkers (1975) described two types of behavioral changes in patients with frontal lesions. The "pseudodepressed" type was associated with lesions in the frontal convexity and was characterized by slowness, indifference, and apathy. The "pseudopsychopathic" type was associated with orbitofrontal lesions and was characterized by lack of adult tact and restraints, coarse, irritable, and facetious behavior, hyperactivity, hypersexuality, antisocial acts, and paranoid or grandiose thinking.

In the present chapter, we will examine the role of frontal lobes in two of the most frequent psychiatric complications of frontal lobe lesions, namely depression and mania. We will demonstrate how the use of a structured psychiatric interview and standardized diagnostic criteria may help to disentangle these affective syndromes from other disorders associated with frontal lobe injury and how clinical-pathologic correlations have begun to illuminate the role of the frontal lobes in these affective disorders.

DEPRESSION FOLLOWING STROKE

The fact that depressive states are frequently the result of brain lesions has been recognized since the beginning of this century (Kraepelin, 1921). In 1951, Bleuler observed that after cerebrovascular infarction, melancholic moods appear frequently, and Adolf Meyer (1904) reported on clinical differences in the presentation of traumatic insanities depending upon the specific locations and causes of brain injury. Differences in emotional symptoms related to hemispheric lesion location were reported by Babinski (1914), Gainotti (1972), Hécaen (1951), and others. Gainotti (1972) found that left hemisphere lesions produced a depressive catastrophic reaction, while right hemisphere lesions were associated with jocularity and euphoria.

In one of our initial studies, we compared 18 patients with left hemisphere stroke lesions with 11 patients with left hemisphere traumatic brain injuries (TBI) for frequency and severity of depression (Robinson and Szetela, 1981). Even though the two groups were comparable in terms of neurologic symptoms, activities of daily living, and cognitive impairments, more than 60% of the stroke patients had clinically significant depressions as compared with only 20% of the TBI patients. Although both groups had similar lesion sizes, lesions in the stroke group were more rostral than lesions in the TBI group. However, when seven patients with stroke lesions were matched for lesion location with seven patients with TBI, there were no significant between-group differences in the frequency of depression. Thus, the finding of a significantly higher frequency of depression in the stroke group was primarily related to the presence of more anterior lesions in the stroke group as compared with the TBI group.

In more recent studies utilizing patients with cerebrovascular lesions, we found a significant association between major depression (as defined by symptoms elicited using the semistructured psychiatric interview in the Present State Examination (Wing et al., 1974) and DSM-III diagnostic criteria (American Psychiatric Association, 1980)) and lesions of the left frontal lobe (Robinson et al., 1984; Starkstein et al., 1987a). Three important variables in this association, side of lesion, proximity to the frontal pole, and region of the frontal cortex, will be discussed in detail.

Side of Lesion

In our patients with lesions restricted to the frontal lobes or with lesions involving the frontal lobes along with other cortical structures, we have consistently found an association between major depression and lesions of the *left* frontal lobe (for review: Starkstein and Robinson 1989a). On the other hand, we found *right* frontal lesions to be associated with an apathetic indifference and cheerfulness that, although not true euphoria, is clearly inappropriate in patients who have suffered a brain injury (Robinson et al., 1984). While other investigators have also found an association between diagnosed cases of depression and left frontal lesions (Eastwood et al., 1989), some studies could not find differences in depression rating scores between patients with left and right hemisphere lesions (Sinyor et al., 1986). Important methodologic issues, such as presence of previous strokes, time between stroke and psychiatric evaluation, and family or personal history of psychiatric disorders (for discussion: Starkstein and Robinson 1989a), may explain these discrepancies.

Proximity to the Frontal Pole

Among patients with frontal lobe lesions, we found that proximity of the anterior border of the lesion to the frontal pole (as determined by computerized tomography (CT) scan) was positively correlated with severity of depression (i.e., more anterior lesions were associated with more severe depressions) (Robinson and Szetela, 1981) (Fig. 15–1). This significant correlation was also found in patients with either restricted cortical lesions or restricted subcortical damage (Starkstein et al., 1987a), left-handed patients (Robinson et al., 1985), patients with bilateral lesions (Lipsey et al., 1983), and patients with TBI (Robinson and Szetela, 1981). Similar correlations between depression scores and proximity of the lesion to the frontal pole have been reported by other authors (Eastwood et al., 1989; Sinyor et al., 1986).

Frontal Areas Involved in Depression after Brain Injury

Very few studies have systematically examined this issue. In one of our recent studies, we found that the left fronto-opercular region was the frontal cortical area most frequently damaged in patients with poststroke major depression (Starkstein et al., 1987a). As mentioned in the introduction, lesions of the frontal lobe convexity have been reported by Blumer and Benson (1975) to produce a mood change they called "pseudodepressed." Lesions of the orbitofrontal cortex, however, have not been associated with depressive disorder.

In support of the finding that dysfunction of the frontal lobes may play an important role in depression, Baxter and colleagues (1989) reported that left prefrontal cortical hypometabolism was the most consistent and severe abnormality found in three different forms of affective disorder (i.e., unipolar major depression, bipolar depression, and major depression with obsessive compulsive disorder).

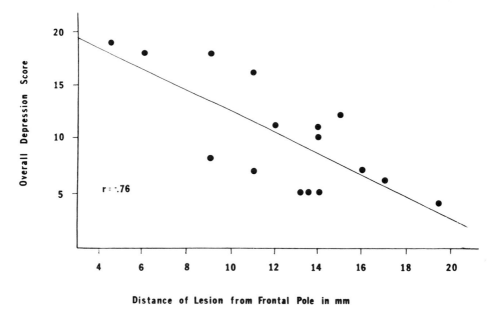

Figure 15-1 Relationship between severity of depression and mean distance of the anterior border of the lesion to the frontal pole for patients with either stroke or traumatic lesions of the left hemisphere. Patients with more anterior lesions (i.e., lesions nearer the frontal pole) had high depression scores (i.e., more severe depressions) (r = −0.76, *p* < .001). (From Robinson and Szetela, 1981, reprinted with permission from *Annals of Neurology*.)

Subcortical Structures

In our study that examined patients with restricted subcortical lesions (no cortical involvement), we found a significant association between depression and left anterior lesions. Major depression occurred in approximately 80% of patients with lesions involving the head of the caudate and the anterior limb of the internal capsule (Starkstein et al., 1987a). In a subsequent study, we compared patients with lesions restricted to either the left or right basal ganglia (primarily head of the caudate nucleus) or left or right thalamus for frequency and severity of depression (Starkstein et al., 1988a). We found that injury to the left head of the caudate produced a significantly higher frequency and severity of depression than either right hemisphere basal ganglia damage or left or right thalamic injury.

In support of these findings, a study that compared patients with functional (i.e., no known brain injury) unipolar major depression and normal controls found a significantly reduced blood flow in the left head of the caudate among patients with major depression (Drevets et al., 1989).

Risk Factors

Although a significant proportion of patients with left frontal lesions develop depression (i.e., approximately 60%), not all patients with these lesions become depressed. In an effort to determine what factors may contribute to this clinical variability, we compared 13 pairs of patients with a similar size and location of lesion (most of them had left frontal or left basal ganglia involvement); one of the pair had major depression, while the other patient was not depressed (Starkstein et al., 1988b). There were no significant between-group differences in demographic variables, education, familial or personal history of psychiatric disorder, or frequency of neurologic deficits. The only significant between-group difference that we could find was a greater amount of subcortical atrophy (as measured by both the third ventricle-to-brain ratio and the lateral ventricle-to-brain ratio) in the major depression as compared with the nondepressed group. On the other hand, there were no significant intergroup differences in measurements of cortical atrophy. We believe that the subcortical atrophy probably pre-existed the stroke because it was present in the acute poststroke CT scan (usually within a day or 2 following the stroke) and it was present in the lateral ventricle contralateral to the lesion. Thus, these findings suggest that preexisting subcortical atrophy may increase the risk of developing a major depression after a left frontal or left basal ganglia stroke.

In comparison with patients with major depression following left frontal or basal ganglia strokes, we found that patients with major depression following right hemisphere lesions had a significantly higher frequency of family history of psychiatric disorders. These major-depressed patients with right hemisphere lesions also had a significantly increased frequency of family history of psychiatric disorder, as compared with nondepressed patients with right hemisphere lesions (differences between depressed and nondepressed patients in personal history of psychiatric disorders were in the same direction but fell short of significance) (Starkstein et al., 1989b). Thus, these findings suggest that a genetic predisposition for depression may play an important role in the production of major depression following right hemisphere lesions and that the etiology and mechanism of all poststroke major depressions are not the same.

Mechanism

Although numerous mechanisms might be proposed to explain why left frontal and basal ganglia lesions lead to depression, we have proposed a mechanism that could account for the finding that proximity of the lesion to the frontal pole correlates significantly with severity of depression. We have hypothesized that frontal cortical lesions may produce depression by disrupting biogenic amine pathways (Starkstein and Robinson, 1989a). These pathways, containing norepinephrine and serotonin, whose cell bodies are located in the brain stem, send axons anteriorly through the hypothalamus and basal ganglia, to the frontal cortex (Morrison et al., 1979). After reaching the frontal pole, these axons arc posteriorly, running through the deep layers of the cortex and sending arborizing terminals to the superficial cortical layers. Thus, lesions that damage these biogenic amine pathways in the frontal cortex would disrupt more terminal fibers than lesions of the same size in the parietal or occipital cortex (i.e., more proximal lesions interrupt more downstream terminals than more distal lesions). This anatomy would explain why we found a significant correlation between proximity of the lesion to the frontal pole and severity of depression.

The fact that biogenic amine pathways have demonstrated asymmetries (e.g., there are different distributions of noradrenergic terminals in the right compared with the left thalamus in humans (Oke et al., 1978)) may explain the higher frequency of depression after left compared with right anterior lesions. Thus, lesions of the left basal ganglia would not only interrupt important frontocaudate connections, but, depending on the distribution of the ascending pathways, could disrupt a greater percentage of the biogenic amine innervation to the frontal cortex than comparable lesions of the right basal ganglia.

MANIA AFTER FRONTAL LOBE LESIONS

Perhaps because of their rather abrupt and sometimes dramatic behavioral effects, euphoria, indifference, disinhibition, and irritability are well-known consequences of frontal lobe lesions. These emotional and behavioral disturbances are usually referred to as "frontal lobe symptoms." The overlap of these symptoms with those found in manic patients raises the question whether this "frontal lobe syndrome" is a manifestation of mania or hypomania as defined by Diagnostic and Statistical Manual of Mental Disorders-Revised (DSM-IIIR) criteria (American Psychiatric Association, 1987), or whether it is a distinct entity. The following symptoms are frequently found in patients with the frontal lobe syndrome: Decreased social concern, jocularity, facetiousness, boastfulness, irritability, coarseness, hyperkinesia, disinhibition, loss of social graces, inappropriate sexual advances, sexual exhibitionism, impulsiveness, restlessness, and grandiose delusions. Thus, it is quite likely that some patients with symptoms that constitute "frontal lobe syndrome" may also meet the DSM-III criteria for mania or hypomania (Table 15-1). Other patients with "frontal lobe syndrome" may have personality disorder, anxiety disorder, dementia, or other clearly defined mental disorder syndromes. Thus, the term "frontal lobe syndrome" probably includes a variety of disorders. Eslinger and Damasio (1985) have suggested that "the frontal lobe syndrome is a misconception that impedes both research and clinical management."

The application of standardized diagnostic criteria as elicited using structured psychiatric interviews to patients with frontal lobe injury may help to clarify the various diagnostic entities that make up "frontal lobe syndrome." Although it seems likely that some patients with behavioral and emotional changes after frontal lesions will not meet criteria for mania, hypomania, personality disorder, or other defined conditions, the disentangling of specific entities from the other disorders may lead to a clearer diagnostic definition of the other syndromes that result from frontal lobe injury. Ultimately, different syndromes associated with frontal lobe injury are likely to have different underlying mechanisms and may therefore require different treatments. This whole issue of

Table 15–1   DSM-IIIR Criteria for Manic Episode

A. Distinct period of abnormally and persistently elevated, expansive, or irritable mood.

B. During the period of mood disturbance, at least three of the following symptoms have persisted (four if the mood is only irritable) and have been present to a significant degree:
   1. Inflated self-esteem or grandiosity
   2. Decreased need for sleep
   3. More talkative than usual or pressure to keep talking
   4. Flight of ideas of subjective experience that thoughts are racing
   5. Distractibility
   6. Increase in goal-directed activity (either socially, at work or school, or sexually) or psychomotor agitation
   7. Excessive involvement in pleasurable activities which have a high potential for painful consequences (e.g., buying sprees, sexual indiscretions, or foolish business investments)

C. Mood disturbance sufficiently severe to cause marked impairment in occupational functioning or in usual social activities or relationships with others, or to necessitate hospitalization to prevent harm to self or others.

D. At no time during the disturbance have there been delusions or hallucinations for as long as two weeks in the absence of prominent mood symptoms.

E. Not superimposed on Schizophrenia, Schizophreniform Disorder, or Psychotic Disorder.

Note: while DSM-IIIR specifies that manic episodes "initiated or maintained" by organic factors should be excluded from this category, we decided to use these criteria because the criteria for "Organic Mood Syndrome" only require the nonspecific symptom of "a prominent and persistent depressed, elevated, or expansive mood."

frontal lobe syndromes, including establishing clear diagnostic criteria, as well as identifying their mechanism and treatment, needs further systematic examination.

In our studies of patients with affective disorder following brain injury, we have examined patients in several studies who met DSM-III diagnostic criteria for mania (Table 15–1). In one study, we compared patients with mania after brain lesions (secondary mania) with patients with primary mania (mania with no known neuropathology) (Starkstein et al., 1987b). We found no significant differences in the frequencies of symptoms such as elation, pressured speech, flight of ideas, grandiose thoughts, insomnia, hallucinations, or paranoid delusions. Although the same diagnostic criteria had been applied to both populations, the study was, nevertheless, consistent with the suggestion that there is a phenomenologic similarity between primary and secondary mania. To illustrate this point, we will briefly describe the case of a patient who developed mania after a frontal lesion (Starkstein et al., 1988c).

The patient was a 63-year-old right-handed man without personal or family history of psychiatric disorder. He had a history of recent onset of progressive blindness, and a CT scan showed a large meningioma extending from the crista galli to the suprasellar cistern. A partial resection of the tumor was carried out, together with most of the right orbitofrontal lobe (Fig. 15–2). After the surgery, the patient showed a marked behavioral change. He boasted of having had the biggest brain tumor in the world, slept very few hours, was euphoric and hyper-

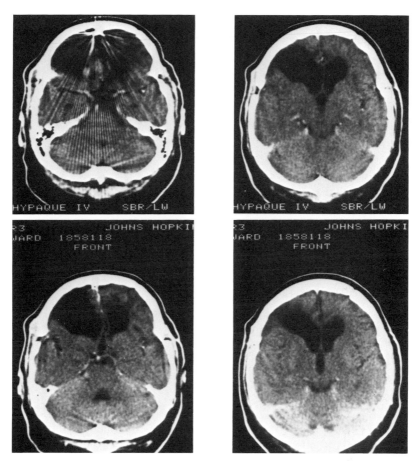

Figure 15–2 After the resection of an orbitofrontal meningioma, a CT scan showed an almost total ablation of the right orbitofrontal lobe. (From Starkstein et al., 1988a, reprinted with permission from Journal of Nervous and Mental Disease.)

active, and showed an excessive and disinhibited interest in sex. He told people that a national celebrity had been talking about him on a television show and he began to mismanage his finances including selling his property for trivial sums of money.

Other patients with frontal lobe lesions may show "sociopathic" behavior (Eslinger and Damasio, 1985) and may meet DSM-IIIR criteria for a personality disorder. The following case has been reported by Goldar and Outes (1972).

The patient was a 40-year-old man who before the frontal lesion was a calm and correct person, generous with his friends, and very skillful in his job. Immediately after a closed head injury, and following a brief confusional state, the patient started to complain about everything, became very aggressive, and frequently used obscene language. He obliged his wife to have sexual intercourse with him in the presence of relatives, and behaved in a brutal way during the sexual act. The patient also showed paranoid ideas and pathologic jealousy,

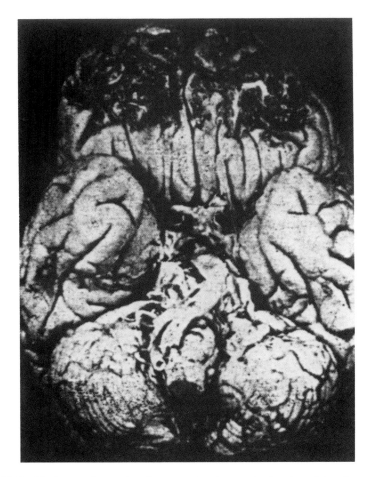

Figure 15–3   Brain specimen showing an extensive contusion involving the entire anterior orbitofrontal cortex. (From Goldar and Outes, 1972, reprinted with permission from Acta Psiquiatrica y Psicologica de America Latina.)

accusing his nephew of having a love affair with his wife. The patient was admitted to a psychiatric hospital where he continued to have frequent aggressive outbursts. He masturbated in public places and in the presence of other people, and started to have homosexual relationships. Following his death several years later, a postmortem examination showed a marked atrophy involving the anterior part of the orbitofrontal cortex (Fig. 15–3).

Lesion Location

In 1888, Welt suggested that damage to the orbitofrontal cortex might cause a change in character expressed by restlessness, euphoria, and overtalkativeness, as well as "lowering of ethical and moral standards." The same year, Jastrowitz (1888) reported elation, pressure of speech, and obscene language in patients with frontal lobe tumors.

Kleist (1931) described euphoria, puerility, and "moral insanity" in patients with orbitofrontal lesions, while loss of psychic and motor initiative, impoverished and stereotyped modes of thinking were associated with lesions of the frontal convexity. Kleist suggested that the orbitofrontal area was the center of the "social self" ("Gemeinschaft Ich"), while area 11 within the orbitofrontal cortex was related to personal and social ego, and area 47, also within the orbitofrontal cortex, was related to mood and emotional sensations.

Manic symptoms have also been described in patients with frontal lobe surgery. Reitman (1946) reported a triad of extroversion, hyperactivity, and euphoria after orbitofrontal leukotomy, and Rylander (1939) described euphoria, hyperactivity, and hypersexuality in a group of patients with frontal lobe surgical resections.

These findings suggest that the orbitofrontal cortex may be a key structure in the production of manic symptoms. The orbitofrontal cortex has efferent connections with diencephalic and midbrain limbic structures such as the septal area, hypothalamus, and mesencephalon (Nauta, 1971). We have suggested that lesions of the orbitofrontal cortex may produce mood and somatic symptoms of secondary mania through disruption of these diencephalic and midbrain connections (Fig. 15–4).

Another brain region that we have found in our studies to be associated with the development of secondary mania is the basolateropolar temporal cortex. In one series of 12 patients with secondary mania, we found that three of seven patients with cortical injury had lesions involving basal portions of the right temporal lobe (Starkstein et al., 1988c), while in a second series of eight patients with mania after brain lesions we found that four of five patients with cortical lesions had involvement of the right basotemporal cortex (Starkstein et al., 1989c).

Subcortical lesions without cortical extension, however, may also produce secondary mania. Cummings and Mendez (1984) reported two patients who developed mania after right thalamic lesions, and in our two series of patients with secondary mania, we found that about 40% of them had subcortical lesions primarily involving the right head of the caudate or the right thalamus. Mania after subcortical lesions, however, could be mediated by distant (diaschisis) effects in orbitofrontal or basotemporal cortex (which are reciprocally connected to one another). We examined this issue in a recent study using [18]fluorodeoxyglucose positron emission tomography ([18]FDG PET) (Starkstein et al., 1989c). Three patients who developed secondary mania after subcortical lesions, (two with ischemic strokes in the head of the caudate and anterior limb of the internal capsule, and one with a small frontal white matter contusion) all showed significant hypometabolism in the right basotemporal cortex compared with similar age normal controls.

Risk Factors

Since not every patient with lesions in limbic areas of the right hemisphere develops mania, we tried to identify risk factors for secondary mania in a group of 11 patients with secondary mania compared with 11 patients with similar lesions but no mood changes (Starkstein et al., 1987b). We found that patients with secondary mania had larger bifrontal ratios (a CT scan measure of subcortical

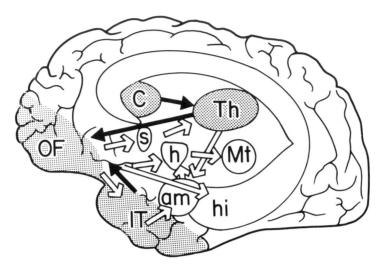

Figure 15–4   Schematic diagram showing the primary areas of injury in patients with secondary mania (shadowed areas) and the central role that the orbitofrontal and baso-temporal cortices play in the interaction of these lesion sites with other limbic structures and brain regions that control somatic functions. Black arrows, afferents to the orbito-frontal cortex; white arrows, orbitofrontal efferents to the limbic system. Th, thalamus; OF, orbitofrontal cortex; IT, inferior temporal cortex; s, septum; h, hypothalamus; am, amygdala; hi, hippocampus; mt, mesencephalic tegmentum; c, caudate. (Modified from Starkstein et al., 1988a.)

atrophy at the level of the frontal lobes) and third ventricle-to-brain ratios (a measurement of atrophy in diencephalic areas) as compared to lesion-matched controls.

Another risk factor for secondary mania identified in our studies was a positive family history of psychiatric disorders. In our first series of patients with secondary mania, manic patients had a significantly higher frequency of psychiatric disorder among their first-degree relatives (predominantly affective disorder) than a demographically comparable group of patients with poststroke depression, or poststroke patients with no mood disorders (Robinson et al., 1988). Interestingly, secondary manics *without* a family history of affective disorders had significantly higher bifrontal ratios than secondary manics with a positive family history, suggesting that *either* subcortical atrophy or genetic loading (but not both) may provide a substrate upon which a specific lesion of the right hemisphere may provoke the pathophysiologic mechanism of mania (Starkstein et al., 1987b).

Mechanism

Several studies have demonstrated that the amygdala, located in the inner or limbic portion of the temporal lobe, has an important role in the production of instinctive reactions and in the association between stimulus and emotional response (Gloor, 1986). In laboratory animals, electrical stimulation of the amygdala may produce flight-or-fight reactions, and in humans, epileptic discharges or electrical stimulation of the amygdala may result in rage or panic attacks (Gloor, 1986).

The amygdala receives its main afferents from two brain areas (Gloor, 1986): (1) The *basal diencephalon,* which in turn receives psychosensory and psychomotor information from the reticular formation, and (2) the *temporopolar* (area 38) and *basolateral* (area 20) cortices, which receive main afferents from heteromodal association areas. These cortical areas receive efferents from modality specific and heteromodal association cortical areas, and through the uncinate fasciculus, they receive a major input from the orbitofrontal cortex (Moral et al., 1987). The main efferent projections of the basolateropolar temporal cortex are directed toward the entorhinal cortex, hippocampus, and amygdala (Moran et al., 1987). By virtue of these connections, the basolateropolar temporal cortex may represent a cortical link between sensory afferents and instinctive reactions, and, in fact, Geschwind (1965) referred to this area as the true association cortex of the limbic system.

The orbitofrontal cortex may be subdivided in two regions. The anterior region, which includes areas 11 and 47, is larger and receives main efferents from the parvocellular dorsomedial thalamic nucleus (Beck, 1949). The posterior region (area 13) is smaller and receives efferents from the magnocellular dorsomedial thalamic nucleus (Hassler, 1948). While the posterior orbitofrontal cortex is restricted to limbic functions and should be considered part of the limbic system, the anterior orbitofrontal cortex exerts a tonic inhibitory control over the amygdala by means of its connection through the uncinate fasciculus with the basolateropolar temporal cortex (Crosby, 1962). Thus, the uncinate fasciculus and the basolateropolar cortex may mediate connections between psychomotor and volitional processes generated in the frontal lobe, and vital processes and instinctive behaviors generated in the amygdala (Goldar and Outes, 1972). It may be hypothesized that, by means of the orbito-temporo-amygdala connections, cognitive functions may influence limbic activity. Thus, a lesion in the orbitofrontal cortex, uncinate fasciculus, or the basolateropolar temporal cortex may release the tonic inhibition exerted by the frontal lobe on the amygdala, which in turn results in emotional disinhibition. The loss of frontolimbic connections may release emotions from intellectual control, and this dissociation results in the cluster of symptoms we identify in secondary mania (Goldar and Outes, 1972).

Another empiric finding that remains to be integrated into the mechanism of secondary mania is the fact that most of the patients with secondary mania have right hemisphere lesions (Starkstein et al., 1988c). In a rat model of focal brain injury, we found that right but not left frontolateral cortical lesions produced locomotor hyperactivity (Robinson, 1979). Moreover, right but not left cortical suction lesions produced bilateral increases in dopaminergic turnover in the nucleus accumbens, which may underlie the production of this asymmetrically elicited hyperactivity (Starkstein et al., 1988d). Thus, it is possible that in the presence of specific risk factors for secondary mania (i.e., subcortical atrophy or genetic vulnerability), changes in biogenic amines produced by right but not left hemisphere lesions may play an important role in the production of secondary mania. This biogenic amine dysfunction may also be most pronounced in the basolateropolar temporal cortex, which is one of the cortical regions with the highest concentration of serotonergic terminals from the raphe nuclei (Moran et al., 1987).

The work of Flor-Henry (1979) and others (Denenberg et al., 1984; Tucker et al., 1981) has suggested that the emotional consequences of right hemisphere lesions may result from the release of transcallosal inhibitory fibers. In the case of mania, it could be hypothesized that a lesion within limbic areas of the right hemisphere may release left limbic areas from tonic inhibition, thus allowing the "positive" tendencies of the left hemisphere to emerge. We have recently tested this hypothesis in a patient with secondary mania who underwent a Wada (amytal) test (Starkstein et al., 1989d). The patient was a 25-year-old man with a negative personal history of psychiatric disorder who developed secondary mania immediately after therapeutic embolization for a right basotemporal arteriovenous malformation. Two months later the patient was still manic, and since the first embolization was only partially successful, a second embolization was scheduled. Before it was conducted, a Wada test was carried out to determine speech dominance, and, during the Wada test, a standardized questionnaire used to elicit manic symptoms was administered. After an amytal injection in the left middle cerebral artery, the patient had a transient period of global aphasia. As the aphasia cleared, however, the patient was elated and irritable, laughed inappropriately, and showed tangential thoughts and pressured speech. A right frontopolar amytal injection was also followed by elation, grandiose delusions, tangential thoughts, and pressured speech. Thus, if secondary mania was explained by the "release" of the "cheerful-prone" left hemisphere after a lesion of the "depression-prone" right hemisphere, the amytal injection of our patient's left hemisphere should have briefly abolished his manic symptoms. Although it could be argued that the manic symptoms returned with the recovery of speech, the left carotid amytal injection produced no obvious changes in the patient's manic symptoms at any time during the Wada test. Thus, this finding is consistent with the hypothesis that secondary mania results from mechanisms within the limbic portions of the right hemisphere, and is not the result of a left hemisphere "release."

CONCLUSIONS

Depression is a frequent finding in patients with frontal lobe lesions. Both hemispheric side of the lesion (i.e., left hemisphere) and site within the frontal lobe (i.e., frontal opercular cortex) seem to be significantly associated with the development of major depression. Risk factors for developing major depression following stroke include subcortical atrophy as evidenced by increased ventricle-to-brain ratios and family history of affective disorder. The fact that genetic vulnerability is significantly associated with major depression following right hemisphere stroke but not left frontal or left basal ganglia stroke suggests that there is more than one etiologic mechanism for these postbrain injury affective syndromes. One possible mechanism to explain the finding that severity of depression in the left hemisphere correlates significantly with proximity of the lesion to the frontal poles is that frontal and basal ganglia lesions interrupt the biogenic amine pathways in more upstream locations leading to greater downstream disruption of function.

Secondary mania is frequently associated with lesions of cortical (orbitofrontal and basolateropolar temporal) and subcortical (head of the caudate and thalamus) limbic and limbic-related regions. Side of lesion also plays an important role, since patients with secondary mania almost always have right hemisphere involvement. Risk factors for secondary mania, just like major depression, include subcortical atrophy or genetic vulnerability. The "release" of limbic structures such as the amygdala and somatic function mediating structures such as the hypothalamus after ipsilateral lesions in the orbitofrontal cortex, uncinate fasciculus, or basolateropolar temporal cortex may underlie the emergence of both affective and autonomic symptoms of mania.

Identification of the mechanisms underlying these affective syndromes and their relationship to frontal lobe function may ultimately lead to more specific and "rational" treatments of these disorders.

ACKNOWLEDGMENTS

This work was supported in part by the following NIH grants: Research Scientist Award MH00163 (RGR), MH40355, NS15080, and a grant from the University of Buenos Aires, Argentina (SES).

REFERENCES

American Psychiatric Association. Diagnostic and Statistical Manual of Mental Disorders (DSM-III). 3rd Edition. Washington DC: APA, 1980.

American Psychiatric Association. Diagnostic and Statistical Manual of Mental Disorders-Revised (DSM-III-R). 3rd Edition, revised. Washington DC: APA, 1987.

Babinski J. Contribution a l'étude des troubles mentaux dans l'hémiplégie organique cérébrale (anosognosie). Revue Neurologique 22:845–848, 1914.

Baxter LR, Schwartz JM, Phelps ME, Mazziotta JC, Guze BM, Selin CE, Gerner RH, Sumida RM. Reduction of prefrontal cortex glucose metabolism common to three types of depression. Archives of General Psychiatry 46:243–250, 1989.

Beck E. A cytoarchitectural investigation into the boundaries of cortical areas 13 and 14 in the human brain. Journal of Anatomy 83:147–157, 1949.

Bleuler EP. Textbook of Psychiatry. New York: Dover Publications, 1951.

Blumer D, Benson DF. Personality changes with frontal and temporal lobe lesions, In Benson DF, Blumer D (eds). Psychiatric Aspects of Neurologic Diseases. New York: Grune & Stratton, 1975.

Crosby E, Humphrey T, Lauer E. Correlative Anatomy of the Nervous System. New York: Macmillan, 1962.

Cummings JL, Mendez MF. Secondary mania with focal cerebrovascular lesions. American Journal of Psychiatry 141:1084–1087, 1984.

Denenberg VH. Behavioral Asymmetry. In Geschwind NE, Galaburda AM (eds), Cerebral Dominance: The Biological Foundations. Cambridge, MA, Cambridge University Press, pp. 114–133, 1984.

Drevets WC, Raichle ME, Fox PT, Preskorn SH, Videen TO. Trait and state cerebral blood flow abnormalities in depression. Society for Neuroscience Abstracts 15:30, 1989.

Eastwood MR, Rifat SL, Nobbs H, Ruderman J. Mood disorder following cerebrovascular accident. British Journal of Psychiatry 154:195–200, 1989.

Eslinger PJ, Damasio AR. Severe disturbance of higher cognition after bilateral frontal ablation: Patient EVR. Neurology 35:1731–1741, 1985.

Flor-Henry P. On certain aspects of the localization of the cerebral systems regulating and determining emotion. Biological Psychiatry 677–698, 1979.

Gainotti G. Emotional behavior and hemispheric side of the brain. Cortex 8:41–55, 1972.

Geschwind N. Disconnexion syndromes in animals and man. Brain 88:237–287, 1965.

Gloor P. Role of the human limbic system in perception, memory and affect: Lessons for temporal lobe epilepsy. In Doane BK, Livingstone KE (eds), The Limbic System: Functional Organization and Clinical Disorders. New York: Raven Press, 1986.

Goldar JC, Outes DL. Fisiopatologia de la desinhibicion instintiva. Acta Psiquiatrica y Psicologica de America Latina 18:177–185, 1972.

Harlow JM. Recovery from the passage of an iron bar through the head. Publications of the Massachusetts Medical Society 2:327–346, 1868.

Hassler R. Uber die Thalamus-Stirnhirn-Verbindungen beim Menschen. Der Nervenarzt 19:9–19, 1948.

Hécaen H, Ajuriaguerra J de, Massonet J. Les troubles visuoconstructifs par lésion pariétooccipitale droit. Encéphale 40:122–179, 1951.

Jastrowitz M. Beitrage zur Localisation im Grosshirn und uber deren praktische Verwerthung. Deutsche Medizinische Wochenschrift 14:81–83, 1888.

Kraepelin E. Manic-Depressive Insanity and Paranoia. Edinburgh: E and S Livingstone, 1921.

Kleist K. Die Storungen der Ichleistungen und ihre Lokalisation im orbital-, innen und Zwischenhirn. Monatsschrift fur Psychiatrie und Neurologie 79:338–350, 1931.

Lipsey JR, Robinson RG, Pearlson GD, Rao K, Price TR. Mood change following bilateral hemisphere brain injury. British Journal of Psychiatry 143:266–273, 1983.

Lishman WA. Organic Psychiatry. Oxford: Blackwell Scientific Publications, 1987.

McLardy T, Meyer A. Anatomical correlates of improvement after leucotomy. Journal of Mental Science 95:182–192, 1949.

Meyer A. The anatomical facts and clinical varieties of traumatic insanity. American Journal of Insanity 60:373, 1904.

Moran MA, Mufson EJ, Mesulam MM. Neural inputs into the temporopolar cortex of the rhesus monkey. Journal of Comparative Neurology 256:88–103, 1987.

Morrison JH, Molliver ME, Grzanna R. Noradrenergic innervation of the cerebral cortex: Widespread effects of local cortical lesions. Science 205:313–316, 1979.

Nauta WJH. The problem of the frontal lobe: A reinterpretation. Journal of Psychological Research 8:167–187, 1971.

Oke A, Keller R, Mefford I, Adams RN. Lateralization of norepinephrine in human thalamus. Science 200:1411–1413, 1978.

Reitman F. Orbital cortex syndrome following leucotomy. American Journal of Psychiatry 103:238–241, 1946.

Robinson RG. Differential behavioral and biochemical effects of right and left hemispheric cerebral infarction in the rat. Science 205:707–710, 1979.

Robinson RG, Szetela B. Mood change following left hemispheric brain injury. Annals of Neurology 9:447–453, 1981.

Robinson RG, Kubos KG, Starr LB, Rao K, Price TR. Mood disorders in stroke patients: Importance of lesion location. Brain 107:81–93, 1984.

Robinson RG, Lipsey JR, Bolla-Wilson K, Rao K, Price TR. Mood disorders in left-handed stroke patients. American Journal of Psychiatry 142:1424–1429, 1985.

Robinson RG, Boston JD, Starkstein SE, Price TR. Comparison of mania with depression following brain injury: Causal factors. American Journal of Psychiatry 145:172–178, 1988.

Rylander G. Personality Changes After Operations on the Frontal Lobes. London: Oxford University Press, 1939.

Sinyor D, Jacques P, Kaloupek DG, Becker R, Goldenberg M, Coopersmith HM. Post-stroke depression and lesion location: An attempted replication. Brain 109:537–546, 1986.

Starkstein SE, Robinson RG, Price TR. Comparison of cortical and subcortical lesions in the production of post-stroke mood disorders. Brain 110:1045–1059, 1987a.

Starkstein SE, Pearlson GD, Boston JD, Robinson RG. Mania after brain injury: A controlled study of causative factors. Archives of Neurology 44:1069–1073, 1987b.

Starkstein SE, Robinson RG, Berthier ML, Parikh RM, Price TR. Differential mood changes following basal ganglia vs thalamic lesions. Archives of Neurology 45:725–730, 1988a.

Starkstein SE, Robinson RG, Price TR. Comparison of patients with and without post-stroke major depression matched for size and location of lesion. Archives of General Psychiatry 45:247–252, 1988b.

Starkstein SE, Boston JD, Robinson RG. Mechanisms of mania after brain injury: 12 case reports and review of the literature. Journal of Nervous and Mental Disease 176:87–100, 1988c.

Starkstein SE, Moran TH, Bowersox JA, Robinson RG. Behavioral abnormalities induced by frontal cortical and nucleus accumbens lesions. Brain Research 473:74–80, 1988d.

Starkstein SE, Robinson RG. Affective disorders and cerebral vascular disease. British Journal of Psychiatry 154:170–182, 1989a.

Starkstein SE, Robinson RG, Honig MA, Parikh RM, Joselyn J, Price TR. Mood changes after right-hemisphere lesions. British Journal of Psychiatry 155:79–85, 1989b.

Starkstein SE, Mayberg HS, Berthier ML, Fedoroff P, Price TR, Dannals RF, Wagner HN, Leiguarda R, Robinson RG. Mania after brain injury: Neuroradiological and metabolic findings. Annals of Neurology 27:652–9, 1990.

Starkstein SE, Berthier ML, Lylyk PL, Casasco A, Robinson RG, Leiguarda R. Emotional behavior after a Wada Test in a patient with secondary mania. Journal of Neuropsychiatry and Clinical Neurosciences 1:408–412, 1989d.

Tucker DM, Starslie CE, Roth RS, Shearer SL. Right frontal lobe activation and right hemisphere performance: Decrement during a depressed mood. Archives of General Psychiatry 38:169–174, 1981.

Ward AA. The anterior cingular gyrus and personality. In: The frontal lobes. Research publications, Assoc for Research in nervous and mental disease 27:438–445, 1948.

Welt L. Ueber Charakterveränderungen des Menschen infolge von Läsionen des Stirnhirns. Deutsche Archiv für Klinische Medizine 42:339–390, 1988.

Wing JK, Cooper JE, Sartorius N. Measurement and classification of Psychiatric Symptoms. London, Cambridge University Press, 1974.

16
Dementia of the Frontal Lobe Type

DAVID NEARY
AND JULIE S. SNOWDEN

Non-Alzheimer forms of primary cerebral atrophy are well documented pathologically but are rarely diagnosed clinically as the cause of dementia. There would appear to be several reasons why this is so. First, there is an absence of adequate clinicopathologic correlation: In pathologic reports citing morphologic findings the neuropsychologic description is insufficient to permit recognition of the corresponding clinical syndrome. Clinical descriptions are often obtained retrospectively from the information available in hospital files and are not based on a prospective analysis of patients' deficits.

Second, there remain uncertainties regarding the nosologic status of pathologically defined conditions. In cases of frontotemporal cerebral atrophy, for example, only a proportion of affected brains exhibit Pick cells with the characteristic neuronal inclusion bodies (Constantinidis et al., 1974; Jervis, 1971), thus conforming to the classic descriptions of Pick's disease (Alzheimer, 1911). While some authors adhere to these strict pathologic diagnostic criteria (Munoz-Garcia and Ludwin, 1986), others utilize the label Pick's disease more loosely to refer to brains exhibiting a circumscribed frontotemporal atrophy, despite the absence of the characteristic cells and inclusion bodies. Where frontotemporal atrophy has been associated with extensive subcortical gliosis in the absence of Pick cells, the designation Pick's disease B was initially employed (Neumann, 1949), but then replaced by the term progressive subcortical gliosis (Neumann and Cohn, 1967), reflecting the predominant histologic change. Similarly, the term "long duration Creutzfeldt-Jakob disease" has been adopted to refer to brains in which spongiform change in the cerebral cortex is prominent (Neumann and Cohn, 1987). In the syndrome of amyotrophic lateral sclerosis (ALS) and dementia, frontotemporal atrophy, neuronal loss, spongiform change, and gliosis in the cortex have been associated with neuronal cell fallout in the substantia nigra and in the hypoglossal nuclei in the brain stem and the anterior horn cells of the spinal cord (Morita et al., 1987). It remains unclear whether these conditions have a similar pathogenesis and differ only with respect to the predominance of specific pathologic features, or whether they represent distinct entities. Such nosologic uncertainties have undoubtedly hindered the identification of affected patients on clinical and, in particular, psychologic grounds.

A third reason for the lack of clinical recognition of non-Alzheimer forms of cerebral atrophy is the nature of psychologic evaluation itself. Neuropsychologic assessment has in the past relied almost entirely on standardized test batteries, which yield quantitative measures of performance at the expense of analytic and qualitative evaluations directed to the characterization of distinct neuropsychologic syndromes. The psychologic emphasis on measurement of the presence and severity of dementia, rather than on an analysis of reasons underlying failure, no doubt derives from the commonly held assumption that dementia represents a uniform breakdown in function and therefore is not amenable to psychologic characterization and differentiation. A further tacit assumption has been that Alzheimer's disease accounts for virtually all cases of primary cerebral atrophy, so that an accurate diagnosis can be made by exclusion, by eliminating specific causes such as cerebrovascular disease, trauma, and alcohol abuse. A corollary of that assumption is that neuropsychologic detection of the presence of dementia is sufficient: There is no need to identify its features. More recently, attempts have been made to refine the diagnosis of Alzheimer's disease. Yet, even when more sophisticated diagnostic criteria are employed (American Psychiatric Association, 1980; McKhann et al., 1984), incorporating inclusion criteria, these are not based on objective correlates of cerebral disorder, and are sufficiently broad that they would be likely to encompass non-Alzheimer forms of primary cerebral atrophy as well as Alzheimer's disease.

It is the purpose of this chapter to demonstrate that when analytic neuropsychologic evaluation is compared with the results of histologic confirmation during life and measures of regional cerebral blood flow and later with the results of autopsy examination, a substantial minority of patients with primary cerebral atrophy emerge who have a condition that is distinct from Alzheimer's disease, and that is associated with frontotemporal cerebral atrophy. That disorder is called dementia of frontal lobe type (DFT).

THE IDENTIFICATION OF DFT

In a study of 24 patients with cerbral atrophy in the presenium who underwent cerebral biopsy, six (25%) did not have the characteristic pathologic or neurochemical hallmarks of Alzheimer's disease (Neary et al., 1986). Nevertheless, they would have fulfilled the conventionally accepted psychiatric criteria for the diagnosis of Alzheimer's disease. These findings support those of an earlier biopsy study (Sim et al., 1966), in which it was demonstrated that a significant proportion of cases of clinically presumed Alzheimer's disease did not have the pathologic features of that disease. The findings of both studies place into question the widely held view that patients with dementia secondary to primary cerebral atrophy will invariably have Alzheimer's disease.

In the study by Neary and colleagues (1986) of patients with non-Alzheimer pathology, of particular interest were four patients who exhibited a neuropsychologic syndrome that appeared quite distinct from that characteristically seen in Alzheimer's disease. Clinically these patients demonstrated striking and progressive change in personality and social conduct, and while historical reports cited memory failure, the latter appeared secondary to attentional and motivational factors rather than an inability to learn and retain information per se. Visuospatial functions were well preserved. In contrast, strikingly poor performance was elicited on psychologic tests sensitive to frontal lobe dysfunction. The clinical picture was strongly suggestive of disease predominantly affecting the frontal lobes.

Increasing numbers of such patients have been recognized since that time, and the development of single photon emission tomography (SPET) using the radioactive tracer ^{99m}Tc-Hm-PAO has made it possible to provide an objective correlate of the purported frontal lobe abnormalities. In patients with the clinical picture of frontal lobe dementia, brain imaging revealed striking and selective reductions in uptake of tracer in the anterior cerebral hemispheres (Neary et al., 1987). Moreover, imaging effectively distinguished patients with frontal lobe dementia from those with pathologically confirmed and clinically presumed Alzheimer's disease, and from those with progressive supranuclear palsy. In Alzheimer's disese the presence of posterior hemisphere abnormalities was characteristic, and in progressive supranuclear palsy the anterior cerebral distribution suggested a subcortical abnormality.

Several patients with the clinical features of DFT have died and their brains have been examined at autopsy. In all cases the absence of histologic hallmarks of Alzheimer's disease, namely, senile plaques and neurofibrillary tangles, has been confirmed. Pathologic evaluation confirmed the presence of frontotemporal atrophy, but in no case were the specific ballooned cells and neuronal inclusions of Pick's disease noted. Thus, the clinically descriptive designation "dementia of frontal lobe type" (DFT) has been retained in preference to a specific pathologic diagnosis.

The identification of DFT as an entity distinct from Alzheimer's disease is supported by the findings of an independent longitudinal investigation of dementia being carried out in Lund, Sweden. Remarkably similar clinical features have been described by Gustafson (1987). Brain imaging findings using xenon inhalation (Risberg, 1987) have revealed striking abnormalities in regional cerebral blood flow in the frontal regions of the brain, consistent with the frontal lobe abnormalities found using SPET (Neary et al., 1987). Pathologic findings in 20 patients (Brun, 1987) have confirmed frontotemporal atrophy and an absence of Alzheimer pathology. It seems likely, then, that DFT is not a condition that arises idiosyncratically in the North West of England. In the British series the ratio of patients with DFT to Alzheimer's disease approached 1:4 (Neary et al., 1988). Although referral biases, including bias toward a presenile patient population, are likely to influence this figure, it nevertheless suggests that DFT may be more common than is generally realized. The clinical differentiation of DFT from Alzheimer's disease is a prerequisite for future researches into the condition's pathogenesis.

CLINICAL FEATURES OF DFT

Historical Presentation

The history of DFT is characterized by personality change and breakdown in social behavior. Patients become unconcerned and lacking in initiative, and they neglect personal responsibilities, leading to mismanagement of domestic and financial affairs and impaired occupational performance. Medical referral may occur following demotion or dismissal from work. Affect is invariably shallow and emotional empathy with others is lost. Rigidity and inflexibility of thinking and impaired judgment are characteristic. Patients vary, however, with respect to certain behavioral features. Some patients present as overactive, restless, highly distractible, and overtly disinhibited. Their affect may appear fatuous and superficially jocular, and they may exhibit stereotyped behaviors such as repeated singing of a ditty, dancing a favored dance, clapping a favored rhythm, producing puns, or reciting verbatim a repertoire of phrases. Other patients present with apathy, inertia, aspontaneity, and emotional blunting. These disparate behaviors are not entirely dissociable. Overactivity and disinhibition may be most marked in patients when they are in the presence of others: Such patients may display little spontaneous activity when left to their own devices. Moreover, overactive patients may show increasing inertia as the disease progresses. Nevertheless, differences in behavioral pattern cannot be attributed entirely to environmental circumstance or time course of illness, and patients tend to polarize in the early and middle stages of disease into the overactive, disinhibited and the underactive, apathetic types.

Neglect of personal hygiene is common in all patients, and incontinence associated with lack of concern may occur. However, hygiene and dress may themselves be the source of stereotyped, compulsive behaviors, which may appear internally contradictory. For example, one patient insisted on repeatedly changing into fresh clothes but refused to wash. Another would wash his hands dozens of times in succession, after visiting the lavatory, or after coming into the house from the garden, but could not be persuaded to take a bath. The compulsive acts are not preceded by evident feelings of anxiety and do not appear to relieve tension. However, if rituals are interrupted or prevented by others then aggression may be provoked. No rational or symbolic meaning can be assigned to stereotypes by the patients or relatives and they bear no obvious relationship to previous personality or proclivities. Toileting may be associated with other idiosyncratic behaviors. One patient would throw all available bathroom objects into the toilet bowl and attempt to flush them away. Another would hoard toilet paper in drawers and in the garden shed.

Hypochondriasis with bizarre somatic complaints may occur, reflecting the patient's apparent obsession with a particular organ of the body. One patient complained constantly of pain in the perineum; another wept profusely while describing her symptom of dry eyes. Such complaints may lead to multiple physical investigations, which invariably yield negative results.

Changes in eating habits are common, and may be an early symptom. Gluttony and especially a relish for sweet foods may lead relatives to ration food to prevent obesity. Excessive and indiscriminate eating may be superseded in middle to late disease by selective food fads, usually involving the favored sweet foods. For example, one patient would eat one brand of chocolate biscuit and refuse all else; another would accept only one brand of peppermints. A total refusal to eat has also been observed in inert patients. Whether this reflects behavioral negativism, or rather a failure to initiate the appropriate motor actions for eating is unclear. Hyperoral traits, involving the mouthing of inedible objects, are observed in some patients, although these would appear to be a relatively late feature.

Changes in sleep pattern may occur, particularly in patients exhibiting the clinical picture of apathy and inertia. Such patients may display increased somnolence, sleeping up to 18 hours a day.

Restlessness in overactive patients may lead to wandering, and patients may walk many miles in a day. In general, patients maintain a fixed route and do not become lost. A fixed routine also characterizes the rest of their daily schedule. Patients frequently clock-watch and will carry out a particular activity at exactly the same time on each day. If their fixed daily routine is not adhered to, irritability and aggression may ensue.

All patients lack insight into their altered character and social misconduct. Despite petty moral and sexual transgressions, major social conflict and criminal offenses are infrequent. Lack of initiative and foresight might be relevant factors in that regard.

Features of personality and behavioral change are prominent presenting symptoms and outweigh specific cognitive symptoms. Reports of memory disturbance are common, although this is frequently thought by relatives to be idiosyncratic and selective in the patient's favor. Speech abnormalities are not prominent early symptoms, although gradual reduction in speech output is noted as the disease progresses, culminating finally in mutism. In addition, incorrect word usage may sometimes be observed. Symptoms of visuospatial disorientation are notably absent. Even in advanced disease patients may negotiate and locate their surroundings accurately, and may carry out stereotyped activities such as repeated careful folding of a handkerchief, which indicate preserved spatial appreciation.

Neuropsychologic Evaluation

Conduct

Economy of mental effort and unconcern regarding accuracy of responses characterizes test performances. Some negativism and lack of compliance occur. However, cooperation and correct answers can often be elicited by cajoling and encouragement. In some patients responses are impulsive and tasks readily abandoned, whereas other patients are slow, inert, and perseverative at the level of single actions.

Language
Spontaneous conversation is characteristically reduced, and responses are brief and unelaborated. Stereotyped remarks may occur and contrast with the prevailing taciturnity. Echolalia and perseveration of responses are common, particularly in the middle stages of disease. Hypophonia and dysprosody may be evident, especially in patients exhibiting a picture of apathy and inertia. However, in overactive, disinhibited patients a press of speech is sometimes noted, with responses being inappropriately constrained by the question. Utterances may represent a stereotyped iteration of a repertoire of overlearned phrases, which is produced essentially verbatim on each occasion. The patient's repertoire of utterances may gradually decrease as the disease progresses. A failure to grasp instructions and irrelevant responses to questions may give the impression of a comprehension impairment. A primary linguistic impairment may not, however, be borne out by specific tests of syntax and semantic understanding, and impairment may reflect concreteness of thinking or inattention to the task. In some patients language error is noted in the form of verbal paraphasias and substitution of generic terms for precise substantives. The extent to which reduced language usage results from linguistic breakdown per se, or is secondary to increasing aspontaneity and a fundamental failure to engage in any mental activity is often difficult to determine. It is suggested, however, that linguistic involvement may be more common in disinhibited, overactive patients than in inert, apathetic individuals. In all patients mutism prevails in the late stage of disease.

Visuospatial Abilities
Behavioral abnormalities, inattention, lack of concerted strategies for carrying out tasks, impersistence, and perseveration compromise performance on visuospatial tasks. Nevertheless, qualitative evaluation of patients' performance suggests an absence of primary visuospatial deficits. Patients can localize objects in space, and their manipulation of objects and clothing indicates preserved spatial orientation. Drawings and block constructions reveal preservation of spatial configuration and the relationship between elements. Spatial disability appears to remain absent even in patients with advanced disease.

Memory
Patients are typically well oriented in place and time, can provide information about current and past autobiographic events, and do not appear clinically amnesic. However, characteristically they perform poorly on formal tests of memory, both recall and recognition. The discrepancy between the clinical impression of well-preserved memory and the demonstrated impairment on formal tests suggests that these patients' amnesia may result from a strategic failure to utilize their memory effectively rather than an inability to acquire and retain new information per se. Relatives' reports of variable and eccentric memory in these patients would seem consistent with this interpretation.

Regulation

Qualitative evaluation of patients' performance suggests poor selective attention, poor use of strategy to accomplish tasks, and poor self-monitoring, so that patients are unaware of errors and do not notice anomalies between their performance and the intended goal. Profound abnormalities in regulatory aspects of cognitive functioning are noted in patients' performance on a variety of tasks, sensitive to frontal lobe dysfunction, which make demands on abstraction, planning, and mental flexibility. Impaired powers of abstraction are noted on card sorting (Nelson, 1976) and block sorting (De Renzi et al., 1966) tasks, and a high proportion of perseverative errors are characteristic. In a picture arrangement test patients typically make no attempt to integrate pictures into a logical sequence and will describe individual cards without reference to an overall narrative. Cards may be moved minimally or even left in their original positions. Verbal fluency is reduced: Patients may abandon the task rapidly, produce items eccentrically, with no systematic strategy for production, and may violate the category or letter instruction. Similarly, design fluency (Jones-Gotman and Milner, 1977) is characterized by violation of the rule that designs should be constructed from four lines, concreteness of responses, and perseveration of a single idea. On a task based on the "20 question" principle (Becker et al., 1986) in which a patient is required to identify a "target" picture from an array, by asking questions yielding a yes or no response, patients show a marked failure to adopt a strategy for eliminating alternatives. They will typically formulate questions pertaining to a single picture only rather than a series of pictures, and they fail to use information gained from one question to influence succeeding ones.

Motor Skills

Patients have normal powers of manipulation, can use feeding implements, dress themselves, and carry out complex sequential acts such as lighting a cigarette until late in the disease. Nevertheless, deficits in motor behavior do occur and are most severe in patients presenting with apathy and inertia. In such patients there may be marked motor perseveration: Patients may perseverate at the level of a completed sequence of actions, such as by writing a complete sentence over and over again, or at the level of a single motor act, such as by reproducing a single pencil stroke. While high level perseveration (complete motor program) tends to be superseded by low level perseveration (single motor act) as the disease progresses, the level at which perseveration occurs would not appear to be entirely determined by time course of disease. Different levels of perseveration may be noted in a single patient, or one type may characterize a patient, apparently regardless of disease severity.

In inert, apathetic patients, failure frequently occurs on motor programming tasks, such as in producing a sequence of three hand postures (slap, fist, cut), alternating hand positions, or tapping of motor rhythms. Such tasks involve implementation of a new motor program, rather than production of an overlearned sequence of actions, such as would be involved, for example, in lighting a cigarette.

There may be a discrepancy between verbal and manual behavior. A patient may read aloud correctly a written instruction, such as "Close your eyes", may acknowledge understanding it, and yet may make no attempt to carry out the motor action required. In the late stages of disease, while the patient may engage in some motor activity spontaneously, it may be impossible to elicit any motor response to verbal command.

Standard Tests of Intelligence

In the early stages scores on formal intelligence tests may be in the normal range. With progression of disease, scores decline, reflecting lack of mental application to tasks. The verbal-performance scale discrepancy noted in Alzheimer's disease, namely, greater decline on performance tests, is not present in DFT.

Neurologic Signs

Patients remain remarkably free from neurologic signs, even in the presence of gross behavioral and cognitive change. Signs are generally limited to the emergence of primitive reflexes, such as grasping, pouting, sucking, and extensor plantar responses.

Investigations

Electroencephalography is normal and remains so in advanced disease. Computed tomography reveals cerebral atrophy. Sometimes a frontotemporal emphasis is recorded but this is not invariable. Single photon emission computerized tomography reveals a selective reduction in uptake of tracer in the anterior cerebral hemispheres.

COMPARISON OF DFT WITH ALZHEIMER'S DISEASE

Clinical differences between DFT and Alzheimer's disease are summarized in Table 16–1. Historically, the major difference lies in the prominence of behavioral and personality change in DFT, contrasting with that of cognitive disorder in Alzheimer's disease. In the latter, social graces are well preserved.

Qualitative differences in pattern of performance are evident on neuropsychologic testing. In Alzheimer's disease, speech becomes hesitant, reflecting word finding difficulty, and patients lose their train of thought. Information content may be limited to social platitudes. Logoclonia develops. The features of concreteness of thinking, economy of effort, echolalia, perseveration, and verbal stereotypies, characteristic of DFT are not features of Alzheimer's disease. In Alzheimer's disease spatial disorientation is an early feature, contrasting with preserved spatial abilities in DFT. The variable memory loss in DFT with preservation of day-to-day memory contrasts with the severe pervasive amnesia of Alzheimer's disease with disorientation, inability to learn, and loss of significant personal and general knowledge.

The desultory performance and lack of concern seen in DFT patients contrasts with the high level of persistence and concern regarding the accuracy of their responses common to patients with Alzheimer's disease.

Table 16–1   Clinical Differences Between Dementia of Frontal Lobe Type and Alzheimer's Disease

	DFT	Alzheimer's disease
History	Personality change	Memory loss
	Social breakdown	Spatial disorientation
		Language failure
Psychological disorder		
Language	Concrete	Aphasia
	Echolalia	Logoclonia
	Perseveration	
	Stereotypes	
Spatial function	Preserved	Disorientation
Memory	Variable	Consistent
		Pervasive
Conduct	Low mental effort	High mental effort
	Unconcerned	Concerned
	Inappropriate	Appropriate
Neurologic signs	Primitive reflexes	Akinesia
		Rigidity
		Myoclonus
EEG	Normal	Slow waves
SPET	Anterior cerebral abnormality	Posterior cerebral abnormality

On neurologic examination patients with Alzheimer's disease develop progressive akinesia and rigidity of the limbs with myoclonic jerking. These features are absent in DFT, where neurologic signs are limited to the presence of primitive reflexes.

In Alzheimer's disease the electroencephalogram shows progressive slowing of wave forms with advancing disease, while in DFT it remains normal. On single photon emission computerized tomography, the presence of abnormalities in the posterior cerebral hemispheres is characteristic of Alzheimer's disease, while in DFT abnormalites are limited to anterior regions.

DEMOGRAPHIC FEATURES OF DFT

DFT appears to be a disease predominantly of the presenium, occurring after the age of 40. There is not a notable female proponderance as occurs in Alzheimer's disease. A family history of dementia in a first-degree relative occurs in approximately half of cases (Gustafson, 1987; Neary et al., 1988). The pattern of inheritance in three extended families with DFT suggests the action of an autosomal dominant gene. Thus, DFT appears to be a more strongly familial condition than is Alzheimer's disease.

The length of illness appears highly variable. In some patients a rapid decline is noted over 2 or 3 years, while in others only minimal change can be detected over a decade. In pathologically verified cases a mean duration of 8 years has been cited (Gustafson, 1987), with a range from 3 to 17 years. It would seem likely that, in general, life expectancy is longer than in Alzheimer's disease, since the dearth of physical signs render patients less vulnerable to intercurrent infection. There is no evident relationship between the rate of disease progression and the pattern of behavioral disorder (i.e., overactive, disinhibited versus aspontaneous, apathetic).

THE PATHOLOGY OF DFT

The four cases who had undergone cerebral biopsy proved on histologic examination to have nonspecific and non-Alzheimer pathology. Three further cases have subsequently come to autopsy examination, and the pathologic changes were closely similar in all three brains. Macroscopically there was gross atrophy of the frontal and temporal lobes. In the frontal lobes the inferior and middle frontal gyri and cingulate gyrus were particularly affected, whereas superior frontal, as well as parietal and occipital cortices, were much less severely atrophied. The inferior, middle, and superior temporal gyri were all affected more severely at the anterior pole. The brain stem and cerebellum appeared grossly normal. The lateral ventricles were grossly dilated with gross atrophy of the caudate nucleus and the putamen. The thalamus and globus pallidus appeared normal. The amygdala and hippocampus were moderately atrophied. The corpus callosum was markedly thinned especially anteriorly. The substantia nigra was well pigmented. Cerebellum and dentate nucleus appeared normal. The major cerebral arteries and those of the Circle of Willis were free from atheroma, and no infarction of the brain was observed.

On microscopic examination the frontal, anterior temporal, insular, and parietal regions revealed severe cortical atrophy characterized histologically by shrinkage and loss of pyramidal neurons particularly at layer III and to a lesser extent at layer V. There was pronounced accompanying status spongiosus and mild astrocytosis in layers I–III, with prominent astrocytosis at the gray/white matter boundary. There was considerable loss of myelin from underlying white matter. Within temporal cortex the inferior and middle temporal gyri were most severely affected, the superior temporal gyrus being only mildly involved. The occipital (calcarine) gyrus was unaffected. The claustrum and caudate nucleus showed similar neuronal atrophy, spongiform change, and gliosis. The hippocampus (Ammon's horn and subicular areas) appeared histologically normal as did the amygdala, although adjacent areas of temporal cortex showed the same histologic appearance as anterior temporal regions. There was also severe loss of cells from the nucleus of Meynert. The globus pallidus, cerebellum, and dentate nucleus appeared normal.

Senile plaques and neurofibrillary tangles were completely absent from the brain and there was no evidence of intraneuronal inclusions of the type associated with Pick's disease. In no areas of the brain were there any abnormalities of the larger extraparenchymal or the smaller intraparenchymal arteries. Similar pathologic changes have been described by Brun (1987).

Understanding of the relationship between DFT and other neurodegenerative disease might throw light on the conditon's pathogenesis. An associative link between DFT and motor neuron disease has been identified and described by Neary and colleagues (1990).

DEMENTIA OF FRONTAL LOBE TYPE AND MOTOR NEURON DISEASE

Four patients who presented with a rapidly progressive dementia of frontal lobe type subsequently developed motor neuron disease. In all four patients personality change with disordered personal and social conduct and stereotyped behaviors were prominent. Reduced verbal output was superseded rapidly by mutism. Profound abnormalities were evident on tests sensitive to frontal lobe dysfunction. Visuospatial abilities were preserved. On neurologic examination, in addition to the finding of primitive reflexes and hyperreflexia, was the presence of widespread muscular fasciculations in the tongue, limbs, and trunk. With progression of disease, muscular wasting increased and bulbar palsy emerged, with dysarthria, dysphagia, and ineffective coughing. None of the patients developed a spastic increase in tone of the limbs. The electroencephalogram in all four patients was normal and remained so on serial investigation. Electrophysiologic studies of neuromuscular function revealed normal nerve conduction studies, multifocal muscular fasciculation, reduced muscular firing rates, and giant motor units, compatible with widespread muscular denervation due to anterior horn cell death.

Three of the four patients died within 3 years of disease onset, and their brains have been examined at autopsy. Each showed frontotemporal cerebral atrophy. On histologic examination three characteristic changes were found: Large neuronal cell loss in the cerebral cortex, spongiform change, and astrocytic gliosis in the cerebral cortex and subcortex. The changes were most marked in the superior and middle frontal gyri and the anterior portion of the cingulate gyrus. Layer III of the cerebral cortex was predominantly affected. In the brain stem there was loss of large pigmented neurons in the substantia nigra with astrocytic gliosis. The hypoglossal nuclei showed extensive cell loss. The cerebellum was normal. In the spinal cord there was marked anterior horn cell loss in the ventral horns of the gray matter. Some preserved neurons contained eosinophilic inclusion bodies. The latter did not stain for ubiquitin. In contrast to the severe loss of cells in the hypoglossal nuclei and anterior columns there was minimal reduction of Betz cells in the motor cortex and little evidence of degeneration of the corticobulbar and corticospinal tracts. There was no evidence of neurofibrillary tangles, senile plaques, or Pick cells. The nature and distribution of pathologic changes are closely similar to those of "dementia and ALS," described by Japanese workers (Morita et al., 1987). Lack of clinical detail from that study prevents a comparison of the respective neuropsychologic syndromes.

A comparison of the pathologic changes of DFT, with and without motor neuron disease, indicates that where DFT is associated with motor neuron disease the frontal and temporal lobes are more selectively affected and the intensity of the pathologic process, especially astrocytic gliosis, is less severe. In cases without motor neuron disease the substantia nigra is spared. The difference in topographic distribution and severity of pathology may reflect the more rapid course of disease to death in patients with motor neuron disease.

CONCLUSIONS

Dementia of frontal lobe type is a degenerative condition that is distinct, both clincially and pathologically, from Alzheimer's disease. It is a disease that is prominent in the presenium, and appears to be under genetic influence, probably through an autosomal dominant mechanism, and to have an association with motor neuron disease. It is characterized by alterations in personality and behavior, and impairment in regulatory aspects of cognition, indicative of disordered frontal lobe function. The clinical picture is not, however, entirely homogeneous. The clinical picture of overactivity and disinhibition resembles that associated with orbitofrontal lesions (Cummings, 1985), while the picture of apathy and inertia is strongly reminiscent of behaviors associated with frontal convexity lesions. Differences in patterns of disorder might then reflect differences in topographic distribution of pathologic change, the diverse clinical manifestations having the same pathogenesis. Alternatively, dementia of frontal lobe type might encompass distinct subtypes.

It is worth speculating in this regard on the relationship between dementia of frontal lobe type and Pick's disease. In a series of 20 patients with frontal lobe degeneration (Brun, 1987) four showed at autopsy pathology consistent with the classic descriptions of Pick's disease, while the remaining 16 differed from that description in terms of a lack of circumscribed knife-blade–type of atrophy and an absence of Pick cells with inclusions and inflated cells. Possible clinical distinctions between patients who conform to Pick's disease and those who do not have been postulated (Gustafson, 1987): It is suggested that symptoms of disinhibiton, oral/dietary hyperactivity, and echolalia may be more common in Pick's disease. Such distinctions must remain circumspect, given the relatively small numbers of patients for comparison. Moreover, in investigations by Neary and colleagues (1988) changes in eating pattern and echolalia were commonly found. Yet, no brain containing Pick cells and bodies has at yet come to autopsy. It remains to be seen whether patients who display the picture of overactivity and disinhibition prove more likely to show Pick pathology than inert, apathetic patients.

In considering the status of Pick's disease it is important to recognize that the Pick bodies that characterize the cells represent degraded protein material without known etiologic significance. It may be fruitful to regard Pick's disease merely as a form of lobar atrophy in which these characteristic inclusion bodies are present within a proportion of neurons. The new pathologic techniques of immunocytochemistry may shed light on the nature of inclusion bodies in Pick's disease and their relationship to the other pathologic changes seen in that disorder and in other forms of lobar atrophy.

DFT accounts for a significant minority of patients with primary cerebral atrophy, yet has been largely unrecognized. Nosologic disagreements, lack of clinicopathologic correlation, and nonanalytic neuropsychologic evaluations have been cited in the introduction as contributory factors. Features of the disorder itself may be of relevance. A frontal lobe syndrome, manifesting in patients in whom there is evidence of alcohol abuse, may be attributed to the effects of alcohol. Yet, excessive alcohol intake may itself be a symptom of patients with DFT, representing one aspect of their change in eating and drinking habits. It is not uncommon for the dementia of an affected relative to be ascribed also to alcoholism, reinforcing the clinical error. A careful history ought to determine whether alcohol abuse preceded or was subsequent to the onset of illness.

The personality change, overactivity, apathy, hypochondriasis, ritualistic behavior, and concreteness of language, symptomatic of DFT patients, may invite a variety of psychiatric diagnoses. The absence of physical signs, normal electroencephalogram, and the ability of patients in the early stages of illness to achieve normal scores on standardized intelligence tests would reinforce such a nonorganic diagnosis. In elderly patients DFT may be thought to be a form of withdrawal or eccentricity. The designation "Diogenes' syndrome" may have been inappropriately appended to patients with DFT.

While taking account of these clinical vagaries, probably the most important force militating against recognition of distinct neuropsychologic syndromes is the widely held misconception concerning dementia. The latter is commonly thought to denote an overall failure of intelligence and memory, manifesting as a disorder of the brain that affects all areas unselectively. To a great extent this formulation owes its legitimacy to the conceptual inheritance of "IQ psychology," in which a measure of "intelligence" is construed as representing the overall power of the mind. Such a theoretic stance inevitably places emphasis on the pass or failure rate on cognitive tasks, and ignores the specific mechanisms underlying pass or failure. Patients with DFT will, with progression of disease, perform poorly on intelligence tests, and will hence conform to the classification of "generalized intellectual failure." Yet, a qualitative analysis of reasons for failure highlights quite specific areas of deficit, which are totally distinct from those seen in Alzheimer's disease. The emergence of DFT as a distinct neuropsychologic syndrome highlights the need for a qualitative and analytic approach to the study of degenerative brain disease. It is by the adoption of a multihierarchic evaluation of the cerebral atrophies and the drawing of correlations between the clinical, neuropsychologic, neurophysiologic, pathologic, genetic, and demographic levels of description that progress can be made into the understanding of dementia and the cerebral atrophies.

ACKNOWLEDGMENTS

We thank Dr. D.M.A. Mann for pathologic analyses.

REFERENCES

Alzheimer A. Über eigenartige Krankheitsfälle des späteren Alters. Z Gesamte Neurol Psychiatr 4:356–385, 1911.

American Psychiatric Association: Diagnostic and Statistical Manual of Mental Disorders, 3rd Edition. Washington: American Psychiatric Associaton, 1980.

Becker JT, Butters N, Rivoira P, Miliotis P. Asking the right questions: problem solving in male alcoholics and male alcoholics with Korsakoff's syndrome. Alcoholism: Clin Exp Research 10:641–646, 1986.

Brun A. Frontal lobe degeneration of non-Alzheimer type. 1. Neuropathology. Arch Gerontol Geriatr 6:193–208, 1987.

Constantinidis J, Richard J, Tissot R. Pick's disease. Histological and clinical corelations. Eur Neurol 11:208–217, 1974.

Cummings JL. Clinical Neuropsychiatry. Orlando, FL: Grune & Stratton, 1985, pp. 57–59.

De Renzi E, Faglioni P, Savoiardo M, Vignolo LA. The influence of aphasia and of the hemisphere side of the cerebral lesion on abstract thinking. Cortex 2:399–420, 1966.

Gustafson L. Frontal lobe degeneration of non-Alzheimer type. II. Clinical picture and differential diagnosis. Arch Gerontol Geriatr 6:209–223, 1987.

Jervis GA. Pick's disease. In Minkler J (ed), Pathology of the Nervous System. Vol 2. New York: McGraw-Hill, 1971, pp. 1395–1401.

Jones-Gotman M, Milner B. Design fluency: The invention of nonsense drawings after focal cortical lesions. Neuropsychologia 15:653–674, 1977.

McKhann G, Drachman D, Folstein M, Katzman R, Price D, Stadlan EM. Clinical diagnosis of Alzheimer's disease: Report of the NINCDS-ADRDA Work Group under the auspices of Department of Health and Human Services Task Force on Alzheimer's disease. Neurology 34:939–944, 1984.

Morita K, Kaiya H, Ikeda T, Namba M. Presenile dementia combined with amyotrophy: A review of 34 Japanese cases. Arch Gerontol Geriatr 6:263–277, 1987.

Munoz-Garcia D, Ludwin SK. Clinicopathological studies of some non-Alzheimer dementing diseases. Can J Neurol Sci 13:483–489, 1986.

Neary D, Snowden JS, Bowen DM, Sims NR, Mann DMA, Benton JS, Northen B, Yates PO, Davison AN. Neuropsychological syndromes in presenile dementia due to cerebral atrophy. J Neurol Neurosurg Psychiatry 49:163–174, 1986.

Neary D, Snowden JS, Mann DMA, Northen B, Goulding PJ, Macdermott N. Frontal lobe dementia and motor neurone disease. J Neurol Neurosurg Psychiatry 53:23–32, 1990.

Neary D, Snowden JS, Northen B, Goulding P. Dementia of frontal lobe type. J Neurol Neurosurg Psychiatry 51:353–361, 1988.

Neary D, Snowden JS, Shields RA, Burjan AWI, Northen B, Macdermott N, Prescott MC, Testa HJ. Single photon emission tomography using 99m Tc-AM-PM in the investigation of dementia. J Neurol Neurosurg Psychiatry 50:1101–1109, 1987.

Nelson HE. A modified card sorting test sensitive to frontal lobe defects. Cortex 12:313–324, 1976.

Neumann MA. Pick's disease. J Neuropathol Exp Neurol 8:255, 1949.

Neuman MA, Cohn R. Progressive subcortical gliosis, a rare form of presenile dementia. Brain 90:405–418, 1967.

Neumann MA, Cohn R. Long duration Jakob-Creutzfeldt disease. Arch Gerontol Geriatr 6:279–287, 1987.

Risberg J. Frontal lobe degeneration of non-Alzheimer type. III. Regional cerebral blood flow. Arch Gerontol Geriatr 6:225–233, 1987.

Sim M, Turner E, Smith WT, Cerebral biopsy in the investigation of presenile dementia. 1. Clinical aspects. Br J Psychiatry 112:119–125, 1966.

17

The Contribution of Frontal Lobe Lesions to the Neurobehavioral Outcome of Closed Head Injury

HARVEY S. LEVIN,
FELICIA C. GOLDSTEIN,
DAVID H. WILLIAMS,
AND HOWARD M. EISENBERG

NEUROPATHOLOGY

The physical proximity of the sphenoid wing to the orbitofrontal region and marked shearing effects in this area (Holbourn, 1943) predispose the frontal lobes to focal lesions after closed head injury (CHI). Utilizing a contusion index that reflects the size and depth of contusions, Adams and coworkers (1980) studied the brains of 151 patients who sustained fatal injuries. As depicted in Table 17–1, the index values were largest for the frontal lobes, followed closely by the temporal lobes. Although caution is advised in extrapolating from these necropsy findings to less severe CHI, investigators and clinicians have implicated frontal lobe damage as an etiologic factor in neurobehavioral sequelae. In this chapter, the results of neuroimaging in patients sustaining nonfatal injuries are reviewed in relation to the neuropsychologic findings.

Magnetic resonance imaging (MRI) has confirmed that the frontal region is the most common location of focal lesions after mild to moderate CHI (Levin et al., 1987). Figure 17–1 shows the neuroanatomic distribution of focal hyperintensities in a series of 20 patients in the Galveston study who underwent MRI within 1 week after injury that produced mild to moderate impaired consciousness. It is seen that frontal lesions in the parenchyma predominated. Although the resolution of these hyperintensities over 1 to 3 months suggests that focal edema may have been the primary (or at least secondary) mechanism, this interpretation awaits corroboration. Positron emission tomography (PET) scanning of a small series of CHI patients has implicated zones of frontal hypometabolism extending beyond the boundaries of morphologic lesions detected by CT or MRI (Langfitt et al., 1986). However, support for this findng also awaits metabolic

Table 17–1 Neuroanatomic Distribution of Contusions in 151 Fatal Cases of Head Injury as Reflected by the Mean Contusion Index (Extent of Lesion Multiplied by the Depth of Lesion)

Locator	MCI
Frontal lobe	5.7
Temporal lobe	5.4
Sylvian fissure	2.7
Occipital lobe	1.2
Parietal lobe	0.7
Cerebellum	0.9
MCI for cerebral hemispheres	15.7
MTCI (whole brain)	16.6

Reproduced from Adams et al., J Clin Pathol 33:1132–1145, 1980.

imaging of a larger series of patients who have undergone concurrent neurobehavioral assessment of frontal lobe functions. Cognitive activation tasks during PET scanning could further elucidate hypofrontal metabolism following head injury (see Weinberger, this volume).

METHODOLOGIC PROBLEMS IN NEUROBEHAVIORAL STUDIES

The extant literature includes studies on groups of CHI patients in whom neuropsychologic tests of purported frontal lobe function have revealed abnormal

Figure 17–1 Neuroanatomic distribution of focal areas of hyperintensity on T_2-weighted magnetic resonance images in patients who sustained mild to moderate closed head injury. (From Levin et al., 1987, with permission.)

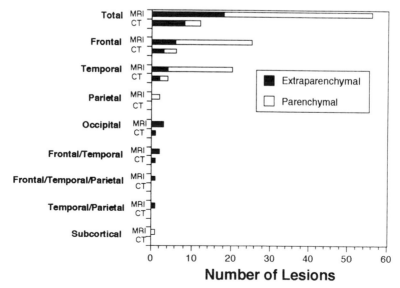

findings (Shallice, 1982; Stuss et al., 1985; Zatorre and McEntee, 1983). Although several reports have documented deficits in CHI patients consistent with widely held concepts of frontal lobe injury, this evidence is largely conjectural because neuroimaging was unavailable or inadequate to document the presumed focal lesions. A potential problem in evaluating the neurobehavioral consequences of traumatic frontal lesions is the frequent presence of concomitant extrafrontal lesions. Localization of focal intracranial abnormalities after CHI is complicated further by the dynamic process in which lesions detected by acute CT (i.e., high or mixed density) frequently resolve (or are surgically evacuated) while discrete areas of increased intensity may evolve on MRI (e.g., degenerative changes in the white matter presumably due to gliosis) at various intervals after injury.

Consequently, detection of a frontal lobe lesion is probably dependent on both the postinjury interval and the type of neuroimaging. This surmise is illustrated in the case study by Levin and colleagues (1985), who found occult bifrontal, parasagittal lesions primarily involving the white matter on MRI in a young woman injured 5 years previously whose acute and follow-up CT scans were consistent with diffuse injury (Fig. 17–2). This patient's MRI also revealed bilateral lesions in the occipitotemporal white matter that were not detected by CT. Another dynamic factor (and potential confounder) in morphologic imaging after CHI is cerebral atrophy that is reflected primarily by lateral ventricular enlargement and less frequently by sulcal prominence (Levin et al., 1981). Levin and coworkers (1981) found lateral ventricular enlargement in about two-thirds of survivors of moderate to severe CHI and showed that this sequel was related to residual cognitive and memory impairment. Notwithstanding the aforementioned problems, CHI does provide an opportunity to investigate the neurobehavioral effects of focal brain lesions in previously intact young patients.

Our intent in raising questions about the classification of frontal lesions is to provoke discussion about the issues that confront investigators rather than to advocate firm guidelines (which would be premature at this point). Strategies might include reporting on a specific type of lesion (e.g., intracerebral hematoma) of minimum size (Levin et al., 1989). In this chapter we summarize previous neurobehavioral research on deficits related to putative frontal lobe injury. In addition, we report the results of a preliminary study in which performance on various tests purported to assess frontal lobe functioning was analyzed according to localization of lesion.

NEUROPSYCHOLOGIC STUDIES IMPLICATING FRONTAL DYSFUNCTION AFTER HEAD INJURY

Language

The literature concerning the lateralization and regional localization of frontal lesions and communication disorders was reviewed by Alexander and associates (1989). However, most of the published studies heretofore have been based on patients with cerebrovascular disease or tumor rather than head injury. Studies

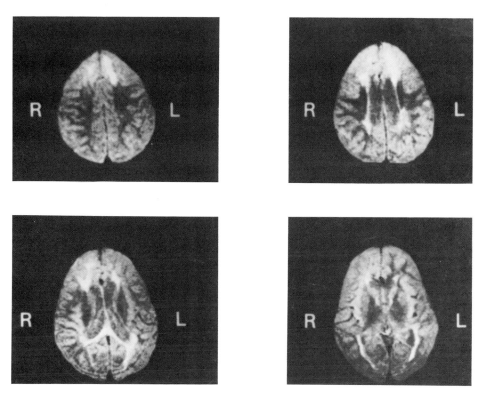

Figure 17–2 Magnetic resonance image showing bifrontal parasagittal lesions primarily involving the white matter in a 24-year-old woman who had sustained a severe closed head injury 5 years previously. Serial computed tomographic scans initially revealed diffuse brain swelling followed by atrophy without evidence of the bifrontal lesions shown here. Occipitotemporal white matter lesions were also visualized by magnetic resonance. (From Levin et al., 1985, with permission.)

of patients with focal hemispheric lesions arising from vascular disease and tumor have demonstrated a relationship between a left anterior site and diminished verbal fluency on a timed test of generating words beginning with designated letters (Benton, 1968). Decreased verbal fluency has been a consistent finding in studies that administered standardized aphasia tests to adults during the initial hospitalization and rehabilitation for moderate to severe CHI (Levin et al., 1976; Sarno, 1980). Although these investigators found no relationship between localization of brain lesion and speech fluency, the studies focused on consecutive admissions (containing insufficient numbers of patients with focal lesions) rather than groups defined by CT scan findings. Moreover, it is likely that MRI could have identified frontal lesions that were undetected by CT in these studies.

Descriptive studies have characterized the discourse of patients surviving severe CHI as tangential with frequent intrusions (Levin et al., 1982). Quantitative linguistic techniques for evaluating narrative discourse have been developed that could elucidate expressive disturbance in frontal lobe patients who exhibit no obvious aphasia. In a study of 21 patients with frontal lesions arising from diverse etiologies (including six head injuries), Novoa and Ardila (1987) evaluated the patients' ability to respond to open-ended questions, to elaborate on an oral composition, and to describe a picture. These investigators found a lack of concordance between the responses of left frontal patients and the questions put forward by the examiners. Moreover, the responses of the left frontal patients were less interpretative. The speech of left frontal patients was frequently contaminated by perseveration and confabulation as compared to the right frontal and control subjects. Overall the amount of spontaneous speech production was reduced in the left frontal patients. Future studies could elucidate the relationship between site of frontal lesion (i.e., dorsolateral versus orbitofrontal) and features of abnormal discourse such as lack of cohesion and reduced capacity for interpretative statements such as deriving a moral from a story (Ulatowska et al., 1983). Inclusion of a group of patients with extrafrontal lesions would provide more compelling evidence for the specificity of frontal injury in producing adverse effects on discourse.

Interference Effects on Attention and Memory

As described in the chapter by Stuss in this volume, studies of other etiologies of frontal lobe damage have implicated increased vulnerability to interference effects on memory and attention. In view of these findings, Stuss and coworkers (1985) postulated that patients who had attained an apparently good recovery from CHI would nevertheless show greater susceptibility to interference with short-term memory produced by a distractor task. Utilizing the Brown-Petersen technique of recalling triads of words, these investigators found that short-term memory under a condition of interference (i.e., counting backwards during the retention interval) was impaired in the head-injured patients relative to a control group. In the absence of group differences on conventional tests of memory and intellectual function that did not involve distraction, Stuss and associates postulated that CHI results in a specific susceptibility to interference. Although the investigators implicated frontal lobe lesions in the increased vulnerability of their head-injured patients to interference, no neuroimaging data were presented to support this interpretation.

Semantic Organization of Memory

Frontal amnesia was described by Baddeley and Wilson (1988) as a dysexecutive syndrome characterized by difficulty in establishing an appropriate retrieval strategy, which was most apparent on tasks that involved semantic processing. These investigators studied a 42-year-old man 6 months after he had sustained a severe CHI complicated by bifrontal lesions. In addition to performing poorly on standard memory tests such as prose recall, this patient had numerous perseverative errors on the Wisconsin Card Sorting Test and he had reduced verbal fluency, features that are widely interpreted as consistent with frontal lobe dysfunction. Baddeley and Wilson's patient also exhibited impaired performance on tasks that involved retrieval of exemplars from a specific category or deciding whether words presented in pairs shared a common category. Moreover, the patient's semantic processing was slow, as reflected by his latencies in verifying sentences such as "rabbits can fly." Baddeley and Wilson inferred that their patient had difficulty in establishing and operating a retrieval strategy rather than an absence of semantic memory.

Converging evidence for inefficient semantic memory performance following frontal lobe injury was reported in a case study by Zatorre and McEntee (1983) who described a 33-year-old man who had sustained a severe CHI with bifrontotemporal contusions 19 years previously. CT at the time of the study revealed focal damage in both frontal lobes, the right temporal lobe, and right basal ganglia. These investigators used the release from proactive interference task in which recall of word triads derived from the same category deteriorates over trials. In contrast to the enhanced recall typically found in normal subjects when the taxonomic category of the words is changed after several trials, this patient's performance did not improve after a shift from articles of clothing to tools. Moreover, this patient's memory also showed no facilitation by semantic processing of words as compared to answering questions about their physical features. Zatorre and McEntee attributed their patient's difficulty in semantic encoding to his frontal lobe lesions and suggested that similar findings in amnesic patients with alcoholic Korsakoff's syndrome reflect frontal dysfunction. However, the extrafrontal lesions in this patient preclude an unambiguous interpretation of the findings.

Further support for the thesis that frontal lobe lesions reduce sensitivity to semantic features of verbal memory was provided by Freedman and Cermak (1986) who studied four amnesic frontal patients and three frontal patients who had normal memory (five of the seven patients had sustained closed or penetrating head injury). Although these investigators confirmed that the amnesic frontal patients failed to exhibit release from proactive interference, there was no comparison group of amnesic patients without frontal lesions. Moreover, failure to release from proactive interference was confined to patients with impaired memory, whereas nonamnesic patients exhibited the effect despite the presence of a frontal lesion.

In contrast to the aforementioned studies employing the release from proactive interference task, Goldstein and colleageus (1989) found preserved sensitivity to semantic features in chronic survivors of severe CHI. The head-injured patients displayed release from proactive interference, which was comparable with the findings in normal control subjects. Moreover, there was no impressive difference in the performance of patients with frontal lesions versus patients who had extrafrontal lesions or diffuse injury according to MRI findings obtained at the time of the study (Fig. 17–3).

To further investigate semantic memory after head injury, our laboratory tested survivors of severe CHI undergoing rehabilitation on a depth of processing task and an encoding procedure that evaluated the capacity to organize semantically related words drawn from three categories and presented in random order. In the level of processing study, Goldstein and associates (1990) showed that facilitation of memory by semantic encoding (as compared with processing physical or phonetic features of the words) was diminished in CHI patients as

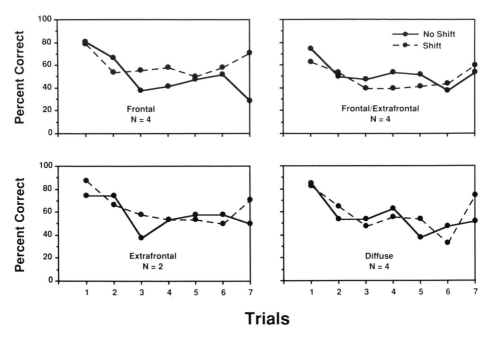

Figure 17-3 Mean percent correct recall as a function of shift versus no shift conditions for closed head injured patients with lesions confined to the frontal region, extending to both frontal and extrafrontal areas (frontal/extrafrontal), lesions outside the frontal lobes (extrafrontal), and the absence of lesions (diffuse) as visualized by magnetic resonance imaging. (From Goldstein et al., 1989, with permission.)

compared with normal controls whose recognition memory markedly improved when they answered questions concerning the meaning of the words presented. However, the reduced enhancement of memory by semantic features in the head-injured patients could not be attributed to deficient semantic knowledge per se. These patients were able to correctly answer questions concerning the categorical features of the words at a rate similar to controls. Review of MRI findings disclosed no relationship between lesion localization and performance.

In a related study that lacked clinicopathologic correlation by MRI, Levin and Goldstein (1986) found that active use of semantic features to guide retrieval was diminished in a similar group of young survivors of severe CHI. In contrast to a control group who organized their recall of related words (presented in random order) into categories, the head-injured patients tended to shift their recall from one category to another without performing an exhaustive search. Taken in combination, our findings implicate difficulty in the use of semantic features to guide recall despite relatively preserved sensitivity to these cues under conditions that involve more passive participation. Although the Galveston studies provide no support for the postulation that inefficient semantic memory is attributable to frontal lobe damage, metabolic imaging to identify areas of focal dysfunction could provide a more definitive test, particularly under an activation condition.

Behavioral Disturbance

Case reports beginning with Harlow's description of increased irritability and obstreperous behavior in Phineas Gage (1848, 1868) have documented marked changes in personality following frontal lobe injury, particularly in patients sustaining bilateral lesions (see Benton's historical review in this volume). Although studies that have characterized posttraumatic behavioral disturbance in groups of CHI patients have documented sequelae (e.g., irritability, immature behavior) traditionally associated with frontal lobe damage, these investigations have generally lacked neuroanatomic correlation (Brooks and McKinlay, 1983). Similarly, the distinction between behavioral changes following orbitofrontal lesions (or connections to this area) which reflect a "psychopathic" personality (i.e., lack of impulse control, irritability, and/or hyperkinesis) and the "pseudodepressed" personality (i.e., slowness, diminished initiative, and indifference) related to frontal convexity lesions rests primarily on clinical case reports (for review: Blumer and Benson, 1975) rather than systematic studies applying more objective measures of psychopathology to groups of patients with focal lesions.

Investigation of servicemen who sustained penetrating missile wounds of the brain has raised the possibility of an interaction between lateralization and localization of frontal lobe lesions in producing behavioral changes. Grafman and coworkers (1986) found that men sustaining right orbitofrontal lesions reported increased edginess, anxiety, and depression as compared with patients with extrafrontal lesions and controls. In contrast, a group with left dorsolateral lesions noted greater anger and hostility.

To characterize behavioral disturbance following CHI, our group employed the Neurobehavioral Rating Scale (Levin et al., 1987), which reflected the clinician's assessment based primarily on findings obtained in an interview and mental status examination. As depicted in Figure 17–4, behavioral features that were prominent in the severely injured patients tended to be characteristic of the constellation of symptoms that clinicians attribute to frontal injury (i.e., disinhibition, poor insight, unrealistic planning). One of the factors to emerge from a principal components analysis of the neurobehavioral data was based on the items that evaluated poor planning, inaccurate self-appraisal, and disinhibition. According to CT findings obtained primarily during the acute stage of treatment, we found that this putative "frontal lobe" factor contributed heavily to the psychopathology documented by the Neurobehavioral Rating Scale in patients with frontal lesions as compared with patients with lesions confined to the extrafrontal region. As in many previous studies, the CT findings were obtained at varying intervals prior to administering the Neurobehavioral Rating Scale and MRI was not available. Although this study raises the possibility of demonstrating qualitative behavioral changes following frontal lobe lesions that are difficult to show using experimental tasks, further research is needed to extend these observations to patients with more clearly defined lesions.

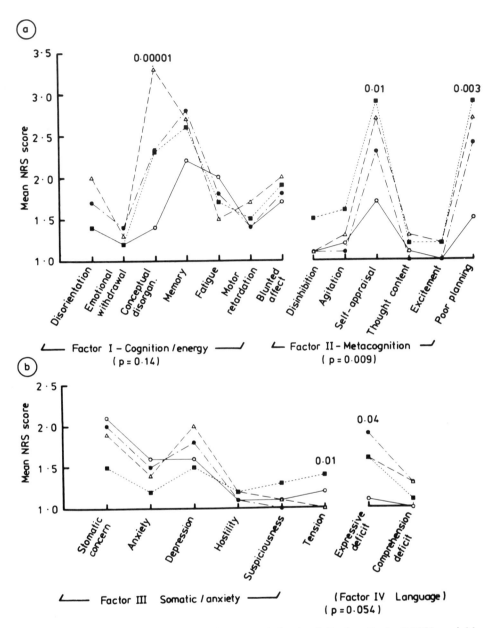

Figure 17–4 Mean scores for the 27 Neurobehavioral Rating Scale (NRS) variables plotted as a function of closed head injury severity. The NRS variables are grouped according to their loadings on the four factors identified by a principal components' analysis. The probability values shown above the variables denote significant effects of head injury severity on the NRS scores. Variables that did not load on a factor are not shown. (From Levin et al., 1987, with permission.)

RECOVERY FROM SEVERE HEAD INJURY: A COMPARISON OF PATIENTS SUSTAINING FRONTAL LESIONS VS NONFRONTAL LESIONS

To explore the contribution of frontal lesions to the neurobehavioral sequelae of severe CHI, we completed a preliminary study in which the patients underwent MRI and were examined by both clinical and experimental neurobehavioral tasks. Thirteen young adult survivors of severe CHI were consecutively selected from the inpatient trainees of the Transitional Learning Community in Galveston provided that they had acute care hospital records documenting a severe CHI at least 1 year earlier (median = 3.1 years), no history of antecedent neuropsychiatric disorder (including substance abuse), no head injury or other neurologic insult subsequent to the CHI, and age at injury between 16 and 30 years. At the time of the study, their median age was 27 years as compared with 26 years in a group of 12 normal control subjects. All subjects consented to undergo testing and MRI.

MRI was performed on a Teslacon system using a 0.6 Tesla magnet operating at a proton resonant frequency of 25.4 MHz. Images were obtained in contiguous 8-mm slices in transaxial and coronal planes using two spin-echo (SE) sequences: (1) A repetition time (TR) of 500 ms and an echo delay time (TE) of 32 ms; and (2) a TR of 2000 ms and a TE of 60 and 120 ms. A board-certified radiologist interpreted the MR images independently of the neurobehavioral data and coded the results on research forms. Intracranial abnormalities were coded as lesions provided that they were present on both the first and second echoes of T2-weighted images.

Sites of lesion, as reflected by increased intensity on MRI, are shown in Figure 17–5. Overlapping lesions are indicated by darker shading. Seven of the CHI patients (54%) had one or more frontal lesions, including the superior frontal gyrus (n = 6), adjacent to the frontal horn of the lateral ventricles (n = 3), the orbitofrontal gyrus (n = 1), and the precentral gyrus (n = 1). We compared the neurobehavioral functioning of this frontal group with the results obtained in the six patients without frontal lesions (including a patient with a right parietal lesion and a case with a left pons lesion).

We selected neuropsychologic procedures that were found in previous research to be differentially sensitive to focal nontraumatic lesions or surgical excisions in the prefrontal versus extrafrontal regions. To assess frontal lobe functioning, cognitive tasks included generation of verbal or nonverbal material under a time limit, flexibility in reasoning, semantic memory, and planning. Other tasks, which we postulated would be more adversely affected by extrafrontal lesions, evaluated nonverbal memory and visual perception.

Following the procedure employed by Benton (1968), verbal fluency was tested by asking the subject to retrieve orally as many words as possible beginning with a specific letter under a 60-second time limit with constraints on using proper nouns and variants of the same stem (e.g., "count" and "counted"). This was repeated for three letters. The measures were total correct words, and percentage of responses that were perseverations. Utilizing the procedure of Jones-Gotman and Milner (1977), figural fluency was tested by asking the subject to draw abstract, novel designs that did not resemble geometric shapes or familiar

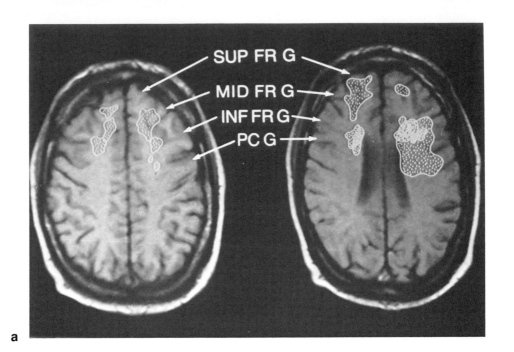

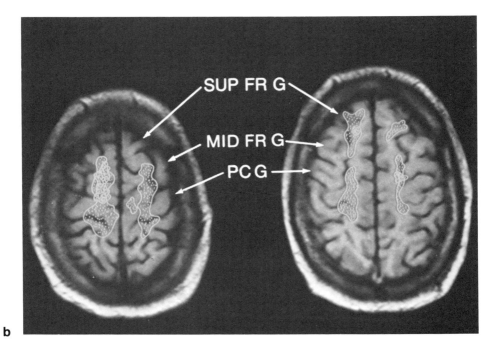

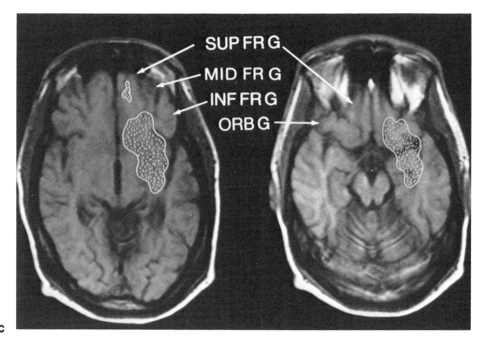

c

Figure 17–5a–5c Location of brain lesions detected by magnetic resonance imaging in a series of 13 young adults studied after a median of 3 years following a severe closed head injury. Based on high intensities found on T_2-weighted images, the lesions were identified and superimposed on a common set of T_1-weighted images. Solid areas indicate overlapping lesions sustained by more than one patient, whereas stippled regions signify nonoverlapping lesions.

objects. Under the free condition the subject was given 5 minutes to generate as many unique designs as possible, whereas the fixed condition had the constraint of using only four lines and a 4-minute time limit. A single reminder was given by the examiner on the first instance of a perseverative error (i.e., exact duplication of a design or a drawing that differed by only one feature).

To evaluate whether frontal lobe lesions disrupt the capacity for semantic organization of memory and increase vulnerability to proactive interference, the California Verbal Learning Test (CVLT) (Delis et al., 1988) was administered. The California Test consists of 16 words derived from four categories (e.g., tools, clothing, spices/herbs, and fruits). Following five recall trials, a second list is presented to produce interference with recall of the first list on the next trial and after a 20-minute delay. Consistent with our focus on the organization of verbal memory, we measured the strategy of clustering words from the same category (i.e., recalling all of the words from one category before shifting to one of the other two categories) and intrusions by extralist words.

The Tower of London task developed by Shallice (1982 and this volume) was used to assess the capacity to "look ahead" in planning moves of dowels on

Initial Position Given to Patient

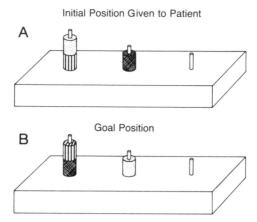

Figure 17-6   A sample Tower of London problem in which the patient was asked to rearrange (in as few moves as possible) the pegs presented in the initial position to match the model (goal position). (Adapted from Shallice, 1982.)

three pegs from an initial position to match the sample provided (Fig. 17–6). Problems of increasing complexity, which ranged from two to five moves for completion, were administered. The Porteus Maze Test (Porteus, 1965) was also used to evaluate planning. To mitigate the contribution of motor slowing, the time required to trace the correct path drawn through each maze was subtracted from the time needed by the patient to reach the goal.

Problem-solving capacity and utilization of feedback provided by the examiner were assessed by the Wisconsin Card Sorting Test (Grant and Berg, 1948) and the 20 Questions procedure (Mosher and Hornsby, 1966). The former, which was administered using a microcomputer, included a measure of perseveration (i.e., sorting cards according to a principle that is no longer rewarded). The 20 Questions procedure used a display of 42 pictures of common objects and living things that could be grouped into categories (e.g, animals, foods, clothing). By asking questions, the patient's task was to guess the target item selected by the examiner. The procedure was repeated for three items. We postulated that patients with frontal lesions would use primarily hypothesis-seeking questions (e.g., is it the carrot?) rather than the more efficient constraint-seeking question (e.g., is it something to eat?). In addition, we analyzed the number of redundant (i.e., perseverative) questions asked.

To investigate the possiblity that patients with extrafrontal lesions would exhibit more severe impairment of visual perception, we tested judgment of the angular orientation of lines (Benton et al., 1983). This task provided an opportunity to evaluate the presence of a dissociation in performance between patients with frontal versus extrafrontal lesions. Finally, intellectual function was estimated by administering the Block Designs and Vocabulary subtests of the Wechsler Adult Intelligence Scale-Revised (Wechsler, 1981).

Both groups of head-injured patients performed below the level of normal control subjects. As summarized subsequently, the most impressive differences

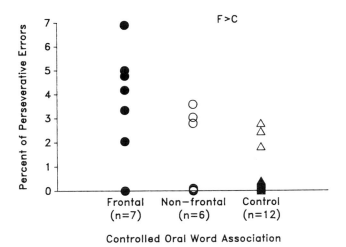

Figure 17–7   Percentage of perseverative errors in retrieving words beginning with specific letters on the controlled oral word association test. Data are plotted for chronic survivors of severe closed head injury who had focal lesions restricted to the frontal region, a comparison group of patients without frontal lesions and normal control subjects.

emerged in comparisons between the patients with frontal lesions and the control group. Several dissociations were found in which the performance of the nonfrontal patients fell below the control subjects and neither of these groups differed significantly from the patients with frontal lesions. Notwithstanding the significant differences between the frontal and nonfrontal groups on several measures, it should be noted that these disparities were fairly modest. It is possible that imposing additional selection criteria such as a minimum lesion size and comparing specific prefrontal locations of lesion might produce more striking differences in performance.

Analysis of the verbal associative fluency data disclosed a higher percentage of perseverative errors in the frontal lesion group as compared to the nonfrontal and control groups (Fig. 17–7), whereas the number of words produced was also lower in the nonfrontal patients than controls. Consequently, the presence of a frontal lesion was related more to the qualitative type of error in word finding rather than to overall productions.

Consistent with the verbal fluency data, attempts to draw unique abstract designs produced a higher percentage of nonperseverative errors in the frontal group (Fig. 17–8a) than in the nonfrontal patients and controls under the free (i.e., unrestricted) condition. In contrast, the perseverative errors did not significantly differ across groups. However, the frontal group difference in perseverative drawings was not present under the fixed condition in which all productions had to consist of four lines. Under the fixed condition the frontal patients exhibited excessive perseverative errors relative to controls (Fig. 17–8b). In contrast, the nonfrontal patients tended to produce more numerous nonperseverative errors than the patients with frontal lesions and controls when the constraint of four lines was imposed.

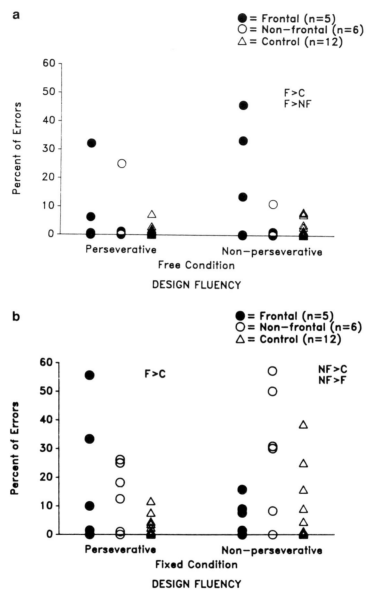

Figure 17–8a and 8b Percentage of perseverative errors incurred while attempting to draw unique, abstract designs under a free **(a)** condition (i.e., no constraints) and a fixed **(b)** condition (each design limited to four lines) in chronic survivors of severe closed head injury who had frontal lesions as compared with patients without frontal lesions and normal controls.

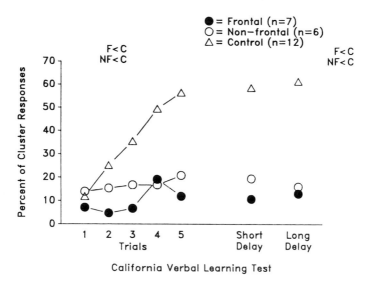

Figure 17-9 Percentage of responses reflecting clustering of words from the same semantic category by patients with frontal lesions as compared with patients without frontal lesions and normal controls.

Analysis of the California Verbal Learning Test (CVLT) revealed a lower level of clustering words from the same category by patients with frontal lesions as compared with both nonfrontal patients and normal controls (Fig. 17–9). Recall by the frontal group tended to be scattered across categories rather than first exhausting all of the words in a single category. However, perseverations and intrusion of extralist words were equally prominent in the CVLT performance by frontal and nonfrontal groups who both differed from the normal subjects. Both groups of CHI patients exhibited impaired recall after a delay as compared with controls.

Problem solving, as reflected by performance on the Wisconsin Card Sorting Test, did not differ between the head-injured patients with frontal lesions and the nonfrontal group. However, both head-injured groups performed below the level of control subjects. Although patients with frontal lesions asked a greater number of redundant questions than control subjects on the 20 Questions Test, the predicted difference in constraint-seeking questions did not occur.

Is there a perseverative tendency in patients with frontal lesions that transcends various tests? Table 17–2 shows a pattern of perseverative errors that is more consistent in the patients with frontal lesions as compared to the nonfrontal group. An excessive number of perseverative errors was defined in relation to the distribution of scores in a group of normal subjects.

To compare planning performance in the three groups, we plotted the percentage of correct responses on the first trial of each Tower of London problem. Figure 17–10 depicts no consistent group differences in performance according to this measure. Other measures of performance on the Tower of London also showed no difference between the frontal and nonfrontal groups.

Table 17-2 Percent Perseverations in Frontal and Nonfrontal Patients

PT	WCST	20 ?s	DFFR	DFFX	COWA	CVLT	Lesion location
Frontal							
1	—	0	0	33.3	6.9	14.4	Bil sup g, Bil periven
2	7	5.7	6.3	33.3	4.2	9.3	Bil sup g, Bil periven
3	12	7.7	0	10	0	1.7	Bil sup g
4	13	0	—	—	0	8.3	L precent g, R sup g
5	31	13.9	32.1	55.6	5.0	5.1	L sup g
6	—	0	—	—	4.8	5	Bil orb g
7	8	12.1	0	0	3.3	6	R sup g
Nonfrontal							
1	12	4.8	25	25	2.8	11.5	None
2	13	0	0	18.2	3.6	0	None
3	18	2.1	0	46.1	0	14.2	R par lobule
4	12	5.4	0	0	0	1.7	L pons
5	—	5.8	0	12.5	3	10.4	None
6	—	0	0	0	0	0	None

Bil = bilateral; COWA = Controlled Word Association; CVLT = California Verbal Learning Test; DFFR = Design Fluency; DFFX = Design Fluency Fixed Condition; g = gyrus; L = left; orb = orbital; par = parietal; periven = periventricular; precent = precentral; R = right; sup = superior; WCST = Wisconsin Card Sorting Test.

Figure 17-10 Percentage of Tower of London problems solved on the first trial plotted as a function of complexity by patients with frontal lesions as compared with patients without frontal lesions and normal controls.

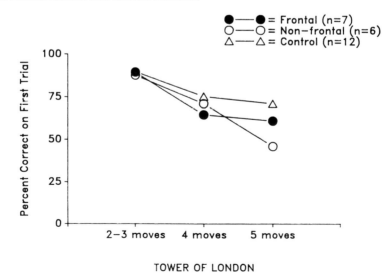

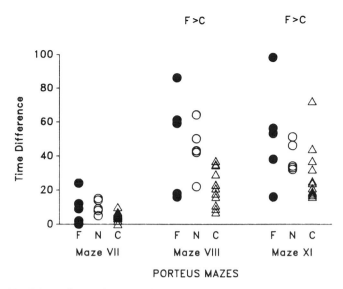

Figure 17–11 Mean time taken to solve Porteus Mazes by chronic survivors of severe closed head injury. The solution time for each patient was obtained by subtracting the time required to trace a correct path previously drawn through the maze. Plotted for patients with frontal lesions, the nonfrontal group, and normal controls.

To isolate the planning component from the motor requirement imposed by the Porteus Mazes, we subtracted the time for tracing a correct path on a similar maze shown to the patient from the total solution time. Figure 17–11 shows the distribution of difference scores (i.e., total solution time − time for tracing) for the three groups. It is seen that maze learning was slower in head-injured patients who sustained frontal lesions than in the nonfrontal and control groups. In contrast to the perseverative pattern of errors in the frontal group, a general tendency toward planning errors on both the Tower of London and the Porteus Mazes was less impressive.

Table 17–3 shows that range of vocabulary was diminished in the nonfrontal head-injured patients, but not in the group with frontal lobe lesions. In contrast, patients with frontal lesions had more difficulty constructing block designs

Table 17–3 Comparison of Performance by Frontal, Nonfrontal, and Control Groups on Other Tests

	Frontal (n = 7)		Nonfrontal (n = 6)		Controls (n = 12)	
	Median	Range	Median	Range	Median	Range
WAIS-R subtests:						
Vocabulary	39	18–51	27[a]	15–42	57[a]	24–69
Block design	26[a]	17–43	19.5[b]	12–37	39.5[a,b]	25–44
Judgment of line						
Orientation	27	18–28	25	15–30	27	22–30

[a,b]Denote a significant difference.

from a two-dimensional model than the control subjects, where the nonfrontal group had relatively preserved performance. Judgment of the angular orientation of lines did not significantly differ across the head-injured and control groups (Table 17–3).

COMMENT

Our preliminary data indicate that deficits presumably reflecting frontal dysfunction were pervasive in both groups of severely head-injured patients. Depending on the task conditions, patients with frontal lesions tended to incur more numerous perseverative errors than patients without frontal lesions. Moreover, the strategy of clustering items according to their semantic relations was underutilized in the frontal group.

In contrast, we found that judgment of the angular orientation of lines in both groups of patients did not differ from the performance of the control subjects. In view of the sensitivity of the line orientation test to posterior parietotemporal lesions, particularly of the right hemisphere (Benton et al., 1983), the relatively preserved performance of both head-injured groups is consistent with their MRI findings. However, how can the negative findings for line orientation be reconciled with the impaired block construction performance in the frontal lesion group? As pointed out previously by Lezak (1983), impulsiveness and failure to monitor errors may detract from construction of block designs by patients with frontal lobe lesions. Although other interpretations of the block design data are possible, a pervasive cognitive impairment is unlikely given the relative preservation of specific abilities.

The present findings corroborate previous work indicating that cognitive functions thought to be subserved primarily by the prefrontal region are vulnerable to the long-term consequences of severe CHI. Although focal frontal lesions appeared to contribute to impairment on several of the cognitive tests, replication using more "control" tasks is necessary to demonstrate dissociations. Potential objections to its interpretation of our findings include concern about the confounding effects of diffuse axonal injury and gray matter damage, and extrafrontal focal lesions.

How should one proceed from this preliminary work? Three strategies are proposed to more definitively characterize brain-behavior relationships after head injury. First, evidence for frontal dysfunction can be adduced by metabolic imaging, which can augment if not replace morphologic lesions as the criterion for localization. It is possible that identifying a group of head-injured patients with frontal metabolic dysfunction (regardless of the presence or site of morphologic lesions) will produce a stronger relationship to neuropsychologic deficits than relying on the localization of structural lesions as the criterion. Second, utilization of the templates developed by H. Damasio (see her chapter, this volume) could facilitate studies relating morphologic lesion sites within the frontal lobes (i.e., dorsolateral versus orbitofrontal) to specific neurobehavioral deficits. This strategy could also determine whether limiting the analysis to intracerebral lesions with distinct margins enhances the specificity of neurobehavioral deficits associated with frontal lobe damage. Finally, parallel studies of patients sustaining traumatic frontal lesions and a comparison group with nontraumatic frontal lesions in similar locations could examine the degree of correspondence in the type and severity of cognitive deficit. Demonstration of similar linkages between lesion site and cognitive deficit in traumatic and other etiologies would buttress our working assumption that investigation of specific groups of head-injured patients can elucidate brain-behavior relationships.

ACKNOWLEDGMENTS

Research described in this chapter was supported by grant NS-21889. We are indebted to Karen Wilkinson, Liz Zindler, and Anita Padilla for assistance in manuscript preparation.

REFERENCES

Adams JH, Graham D, Scott G, Parker LS, Doyle D. Brain damage in fatal non-missile head injury. J Clin Pathol 33:1132–1145, 1980.

Alexander MP, Benson DF, Stuss DT. Frontal lobes and language. Brain Lang 37:656–691, 1989.

Baddeley A, Wilson B. Frontal amnesia and the dysexecutive syndrome. Brain Cogn 7:212–230, 1988.

Benton AL. Differential behavioral effects in frontal lobe disease. Neuropsychologia 6:53–60, 1968.

Benton AL, Hamsher K deS, Varney NR, Spreen O. Contributions to Neuropsychological Assessment. A Clinical Manual. New York: Oxford University Press, 1983.

Blumer D, Benson DF. Personality changes with frontal and temporal lesions. In Psychiatric Aspects of Neurologic Disease. Benson DF, Blumer D (eds). New York: Grune & Stratton, 1975.

Brooks DN, McKinlay WW. Personality and behavioural changes after severe blunt head injury: The relative's view. J Neurol Neurosurg Psychiatry 46:336–344, 1983.

Delis DC, Kramer JH, Freeland J, Kaplan E. Integrating clinical assessment with cognitive neuroscience: Construct validation of the California Verbal Learning Test. J Consult Clin Psychol 56:123–130, 1988.

Freedman M, Cermak LS. Semantic encoding deficits in frontal lobe disease and amnesia. Brain Cogn 5:108–114, 1986.

Goldstein FC, Levin HS, Boake C. Conceptual encoding following severe closed head injury. Cortex 25:541–554, 1989.

Goldstein FC, Levin HS, Boake C, Lohrey JH. Facilitation of memory performance through induced semantic processing in survivors of severe closed head injury. J Clin Exp Neuropsychol 12:286–300, 1990.

Grafman J, Vance SC, Weingartner H, et al. The effects of lateralized frontal lesions on mood regulation. Brain 109:1127–1148, 1986.

Grant DA, Berg EA. A behavioral analysis of degree of reinforcement and ease of shifting in new responses in a Weigl-type card-sorting problem. J Exp Psychol 38:404–411, 1948.

Harlow JM. Passage of an iron bar through the head. Boston Med Surg J 39:389–393, 1848.

Harlow JM. Recovery from the passage of an iron bar through the head. Pub Mass Med Soc 2:327–347, 1868.

Holbourn AHS. Mechanics of head injuries. Lancet 2:438–441, 1943.

Jones-Gottman M, Milner B. Design fluency: The invention of nonsense drawings after focal cortical lesions. Neuropsychologia 15:653–674, 1977.

Langfitt TW, Obrist WD, Alavi A, Grossman RI, Zimmerman R, Jaggi J, Uzzell B, Reivich M, Patton DR. Computerized tomography, magnetic resonance imaging, and positron emission tomography in the study of brain trauma. Preliminary observations. J Neurosurg 64:760–767, 1986.

Levin HS, Amparo E, Eisenberg HM, et al. Magnetic resonance imaging and computerized tomography in relation to the neurobehavioral sequelae of mild and moderate head injuries. J Neurosurg 66:706–713, 1987.

Levin HS, Benton AL, Grossman RG. Neurobehavioral Consequences of Closed Head Injury. New York: Oxford University Press, 1982.

Levin HS, Gary HE, Jr, Eisenberg HM, NIH Traumatic Coma Data Bank Research Group. Duration of impaired consciousness in relation to lateralization of intracerebral lesion after severe head injury. Lancet 1:1001–1003, 1989.

Levin HS, Goldstein FC. Organization of verbal memory after severe closed-head injury. J Clin Exp Neuropsychol 8:643–656, 1986.

Levin HS, Grossman RG, Kelly PJ. Aphasic disorder in patients with closed head injury. J Neurol Neurosurg Psychiatry 39:1062–1070, 1976.

Levin HS, Grossman RG, Sarwar M, Meyers CA. Linguistic recovery after closed head injury. Brain Lang 12:360–374, 1981.

Levin HS, Handel SF, Goldman AM, Eisenberg HM, Guinto FC, Jr. Magnetic resonance imaging after "diffuse" nonmissile head injury. Arch Neurol 42:963–968, 1985.

Levin HS, High WM, Goethe KE, et al. The neurobehavioral rating scale: Assessment of the behavioral sequelae of head injury by the clinician. J Neurol Neurosurg Psychiatry 50:183–193, 1987.

Levin HS, Meyers CA, Grossman RG, Sarwar M. Ventricular enlargement after closed head injury. Arch Neurol 38:623–629, 1981.

Lezak MD. Neuropsychological Assessment. New York: Oxford University Press, 1983.

Mosher FA, Hornsby JR. On asking questions. In Studies in Cognitive Growth. Bruner JS, Olver RR, Greenfield PM, et al (eds). New York: John Wiley & Sons, 1966.

Novoa OP, Adrila A. Linguistic abilities in patients with prefrontal damage. Brain Lang 30:206–225, 1987.

Porteus SD. Porteus Maze Test. Fifty Years' Application. Palo Alto, Calif.: Pacific Books, 1965.

Sarno MT. The nature of verbal impairment after closed head injury. J Nerv Ment Dis 168:685–692, 1980.

Shallice T. Specific impairments in planning. Philos Trans R Soc Lon [Biol] 298:199–209, 1982.

Stuss DT, Benson DF. The Frontal Lobes. New York: Raven Press, 1986.

Stuss DT, Ely P, Hugenholtz H, et al. Subtle neuropsychological deficits in patients with good recovery after closed head injury. Neurosurgery 17:41–47, 1985.

Ulatowska HK, Freedman-Stern R, Doyel AW, Macaluso-Haynes S, North AJ. Production of narrative discourse in aphasia. Brain Lang 19:317–334, 1983.

Wechsler D. WAIS-R Manual. New York: Psychological Corporation, 1981.

Zatorre R, McEntee W. Semantic encoding deficits in a case of traumatic amnesia. Brain Cogn 2:331–345, 1983.

18

Guidelines for the Study of Brain-Behavior Relationships During Development

ADELE DIAMOND

One way to study the relationship of brain maturation to the elaboration of cognitive abilities during development is to use a two-pronged approach: (1) Study the developmental progression of children's performance on behavioral tasks, and (2) link successful performance on those tasks uniquely to specific neural systems. I would like to suggest a set of guidelines for the conduct and evaluation of such research. I will use the work of myself and others on the development of cognitive abilities linked to dorsolateral prefrontal cortex to illustrate these guiding principles.

A Brief Overview of the Anatomical Connections and Functions of Dorsolateral Prefrontal Cortex

Dorsolateral prefrontal cortex is located between the frontal pole and the arcuate sulcus in the monkey brain (see Fig. 18–4). It is centered around the principal sulcus (Walker's area 46) and is immediately anterior to the supplementary motor area (SMA) and premotor cortex. SMA and premotor cortex, like dorsolateral prefrontal cortex, are among the subregions of frontal cortex. Dorsolateral prefrontal cortex is defined anatomically, in part, by its reciprocal connections with the **parvocellular portion of the mediodorsal nucleus of the thalamus** (Rose and Woolsey, 1948; Johnson et al., 1968; Leonard, 1969). It also has strong reciprocal connections with **parietal cortex,** and the dorsolateral prefrontal and parietal cortices appear to be coupled in their projections throughout the brain (Pandya and Kuypers, 1969; Goldman and Nauta, 1977; Goldman-Rakic and Schwartz, 1982; Schwartz and Goldman-Rakic, 1984; Selemon and Goldman-Rakic, 1985a,b; 1988; Johnson et al., 1989). The same may be true of the dorsolateral prefrontal and **premotor** cortices to a lesser extent (Pandya and Vignolo, 1969; 1971; Haaxma and Kuypers, 1975; Pandya and Kuypers, 1969; Goldman and Nauta, 1977; Kunzle, 1978). One of the major output structures of dorsolateral prefrontal cortex is the **caudate nucleus** (Nauta, 1964; Johnson et al., 1968; Kemp and Powell, 1970; Goldman and Nauta, 1977). Other output sites include the **superior colliculus** (Goldman and Nauta, 1976; Kunzle, 1978) and the **cingulate gyrus** (Johnson et al., 1968; Pandya and Vignolo, 1969; Goldman and Nauta, 1977; Kunzle, 1978).

Frontal cortex is the largest area of cortex in the human brain; it has increased the most in size (and in the proportion of brain mass devoted to it) over the course of evolution; and it has an unusually protracted period of maturation (probably only reaching full maturity during puberty). There is general agreement that the most anterior regions of frontal cortex (i.e., prefrontal cortex) subserve our highest cognitive abilities. Dorsolateral prefrontal cortex has been most closely associated with functions of memory and inhibitory control (see discussion of the critical abilities thought to be dependent on dorsolateral prefrontal cortex toward the close of this paper). The role of dorsolateral prefrontal cortex in helping us relate information separated in time or space, and in helping us gain control over our actions so we can choose what we want to do and not simply react, makes this area of the brain of great importance for complex cognitive operations.

The classic test for dorsolateral prefrontal cortex function in nonhuman primates is the delayed response task (Jacobsen, 1935; 1936; for reviews: Nauta, 1971; Warren and Akert, 1964; Rosvold, 1972; Markowitsch and Pritzel, 1977; Diamond, 1991a). This hiding task requires both memory and the ability to inhibit merely repeating the last rewarded response. The classic test for dorsolateral prefrontal cortex function in human adults is the Wisconsin Card Sorting Test (Milner, 1963; 1964). Here, as in delayed response, the subject must flexibly switch to a new response after having been rewarded for a particular response. The subject must remember which sorting criteria were most recently tried and found incorrect, and which sorting criterion is now correct.

The guiding principles I would like to suggest for research on brain-behavior relations in development are as follows:

1. Convergent Validity. Use *more than one task* linked to a given neural circuit and on which performance improves during a given period of development

It is important to look for converging evidence from diverse tests all linked to the same neural system. An impairment, or an improvement, on one test might be due to diverse causes; converging evidence from diverse tests is more convincing. These converging results are more powerful the more dissimilar the tasks.

Thus, in our work on the developmental progression during infancy of abilities dependent on dorsolateral prefrontal cortex, for example, we have used two hiding tasks (A$\overline{\text{B}}$ and delayed response), which require subjects to keep track of where the reward has been hidden in the absence of visible cues, and a transparent barrier detour task (object retrieval), where nothing is hidden and the reward is always visible, but a circuitous route to the goal is required (see e.g., Diamond,

1988; 1991a). AB̄ and delayed response are almost identical tasks. They were chosen because delayed response has been so firmly and convincingly linked specifically to dorsolateral prefrontal cortex, and because AB̄ has been repeatedly shown to be a clear marker of developmental change during infancy (e.g., Gratch, 1975; Wellman et al., 1987). The object retrieval task was chosen because it is very different from AB̄ and delayed response, and yet work by Moll and Kuypers (1977) has linked it, too, to frontal cortex.

In the AB̄ and delayed response tasks, the subject is centered between two identical hiding wells, one to the left and one to the right. The experimenter holds up an object of keen interest to the subject, and *as the subject looks on* the experimenter places this object in one of the two hiding wells. The experimenter then covers both hiding wells simultaneously with identical covers and a brief delay of 0–10 seconds is imposed during which the subject is prevented from looking at, or moving or straining toward, the correct well. After the delay, the subject is allowed to reach. In these details the AB̄ and delayed response tasks are identical. The tasks differ solely in the rule for deciding where the reward is to be hidden. In AB̄, the reward is hidden in the same well until the subject is correct to a specified criterion (typically, two consecutively correct responses), then the reward is hidden in the other well and the procedure repeated.[1] In delayed response, the hiding location of the reward is varied randomly by a predetermined schedule.

For the object retrieval task, a plexiglass box open on one side is used. A reward is placed in the box; the subject's task is to retrieve the reward. There is no delay nor time limit; a trial ends when the subject retrieves the reward or stops trying. Experimental variables include (1) which side of the box is open (front, top, left, or right), (2) distance of the reward from the opening (ranging from partially outside the box to deep inside the box), and (3) position of the box on the testing surface (near the front edge of the table or far; far to the left, at the midline, or far to the right). The reward is always visible when the box is transparent, but the experimental variables jointly determine whether the reward is seen through a closed side of the box or through the opening. (For greater detail see Diamond, submitted.) Object retrieval requires inhibition of the strong pull to reach straight to the visible reward (rather than detouring around the barrier), and like delayed response, AB̄, and the Wisconsin Card Sorting Test, it requires the subject to remember which responses were most recently tried and found incorrect (in this case, which sides of the box were tried and found closed) and to flexibly switch to a new response.

The converging evidence one would like from the different tasks is that (1) they are all linked to the same neural circuit, and (2) developmental improvements in performance on the tasks occur during the same age period. It is important to be as precise as possible here. For example, different regions of frontal cortex (even different regions within prefrontal cortex) participate in different neural circuits (e.g., Goldman and Rosvold, 1970; Bachevalier and Mishkin, 1986). It is not sufficient, then, to use tasks linked simply to frontal cortex, nor even all linked to prefrontal cortex; they must be linked to the same functional region.

The work by Moll and Kuypers (1977), upon which our choice of the object

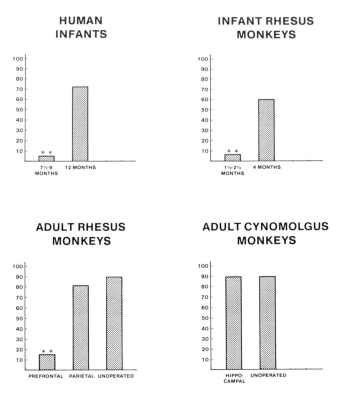

Figure 18–1   Percentage of trials during object retrieval testing where subjects reached to the box opening without ever having looked into the opening on that trial. Human infants of 7½–9 months, adult monkeys with lesions of dorsolateral prefrontal cortex, and infant monkeys of 1½–2½ months almost never reach to the opening unless they have looked into the opening on that trial. On the other hand, 12-month-old human infants, 4-month-old infant monkeys, unoperated adult monkeys, and adult monkeys with lesions of parietal cortex or the hippocampus often reach to the opening without ever having looked into the opening on that trial. (This figure summarizes work from Diamond 1990b; submitted; Diamond and Goldman-Rakic, 1985; 1986; and Diamond et al., 1989b.)

retrieval task was based, had relied on very large lesions, spanning the supplementary motor, premotor, and dorsolateral prefrontal regions of frontal cortex. Our work, however, has shown that lesions restricted specifically to dorsolateral prefrontal cortex disrupt performance on the object retrieval task (Diamond and Goldman-Rakic, 1985) (Fig. 18–1).[2] Previous work had linked delayed response to dorsolateral prefrontal cortex; our work confirmed this (Diamond and Goldman-Rakic, 1989). Given the marked similarity between A$\overline{B}$ and delayed response it seemed likely that success on A$\overline{B}$, too, would depend on involvement of dorsolateral prefrontal cortex. Our work confirmed this suspicion; lesions restricted to dorsolateral prefrontal cortex disrupt performance on the A$\overline{B}$ task (Diamond and Goldman-Rakic, 1989) (Table 18–1).

Moreover, our work has shown that performance on all three tasks improves during the same period of development in both human infants and

Table 18–1   Percentage Correct on the A$\overline{\text{B}}$ Task by Delay and by Experimental Group

Experimental groups	Delay (in seconds)		
	2	5	10
Adult rhesus monkeys with lesions of dorsolateral prefrontal cortex			
F1	45		
F2	71	63	58
F3	67	67	64
F4	67	63	59
Mean	63	64	60
Adult rhesus monkeys with lesions of parietal cortex			
P1	97	94	92
P2	100	100	99
P3	98	99	98
Mean	98	98	96
Unoperated adult rhesus monkeys			
U1	99	98	98
U2	96	98	96
U3	99	96	97
Mean	98	97	97
Adult cynomolgus monkeys with lesions of the hippocampal formation			
H1	98	93	87
H2	100	88	86
H3	95	95	80
Mean	98	92	84
Unoperated adult cynomolgus monkeys			
C1	92	96	95
C2	99	91	91
C3	87	95	85
Mean	92	92	90
5-month-old infant rhesus monkeys with lesions of dorsolateral prefrontal cortex at 4 months			
I1	81	75	65
I2	75	73	71
Mean	78	74	68
Unoperated 5-month-old infant rhesus monkey			
I3	97	97	97

infant monkeys. In human infants, performance improves on A$\overline{\text{B}}$, delayed response, and object retrieval between 7½ and 12 months of age (Diamond, 1985; Diamond and Doar, 1989; Diamond, submitted) (Figs. 18–2 and 18–3). In infant monkeys, performance improves on all three of these tasks between 1½ and 4 months of age (Diamond and Goldman-Rakic, 1986) (see Fig. 18–1 and Table 18–1).

2. Divergent Validity, 1: Study the role of *other neural regions* in performance of these tasks

To determine that the tasks of interest are linked specifically to one neural circuit it is important to demonstrate that the functioning of other neural regions is not also related to performance of these tasks.[3] For example, is improved perfor-

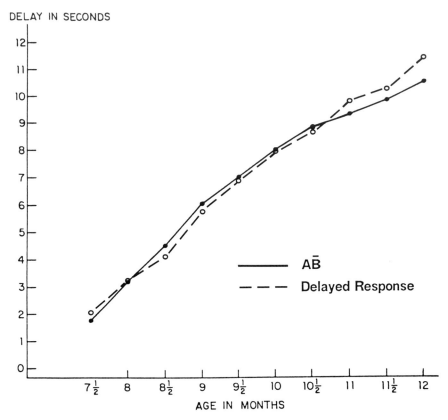

Figure 18–2 Developmental progression in the delay human infants can tolerate on the AB̄ and delayed response tasks. AB̄ results are usually reported in term of the age at which the AB̄ *error* occurs. In an attempt to use a comparable measure for the delayed response task, results are plotted here in terms of the delay at which errors occurred (i.e., the delay at which performance was below the criterion of 88% correct). The AB̄ results are shown by the solid line and are based on the infants studied longitudinally in Cambridge, MA by Diamond (1985). The delayed response results are shown by the dashed line and are based on the infants studied longitudinally in St. Louis, MO by Diamond and Doar (1989). (From Diamond and Doar, 1989, with permission. © John Wiley & Sons, Inc., 1989.)

mance simply due to general brain development? Is impaired performance a sequela that follows damage anywhere in the brain?

To address these kinds of questions, Diamond and Goldman-Rakic investigated the role of parietal cortex in performance of the AB̄, delayed response, and object retrieval tasks. Parietal cortex is involved in the processing of spatial information and the programming of movements in space (see, e.g., LaMotte and Acuna, 1978; Van Essen, 1979; Andersen, 1988). These abilities would appear to be relevant to all three tasks: In AB̄ and delayed response the hiding wells differ only in spatial location, and in object retrieval the subject must reach around a spatial barrier. Removing all of inferior parietal cortex (Brodmann's

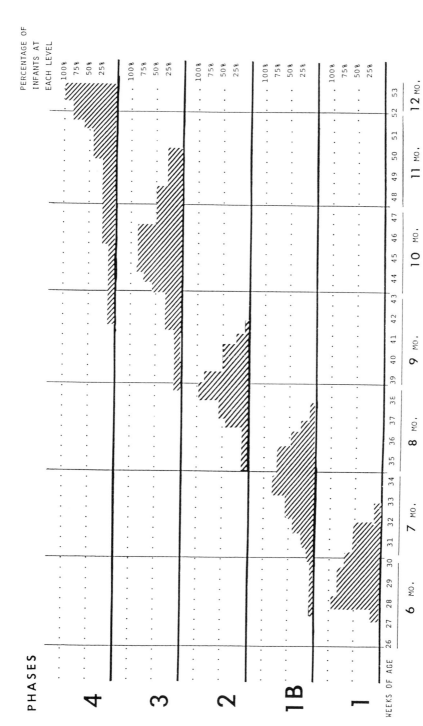

Figure 18-3 Developmental progression of the performance of human infants on the object retrieval task with transparent barrier, showing histograms for the age distribution of each phase. (From Diamond, submitted.)

area 7), however, had no observable effect on performance of A$\overline{\text{B}}$ and delayed response, and while the monkeys with lesions of parietal cortex showed some initial misreaching errors in aiming their hand to clear the box opening on object retrieval, they showed none of the errors on the task characteristic of monkeys with lesions of dorsolateral prefrontal cortex, infant monkeys, or human infants (Diamond and Goldman-Rakic, 1985; 1986; 1989) (see Table 18–1 and Fig. 18–1).

The abilities most generally considered essential for A$\overline{\text{B}}$ and delayed response are memory and inhibition; the latter is also thought essential for object

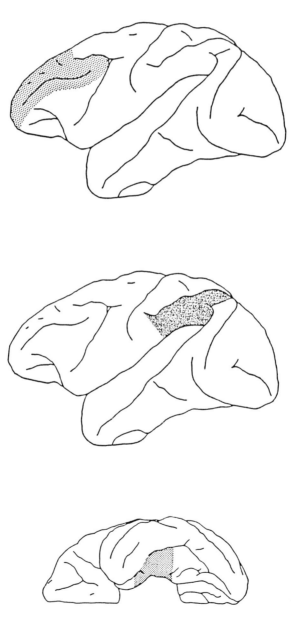

retrieval (see, e.g., Diamond, 1985; 1988; 1991a). These abilities are frequently associated with the hippocampus (see, e.g., Squire and Zola-Morgan, 1983; Douglas, 1967). Therefore, Diamond and colleagues (1989b) went on to investigate the role of the hippocampus in performance of these tasks. As was found with parietal cortex, however, the presence or absence of the hippocampus appeared to have no effect on performance of A$\overline{\text{B}}$ or delayed response at the brief delays at which monkeys with lesions of dorsolateral prefrontal cortex, infant monkeys, or human infants fail, and no effect on object retrieval performance (see Table 18-1 and Fig. 18-1). This was true even though (1) the lesions of the hippocampus included not only the hippocampus proper (Ammon's horn) but also the dentate gyrus, subiculum, 90% of the parahippocampal gyrus (area TF-TH of von Bonin and Bailey, 1947), and the posterior half of the entorhinal cortex (Fig. 18-4); and (2) the monkeys with these hippocampal lesions were profoundly impaired on delayed nonmatching to sample, a classic memory test closely linked to hippocampal function.

Delayed alternation bears some resemblance to delayed response, and performance on it, too, is impaired following lesions of dorsolateral prefrontal cortex. It was not chosen for study, however, because of questions of divergent validity—for delayed alternation is sensitive to damage to diverse regions of the brain (e.g., performance is impaired by lesions of the hippocampus or by lesions of dorsolateral prefrontal cortex). On this task, the reward is hidden (out of sight,

---

← ———————————————————————————————

Figure 18-4 Sites of the brain lesions. From top to bottom: dorsolateral prefrontal cortex lesion, inferior parietal cortex lesion, and hippocampal formation lesion (including the subiculum and posterior portion of the entorhinal cortex). The prefrontal and parietal lesions are shown on lateral views of the brain. The hippocampus is a deep structure that cannot be seen from the brain's surface. In the ventral view of the brain, the shaded area indicates the cortex that was removed in the hippocampal formation lesion. The hippocampus itself is buried deep beneath this region of cortex.

The dorsolateral prefrontal cortex lesions included cortex in both banks of the principal sulcus, the anterior bank of the arcuate sulcus, and all tissue on the dorsolateral surface rostral to the arcuate sulcus. This area corresponds most closely to area 46 of Walker, including Walker's areas 8 and 9 as well. In the terminology of Brodmann's map of the macaque brain, it corresponds to most of Brodmann's area 9, area 8, and some of area 10.

The parietal cortex lesions included the posterior bank of the intraparietal sulcus, the posterior bank of the superior temporal sulcus for about 10 mm, and all cortex between the two sulci including roughly 4 mm of the Sylvian fissure (i.e., most of Brodmann's area 7).

The hippocampal formation lesions included fields CA1-4 of the hippocampus proper, the dentate gyrus, the subiculum, 90% of the parahippocampal gyrus (area TF-TH of von Bonin and Bailey), and the posterior half of the entorhinal cortex. Inadvertent damage to area TE of von Bonin and Bailey also occurred. The caudate nuclei, lateral geniculate nuclei, amygdaloid nuclei, and the temporal stem were undamaged in all animals. There was some shrinkage and gliosis in the mammillary bodies, and extensive gliosis bilaterally throughout the fornix.

All lesions were bilateral, symmetric, and performed in one stage.

during a brief delay of 5 seconds or so) in the well to which the subject did not reach last time. Note that if a subject reaches perseveratively to one well, the reward will continue to be hidden in the other well, and the subject will continue to be wrong on one trial after another. Perseveration is a frequent consequence of damage to diverse areas of the brain. Any subject who tends to perseverate will tend to do poorly on delayed alternation. However, subjects can perseverate because of diverse reasons and the delayed alternation task tends not to discriminate between these different etiologies.

3. Demonstrate that success on the tasks in question depends specifically on a given neural circuit in the *infant,* as it does in the adult

3A. Damage to a mature system may produce different effects than damage to a developing, or immature, system

There are three issues here. One, it is possible that different neural systems may subserve similar functions at different ages. It has been suggested that lower areas of the brain might mediate infants' performance on a task, even though performance of that task by adults is mediated by a later maturing area of the brain. Thus, if a neural region is late maturing, lesions of that region may produce deficits in the adult, but not in the infant (for examples see Divac et al., 1967; Goldman, 1971; 1974).

Although successful performance on A$\overline{B}$, delayed response, and object retrieval depends on dorsolateral prefrontal cortex in the adult, this would not necessarily have to be true in the infant. For this reason it is important to investigate directly the effects of lesions in infant monkeys, and not only in mature animals. Diamond and Goldman-Rakic (1986) investigated this for the A$\overline{B}$ and delayed-response tasks, and found the same impairment in infant monkeys operated at 4 months and tested at 5 months as is found in adult monkeys following lesions of dorsolateral prefrontal cortex (see Table 18–1). This was true despite extensive preoperative training on the tasks given to the infant monkeys, and despite their excellent performance even at long delays prior to surgery. The effect of lesions of dorsolateral prefrontal cortex on object retrieval performance in infant monkeys has yet to be investigated, but it is important that this be tested as well.

Table 18–2 summarizes this body of work looking at the performance of human infants, infant monkeys, and monkeys with selective brain lesions on three behavioral tasks (A$\overline{B}$, delayed response, and object retrieval):

3B. The effects of destruction, or the characteristics of breakdown, are not necessarily a mirror-image of the characteristics of maturation

The second issue is that deficits following destruction or breakdown of a system are by no means an infallible guide to what happens during maturation of that system. Lesion studies, even in the infant, are not sufficient. First, impairments that result from the improper functioning, or lack of functioning, of a part do not necessarily tell you the functions of that part. In addition, of course, deficits may not even be due to damage to that part but might be due to damage to fibers

Table 18–2 Studies of the Developmental Progression of Human Infants, the Developmental Progression of Infant Monkeys, and the Effects of Lesions in Infant and Adult Monkeys on the Same Three Behavioral Tasks.

	A$\overline{\text{B}}$	Delayed response	Object retrieval
Human infants show a clear developmental progression from 7½ to 12 months.	Diamond, 1985	Diamond & Doar, 1989	Diamond, submitted
Adult monkeys with lesions of frontal cortex fail.	Diamond & Goldman-Rakic, 1989	Diamond & Goldman-Rakic, 1989	Diamond & Goldman-Rakic, 1985
Adult monkeys with lesions of parietal cortex succeed.	Diamond & Goldman-Rakic, 1989	Diamond & Goldman-Rakic, 1989	Diamond & Goldman-Rakic, 1985
Adult monkeys with lesions of the hippocampus succeed.	Diamond, Zola-Morgan, & Squire, 1989	Squire & Zola-Morgan, 1983	Diamond, Zola-Morgan, & Squire, 1989
Infant monkeys show a clear developmental progression from 1½ to 4 months.	Diamond & Goldman-Rakic, 1986	Diamond & Goldman-Rakic, 1986	Diamond & Goldman-Rakic, 1986
5-month-old infant monkeys, who received lesions of frontal cortex at 4 mo, fail.	Diamond & Goldman-Rakic, 1986	Diamond & Goldman-Rakic, 1986	

of passage or to overlying cortex (in the case of a deep structure such as the hippocampus). Second, the way a system deteriorates from damage or old age is by no means necessarily the reverse of how that system is built up during development, although there are often parallels. For example, the last abilities to develop are often the first to deteriorate, but the order of development is not always exactly the opposite of the order of deterioration. Research must be done on functioning in the intact brain of infants (both monkey and human), and linking maturational changes in the neural circuit in question to improved performance on the behavioral measures.

For this reason, the kind of work being done in the laboratories of investigators such as Fox and Chugani is of great importance. In a longitudinal study of A$\overline{\text{B}}$ and object retrieval performance, Fox and Bell (in press) found increased frontal electroencephalogram (EEG) activity in individual infants at the time that each infant was improving on the tasks. The relation between increased frontal cortex activity and improved performance was significant for each task. Using 2-deoxy-2-[^{18}F]fluoro-D-glucose and positron emission tomography (PET), Chugani and associates (1987) have been able to measure metabolic rates for glucose uptake in localized regions of the brain in healthy, awake infants at rest, as young as 5 days of age. The more active a neural region, the more glucose it will need to use. Chugani and coworkers (1987) found that beginning around

8 months, glucose utilization increases specifically in frontal cortex (i.e., activity in frontal cortex appears to increase just before and during the period when infants are improving on the AB̄, delayed response, and object retrieval tasks).

Much work remains to be done, however, especially on the role that specific maturational changes in dorsolateral prefrontal cortex play in the age-related changes in performance of AB̄, delayed response, and object retrieval. What exactly is changing in the prefrontal neural system over these months that permits the system to subserve functions it had earlier been incapable of supporting?

One likely maturational change is increasing levels of dopamine in the prefrontal neural system. Dopamine is a particularly important neurotransmitter in prefrontal cortex, where its concentrations are higher than in any other cortical region (Brown et al., 1979). There are two main dopaminergic systems in the brain. One originates in the ventral tegmental area and projects heavily to prefrontal cortex (Divac et al., 1978; Porrino and Goldman-Rakic, 1982). The other originates in the substantia nigra and projects heavily to the caudate nucleus (Anden et al., 1964). The caudate is a major output structure of dorsolateral prefrontal cortex (Selemon and Goldman-Rakic, 1985a). Thus, both cortical and subcortical components of the prefrontal system receive strong dopaminergic input.

High levels of dopamine in dorsolateral prefrontal cortex are essential for proper functioning: (1) If dorsolateral prefrontal cortex is selectively depleted of dopamine by local injection of 6-OHDA, monkeys show impairments on delayed response as large as those found after dorsolateral prefrontal removal (Brozoski et al., 1979). (2) Monkeys treated with MPTP (1-methyl-4-phenyl-1,2,3,6-tetra-hydropyridine) show deficits on object retrieval similar to those seen following dorsolateral prefrontal cortex lesions and similar to those seen in young infants (Taylor et al., 1990; Saint-Cyr et al., 1988). MPTP injection results in reduced levels of dopamine in the substantia nigra and in the frontal-striatal system (Elsworth et al., 1987; Mitchel et al., 1986) and is thought to produce behavioral deficits similar to those seen in patients with Parkinson's disease (Burns et al., 1983; Stern and Langston, 1985). Here, depletion of dopamine in the neural circuit appears to produce the same deficits on object retrieval as do lesions to the circuit.

The level of dopamine in the brain increases markedly during the period when performance on AB̄, delayed response, and object retrieval is improving in infant monkeys (Diamond and Goldman-Rakic, 1986; Goldman-Rakic and Brown, 1982).[4] Given the importance of dopamine for dorsolateral prefrontal cortex function and given the increases in brain dopamine levels during the period when tasks dependent on dorsolateral prefrontal cortex are first mastered, it is reasonable that increases in dopamine levels over age may play a causal role in the developmental improvements on these tasks. This remains to be directly demonstrated, however.

3C. Although work with animals or adult patients is important, evidence must, at some point, be obtained directly in children

Work with nonhuman primates is useful because the most precise information on brain function comes from invasive procedures that cannot be used with humans. Adult patients enable the investigator to study the effects of brain damage that one would never want, nor would one be allowed, to impose solely for the purposes of research. However, work with animals or adults needs to be complemented by work with children. There is an inescapable inferential leap when drawing conclusions about development in children from studies of animals or adults. At some point, children themselves must be studied.

One way to do this is to study the performance of children with well-localized, verifiable brain damage, much as adult patients are studied. Another valuable approach is to use noninvasive measures of brain function, such as EEG, event related potential (ERP), and magnetoencephalography, to study functioning in intact, healthy children. Yet another approach is to study children with lower levels of dopamine but who appear to have no structural damage to the brain. Children with early-treated phenylketonuria (PKU) may fall in this latter category, as they are thought to a functional deficit in frontal cortex function due to dopamine depletion with no structural damage. We are now investigating whether these children are impaired specifically on tasks linked to dorsolateral prefrontal cortex function in the face of otherwise preserved cognitive functioning, and whether there is a relationship between their performance and their levels of dopamine.

If PKU is untreated, it results in severe mental retardation (Primrose, 1983; Tourian and Sidbury, 1978). Dietary regulation, begun early and consistently maintained, results in IQs within the normal range and no gross cognitive impairments (Dobson et al., 1977; Holtzman et al., 1986; Hudson et al., 1970; Koch et al., 1984; Williamson et al., 1977). There are reports, however, that even when a special diet is followed, children with PKU may have residual frontal lobe signs (Cowie, 1971; Pennington et al., 1985; Welsh et al., 1990). It would make sense that these children might have such a selective impairment given the tendency of PKU patients, even when they have been maintained on diet from shortly after birth, to have lower dopamine levels (Krause et al., 1985), and given the importance of dopamine for frontal cortex function.

At least for the present, however, studies of children need to be complemented by more precise, invasive procedures with animals. Too often, studies of brain-behavior relationships in children are able to be correlational only. For example, the research with children with early-treated PKU needs to be complemented by work with infant monkeys where the relation between maturational changes in dopamine levels within dorsolateral prefrontal cortex and the emergence of cognitive functions subserved by dorsolateral prefrontal cortex can be studied directly, and where the nature and underlying mechanisms of the causal relation can be explored. Thus, while studies of animals must be complemented by studies of brain-behavior relations in children, so too must studies of children be complemented by studies of brain-behavior relations in animals.

4. Use *the same tasks* when studying the developmental progression in children and when studying the neural basis in other populations, rather than tasks that are simply similar.

Tasks that appear to be similar, or appear to require similar abilities, often turn out to depend on quite different neural systems. Small changes in a task, which one might have thought would be inconsequential, often turn out to be critical.

For example, dorsolateral prefrontal cortex is not required if the rule is to reach to a *different* object than the one you just saw, but it apparently *is* required if the rule is to reach to the *same* object you just saw (Mishkin et al., 1962). As the delay increases on AB̄ and delayed response, these tasks change from being sensitive selectively to dorsolateral prefrontal cortex function at delays of 2–5 seconds to being sensitive to hippocampal function as well at delays of 15 seconds or more (Diamond et al., 1989b). Patients with frontal lobe damage are selectively impaired in producing as many words as they can think of beginning with a given letter (*F, A,* or *S*; e.g., Benton, 1968), but they are not selectively impaired in producing as many words as they can think of belonging to a given category (e.g., animals or clothing). The neuropsychological literature is replete with such fascinating dissociations. Similarly, any ability such as memory, attention, or inhibition can be shown to be present in very young children on one test but absent in much older children on a different test, even though both tests are considered measures of "memory" or "inhibition." The exact manner in which something is assessed is terribly important.

For this reason, in our work with human infants, infant monkeys, and adult monkeys, we have used the same tasks, not simply analogous ones. AB̄, delayed response, and object retrieval were administered to all subjects. Accommodations were made for species differences: e.g., toys served as the reward for human infants; peanuts and raisins served as the reward for monkeys. Aside from these small adjustments, however, children and monkeys were tested in the same way on all three tasks.

This guideline raises a problem, however, in studying brain-behavior relations in development during the preschool and early elementary school years. After 1–2 years of age, children need more sophisticated tasks than can be used with monkeys, but not until 8–12 years of age can they succeed on tests of frontal cortex function used with adult patients. With children 3–8 years of age, we have used modifications of the tasks used with adults (e.g., the Wisconsin Card Sorting Test [Diamond and Boyer, 1989] and the Stroop Test [Diamond et al., in prep.]). It is possible, however, that we have modified the tests in ways that we did not realize were crucial, and this is of great concern to us. Evidence directly linking the versions of the tests we have used to frontal cortex function is critically needed.

Two caveats are in order concerning guideline #4. First, sometimes a task must be modified *in order* for it to measure the same ability in a different population. An obvious example would be that a test of memory given in English to English-speaking children should be administered in French to French-speaking children if one is interested in testing memory. Similar modifications are sometimes needed to accommodate age or species differences in subjects. Some of the early work in child development foundered because experimenters tried to use the same tasks with children that had been used with animals without modifying the tasks to make them appropriate for children (for some examples, see Donaldson, 1978). Sometimes a task must be modified in order to keep it equivalent for two different populations.

The second caveat is that sometimes using the same task, even when it appears to be appropriate for each population, is not a guarantee that one is

Table 18-3 Performance on Delayed Nonmatching to Sample by Age and Delay

	5-sec delay			30-sec delay
Ages	Mean number of trials to criterion[a]	Percent passing criterion	Percent correct	Percent correct
12 months[b]	17	50	66	65 (N = 6)[c]
15 months	16	67	67	65 (N = 8)
18 months	16	67	71	81 (N = 8)
21 months	11	92	80	80 (N = 11)
24 months	9	92	87	86 (N = 11)
27 months	7	100	85	90
30 months	8	100	84	86
3 years	6	100	93	96
4 years	5	100	98	99
5 years	5	100	94	95

[a]Criterion = 5 correct responses in a row. For subjects who never reached criterion (6 subjects at 12 months, 4 subjects each at 15 and 18 months, and 1 subject each at 21 and 24 months) the total number of trials they were tested (25) is entered here.
[b]N = 12 for all ages.
[c]Only subjects who passed criterion at 5 sec were tested at 30 sec.

tapping the same ability in two different populations. The delayed nonmatching to sample task[5] is a test of memory sensitive to hippocampal damage in adult monkeys (e.g., Zola-Morgan and Squire, 1986) and sensitive to amnesia in human adults (Squire et al., 1988). It is also a task appropriate for testing young children, and on which they show a developmental progression between 12 and 30 months of age (Diamond, 1990a; Overman, 1990).[6] However, while this task is a measure of memory ability in adult monkeys and human adults, sensitively reflecting damage to neural structures important for memory, the developmental progression of improved performance on delayed nonmatching to sample *in infants* does *not* chart the maturation of this memory function or of the hippocampal neural circuit, even though the same task is used with infants, adults, and monkeys.

Until about 21 months of age, children fail this task even at delays of only 5 seconds (Table 18-3), although it is well established that infants can remember for far longer than 5 seconds well before 21 months (there is evidence of such memory by at least 2-3 months of age: e.g., Werner and Perlmutter, 1979; Rovee-Collier, 1984). Indeed, emerging anatomical and biochemical evidence indicates that the hippocampus develops quite early in humans and monkeys (e.g., Rakic and Nowakowski, 1981; Eckenhoff and Rakic, 1988; Bachevalier et al., 1986; Kretschmann et al., 1986; see Diamond, 1990a). Moreover, in the same session in which children first succeed on delayed nonmatching to sample with a 5-second delay they typically succeed with 30-second delays as well (see Table 18-3). One might expect success at a delay of 30 seconds to come in later if the task were assessing the development of memory. In adult monkeys or humans, in whom other abilities are fully mature, disturbance of the memory system produces errors on the task—for memory is, indeed, one of the abilities required for success, but it is only one of the required abilities. The slow developmental progression in performance of the delayed nonmatching to sample task is due to the late maturation of some other ability. We tested whether this late-developing ability might be the ability to deduce an abstract rule, the ability to quickly encode visual stimuli (speed of processing), or the ability to tolerate retroactive interference (Diamond, 1990a; Towle and Diamond, 1991). Telling the children the rule or giving them a long time to encode the stimulus only marginally improved performance. However, reducing retroactive interference (by not introducing a reward after subjects displaced the sample when the sample was presented alone during familiarization) had a dramatic effect: It enabled children to succeed almost 12 months earlier (Towle and Diamond, 1991).

Here is a case where a task has been linked specifically to a discrete neural circuit, and where the same task has been used with children and the developmental progression documented, yet it is incorrect to conclude that the developmental progression in children's performance of the task reflects maturation of that neural circuit. Thus, while it is true that success on delayed nonmatching to sample requires hippocampal involvement, and it is true that success on delayed nonmatching to sample appears relatively late in development, it is not true that the late emergence of success on this task is due to late maturation of the hippocampus, or of the memory ability it subserves. This illustrates why caution must be used in drawing conclusions about brain-behavior relations in development. In this case important clues came from two sources: (1) Infant monkeys also show a protracted developmental progression in performance of the task despite evidence of early hippocampal maturation in the monkey (Bachevalier and Mishkin, 1984; Brickson and Bachevalier, 1984; Bachevalier, 1990 and (2) the qualitative aspects of the performance of infant monkeys and human infants on the task are different from those of adult monkeys and human patients (e.g., adult monkeys and humans succeed at the shortest delays and perform progressively more poorly as the delay increases; human infants and infant monkeys perform at chance even at the very shortest delay; their performance does not worsen as delay increases). This leads directly to guideline #5.

5. Compare the *qualitative,* as well as quantitative, aspects of children's performance on the tasks to that of brain-damaged populations

Because someone may fail a task for a variety of reasons, it is important to determine the reasons for failure. The qualitative aspects of performance should be investigated, and not simply rate of success or failure. If one is comparing the performance of children with the performance of animals with selective lesions, then the younger children should fail under the same conditions and in the same ways as do the animals with lesions to the relevant neural system. Changes in task parameters should affect both the young children and the lesioned animals in the same ways. It becomes more likely that the performance of the children and lesioned animals reflects the presence or absence of the same abilities and depends upon the same neural system, the more parameters on which their performance matches and the more identical the circumstances under which these behaviors are elicited.

For example, in comparing human infants and monkeys with lesions of dorsolateral prefrontal cortex we have looked not only at their overall success rates but also at the conditions under which they err and what their errors look like. Figures 18-5 and 18-6 illustrate this. On the A$\overline{B}$ and delayed response tasks, human infants of 7½–9 months fail at delays of only 2–5 seconds. The only group of adult monkeys to fail at such brief delays are those with lesions of dorsolateral prefrontal cortex. Monkeys with lesions of parietal cortex or the hippocampus perform as well as unoperated controls here.

Moreover, at these delays infants show a characteristic pattern of performance: Their errors are confined to trials on which side of hiding is reversed and to the next few trials at that new location. Their performance is excellent when the reward is hidden in the same well as on the previous trial and they were correct on the previous trial (Repeat-following-correct trials; see Fig. 18-5). The only group of adult monkeys to show this pattern of performance are monkeys with lesions of dorsolateral prefrontal cortex (see Fig. 18-5), and they show this pattern at the same delays as do 7½–9-month-old human infants. At long delays monkeys with lesions of the hippocampal formation also fail A$\overline{B}$, but they never show this differential pattern of performance by type of trial. At delays of 15–30 seconds, they have difficulty remembering where the reward has been hidden and their performance declines, but it does not decline selectively for reversal trials. When monkeys with hippocampal lesions reach incorrectly, they show some tendency to repeat that error on the next trial, but where these strings of errors begin is randomly distributed over a testing session (Diamond et al., 1989b).

On the object retrieval task, human infants of 8½–9 months lean all the way over to look in the opening when the left or right side of the box is open. When they do this they reach with the hand contralateral to the opening, which though easier from this position than reaching with the ipsilateral hand, looks very contorted and is therefore termed an "awkward reach." The awkward reach is not the result of a hand preference, as it is seen on both sides of the box (Diamond, submitted; Bruner et al., 1969; Gaiter, 1973; Schonen and Bresson, 1984). One group of adult monkeys also shows this strange awkward reach—monkeys with lesions of dorsolateral prefrontal cortex (Fig. 18-6).

6. Divergent Validity, 2: Study performance on *other tasks linked to other neural circuits*

It is also important to establish a second kind of divergent validity by determining that performance on tasks linked to other neural circuits and requiring other abilities (1) does not improve over the same age period as does performance on tasks linked to the neural system of interest, and (2) is not affected by disruption of functioning in the neural system of interest. (The first kind of divergent validity discussed previously was that disruption of functioning in other neural systems should not affect performance on tasks linked to the neural system of inter-

AB̄ PERFORMANCE WITH DELAY OF 2-5 SEC

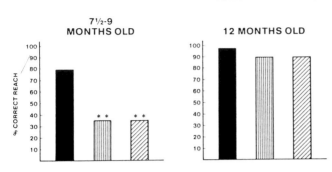

1 HUMAN INFANTS

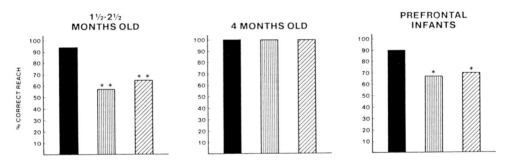

2 INFANT RHESUS MONKEYS

Figure 18–5 Percentage correct by type of trial at delays of 2–5 sec for human infants, infant monkeys, and monkeys with lesions to prefrontal cortex, parietal cortex, and the hippocampal formation. **Row 1:** Human infants of 12 months perform perfectly. Human infants of 7½–9 months perform well on repeat-following-correct trials, but perform significantly worse on reversal trials and on repeat-following-error trials in both the AB̄ task (Diamond, 1985) and the delayed-response task (Diamond and Doar, 1989). **Row 2:** Infant rhesus monkeys of 4 months perform perfectly. Infant monkeys of 1½–2½ months and infant monkeys who have received bilateral lesions of dorsolateral prefrontal cortex at 4 months and were retested at 5 months show a similar pattern of differential performance over trials as do 7½–9-month-old human infants (Diamond and Goldman-Rakic, 1986).

est.) This is important for determining whether improvements, or impairments, are general or specific. For example, are all abilities improving at the same time, at the same rate, or are developmental changes more pronounced in different abilities during different age periods?

For instance, while human infants improve on AB̄, delayed response, and object retrieval (tasks all linked to dorsolateral prefrontal cortex) between 7½ and

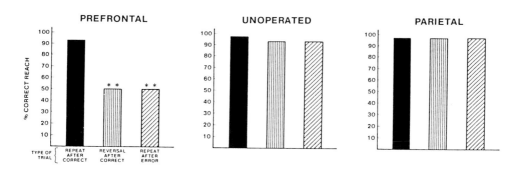

3   ADULT RHESUS MONKEYS

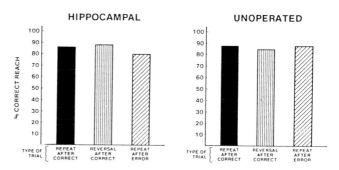

4   ADULT CYNOMOLGUS MONKEYS

Figure 18–5 (continued)   Row 3: Unoperated adult rhesus monkeys and those with bilateral lesions of inferior parietal cortex perform perfectly. Adult rhesus monkeys with bilateral lesions of dorsolateral prefrontal cortex, however, show the same pattern of differential performance over trials as do 7½–9-month-old human infants (Diamond and Goldman-Rakic, 1989). **Row 4:** Unoperated adult cynomolgus monkeys and those with bilateral lesions of the hippocampal formation perform perfectly at delays of 2–5 sec (Diamond et al., 1989b). (At delays of 15–30 sec hippocampal monkeys no longer perform well on the task, but at these delays they still do not show the pattern of differential performance by type of trial seen in 7½–9-month-old human infants, 1½–2½-month-old rhesus monkeys, and in infant and adult rhesus monkeys following lesions of dorsolateral prefrontal cortex).

12 months of age, they improve on visual paired comparison (a task linked to the hippocampal-amygdala system) (Brickson and Bachevalier, 1984; Saunders, 1989) between 2 and 9 months of age (Diamond, 1990a; Fagan, 1990). In the visual paired comparison task, subjects look at a stimulus for a fixed familiarization period or until habituated, a delay is imposed, and then memory of the sample is tested by pairing the sample with another stimulus. Preferential looking at the new stimulus is taken as evidence of memory of the sample, since infants have a natural preference for novelty (Fagan, 1970; Diamond, 1990a).

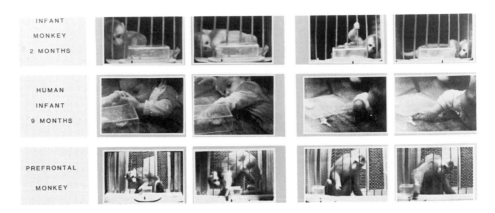

Figure 18–6 The "awkward reach" in an infant monkey of 2 months, a human infant of 9 months, and an adult monkey with bilateral lesion of dorsolateral prefrontal cortex. **Frame 1:** Subject leans and looks at bait through opening of box. **Frame 2:** Subject reaches in awkwardly with the far hand. **Frame 3:** Opening is on the other side of the box. Performance is the same. Subject leans and looks into the opening. **Frame 4:** Subject reaches in awkwardly with the far hand.

The visual paired comparison task presents some of the same task requirements as do A$\overline{\text{B}}$ and delayed response: All require that memory be updated on each trial (to remember where the reward was just hidden or which stimulus was just presented). All present the to-be-remembered information visually and only once. All impose the delay within a trial, as opposed to between trials or between testing sessions. However, the visual paired comparison task also differs considerably from A$\overline{\text{B}}$ and delayed response. For example, A$\overline{\text{B}}$ and delayed response require a reaching response; visual paired comparison does not. The to-be-remembered information is presented much longer in visual paired comparison. In A$\overline{\text{B}}$ and delayed response the same two hiding wells are used throughout, presenting possible problems of proactive interference; in visual paired comparison, on the other hand, new stimuli are used on each trial (rather than using the same two stimuli repeatedly, varying only which is the sample on a given trial). Subjects must remember spatial location information for A$\overline{\text{B}}$ and delayed response, but not for visual paired comparison.

As more tasks are studied, a better understanding emerges of the abilities developing during each age period and depending on the different neural circuits.

REMAINING QUESTIONS

What Happens After 12 Months of Age in the Neural Circuit of Interest?

The work on A$\overline{\text{B}}$, delayed response, and object retrieval appears to provide a window into dorsolateral prefrontal cortex development between 7½ and 12 months of age. Neither dorsolateral prefrontal cortex, nor the abilities it subserves, are fully mature by 12 months of age, however. Indeed, frontal cortex is not thought to be fully mature until puberty. For example, children do not perform at adult levels on the Wisconsin Card Sorting Test (a criterial test of frontal cortex function in adults [Milner, 1963]) until about 9–10 years of age (Chelune and Baer, 1986). What changes occur in the dorsolateral prefrontal neural circuit, and when, after 12 months? In what ways do the abilities dependent on frontal cortex change and improve over these years? Is the improvement simply quantitative, or is it qualitative as well? Is the improvement gradual, or are there growth spurts and plateaus? When are critical points in the development of frontal cortex reached?

We have begun to investigate these questions. In a study of 72 children (12 each at 3, 4, 5, 6, 7, and 8 years of age) we have found a significant improvement from 3–6 years on seven different measures of abilities associated with frontal cortex, with a leveling off from 6–8 years (Diamond et al., in prep.) (Fig. 18–7). On all tests we found this same pattern; there were no exceptions. This suggests that the age of 6 may be something of a watershed; on a host of tests linked to frontal cortex, children either reach ceiling performance by 6 years of age or reach a plateau where they remain for at least the next 2 years. Five of our tests assessed inhibitory control of action, one assessed the ability to execute a sequence of actions, and one assessed the ability to remember sequential information. The tests of inhibition were: tapping (Luria, 1973), Stroop (Stroop, 1935), three pegs (Wozniack et al., 1987), Simon Says, and simultaneous switch (Luria, 1973). The test of sequential action was flat-fist-edge (Luria, 1973). The memory task was multiple boxes (Petrides & Milner, 1982; Passingham, 1985; Petrides, 1988).

On the tapping task, a subject must tap twice when the experimenter taps once, and then tap only once when the experimenter taps twice. This requires inhibiting the pull to do what the experimenter does. Frontal patients fail because, while they may start out correctly, they shortly begin to mirror the experimenter's behavior, rather than following the rule. Similarly, children under 6 years tend to match what the experimenter does rather than follow the rule. Only by 6 years could children consistently succeed on the task (Fig. 18–7A).

In the adult version of the Stroop test, the names of colors are printed in the ink of another color (e.g., the word "blue" is printed in red ink). Subjects are instructed to report the color of the ink. This requires inhibiting the customary response when reading, which is to ignore the ink and attend instead to the meaning of the word. Frontal patients fail the test, as they tend to recite the words and not the color of the ink (Perret, 1974). In our version of the Stroop test for children we use a deck of cards. The front of half the cards is black with a yellow moon and several stars; the front of the other cards is white with a bright sun. Subjects are to say "day" when the experimenter turns over a black card and "night" when a white card appears. This is similar to a modified Stroop test used by Passler and associates (1985) where plain black and white cards were used. Passler and colleagues found on their version that children were at ceiling by the youngest age they tested (6 years). We found that most children ≥ 6 years

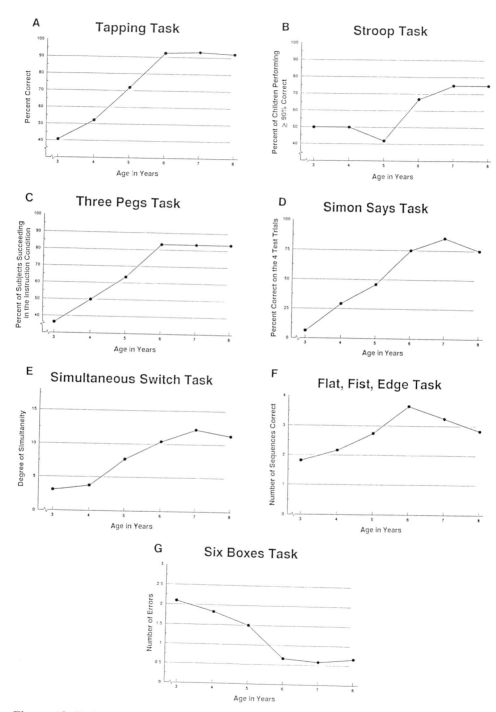

Figure 18-7 Developmental progression in children aged 3–8 years on eight tests of abilities associated with frontal cortex.

succeeded, but not most children at younger ages. Indeed, there was little change in the number of children succeeding from 3 to 5 or from 6 to 8 years, but there was a dramatic improvement from 5 to 6 years.

On the three pegs test, the subject is to hammer in a row of pegs (red, yellow, and green) in the order: red, green, and then yellow. The subject must inhibit the tendency to hammer the pegs in spatial left-right order, and instead follow the rule. Performance improved steadily from 3–6 years, and remained at ceiling thereafter (Fig. 18–7C).

Simon Says is a common children's game. The trials of interest here are where the experimenter fails to say "Simon Says." On these trials, the child is not supposed to do anything. This requires inhibiting the tendency to carry out the command anyway. On other trials, the child is to touch his or her nose or eyes, for example, as instructed by "Simon." Before 6 years, children are much more likely to act when they should refrain from acting than are children ≥ 6 years.

In the simultaneous switch: fist–flat task, the subject starts with one hand in a fist on the table, and the palm of the other hand flat on the table. The subject is then to switch these hand positions simultaneously back and forth six times. This requires inhibiting one hand from doing what the other is doing. Younger subjects, like frontal patients, tend to err by doing the same thing with both hands or by switching the position of one hand and then the other. We found a marked increase between 4 and 6 years in the degree of simultaneity children showed in switching one hand to one position while simultaneously switching the other hand to the other position. At the 2 extremes of the age range there was little change: Performance did not significantly improve between ages 3 and 4, nor between ages 6 and 8 (Fig. 18–7E).

In the flat–fist–edge task, the subject must change the position of one hand in the following sequence: palm flat on the table, closed fist on the table, and palm at right angles to the table (edge). This sequence is repeated 4 times. Here, the children appeared to reach ceiling at 6 years and thereafter their performance declined slightly.

In the Multiple Boxes task, the subject watches as the experimenter hides a sticker in each of six boxes. All boxes are then closed. The subject is permitted to open one box at a time, in any order he or she chooses. A 10-second delay is imposed between reaches. The goal is to open all the boxes without repeating a choice. The number of reaches needed to open all the boxes progressively decreased until age 6 where it plateaued.This task is selective for dorsolateral prefrontal cortex damage in both monkeys (Passingham, 1985; Petrides, 1988) and human adults (Petrides and Milner, 1982). In short, on all seven of the tasks used, a significant improvement was found up to 6 years. There was little further change from 6–8 years, either because the tests were not sensitive enough to pick up such changes, or because the abilities tapped by these tests remain relatively constant during the 6–8 year age period.

It should be noted, however, that the Stroop test had to be modified for use with children, as those at the younger end of the age range cannot read, and the three pegs test and Simon Says have never been directly linked to frontal cortex function in children or adults. Such evidence, directly linking the modified

Stroop test, the three pegs test, and Simon Says to frontal cortex function, is needed. Moreover, even though there is evidence linking performance on the tapping test, the adult version of the Stroop test, and the simultaneous switch tests to the integrity of frontal cortex, information on the role of localized regions within frontal cortex in supporting performance on these tasks is lacking. Such information is needed.

What Happens Before 7½–8 Months of Age in the Neural Circuit of Interest?

Development does not begin at 7½–8 months. Indeed, it is only because of the developmental accomplishments present by 7½–8 months that testing on A$\overline{B}$, delayed response, and object retrieval can begin at roughly those ages. For example, hiding tasks are not possible with younger infants because they will not search for a hidden object. What abilities are developing before 7½–8 months, and what are the neural bases for these accomplishments? What is happening in frontal cortex up until this age? I have suggested (Diamond, 1990b; 1991b) that some of the accomplishments between 5 and 8 months of age may be made possible by maturational changes in the supplementary motor area (an area of frontal cortex immediately posterior, and medial, to dorsolateral prefrontal cortex). The inhibition of the reflexes of the hand (the grasp and avoidance reactions) and the ability to link two action sequences together into a larger means-end sequence (e.g., removing a cloth in order to then retrieve the reward underneath it) may require involvement of the supplementary motor area. More work is needed in testing this hypothesis and in exploring when and where other neural changes are occurring.

What Abilities Are Dependent on the Neural Circuit of Interest and in What Ways Do These Abilities Change Over Age?

For example, if success on A$\overline{B}$, delayed response, and object retrieval depends on involvement of dorsolateral prefrontal cortex, as it now appears, what ability(s) are required by these tasks that accounts for this dependence?

Many of the tasks dependent on dorsolateral prefrontal cortex and on which infants show a developmental progression between 7½ and 12 months (e.g., A$\overline{B}$ and delayed response) appear to require memory. For instance, monkeys with dorsolateral prefrontal cortex lesions and human infants perform well if there is no delay but fail with a delay, all other conditions being equal. What are the characteristics of this memory ability?

Spatial Memory
One prominent theory is that the memory ability subserved by dorsolateral prefrontal cortex is memory of spatial information in particular (e.g., Goldman-Rakic, 1987). Evidence for this view includes: Monkeys with lesions of dorsolateral prefrontal cortex are less impaired on some nonspatial memory tasks (e.g., delayed object alternation) than they are on comparable spatial memory

tasks (e.g., delayed spatial alternation) (Mishkin et al., 1969). Monkeys with lesions of the principal sulcus (the "heart" of dorsolateral prefrontal cortex in the monkey) perform well on spatial tasks that do not require memory but fail spatial tasks that require memory (Goldman and Rosvold, 1970). There are cells in dorsolateral prefrontal cortex that increase firing after a cue is presented and maintain that level of activity throughout the delay (i.e., they appear to serve a memory function); moreover, a subset of these cells is direction-selective, i.e., they fire more if the cue was on the right or left (Fuster and Alexander, 1971; Niki, 1974; Funahashi et al., 1989).

In addition, the anatomical connections between dorsolateral prefrontal cortex and inferior parietal cortex (Brodmann's area 7) are particularly strong (e.g., Schwartz and Goldman-Rakic, 1984). Indeed, not only are there heavy reciprocal connections between these two areas, but throughout diverse areas of the brain, wherever dorsolateral prefrontal cortex projects so does inferior parietal cortex, and in each case their projections interdigitate (i.e., columns of cells receiving projections from prefrontal cortex alternate with columns of cells receiving projections from parietal cortex) (e.g., Goldman-Rakic and Schwartz, 1982; Selemon and Goldman-Rakic, 1985; 1988). This is relevant because parietal cortex participates in that portion of the visual system specialized for the perception of motion rather than the perception of form or texture. It is conceivable that through its connections with parietal cortex, dorsolateral prefrontal cortex might specialize in the memory of spatial information rather than memory of object features.

However, lesions of inferior parietal cortex leave $A\overline{B}$ and delayed response performance undisturbed. Subjects are evidently able to succeed at these tasks without the perceptual information processed in parietal cortex. Problematic for the spatial memory view is that infants and prefrontally operated monkeys generally perform well at the first location (well A), even though spatial memory is required here as elsewhere. Errors generally first appear only when the location of the reward changes. Some of the cells in dorsolateral prefrontal cortex (and within the principal sulcus itself) that increase firing after a cue is presented and maintain that level of activity throughout the delay fire selectively depending on the *color* of the cue, just as other cells there fire selectively depending on the location of the cue (Quintana et al., 1988; Wilson and Goldman-Rakic, 1989).

Moreover, most tasks diagnostic of frontal cortex damage in human adults do not appear to have a spatial component. For example, in the Wisconsin Card Sorting Test the sorting criterion (color, shape, or number) changes during testing, and the subject must stay attentive to which criterion is currently correct, but spatial position is irrelevant to the task. Similarly, spatial position is irrelevant on the self-ordered pointing task, which requires subjects to keep track of what stimuli they have already pointed to (Petrides and Milner, 1982). Here, the spatial locations of the stimuli are scrambled after each reach. Indeed, when the stimuli are left stationary, so that the task can be solved by spatial memory, patients with frontal cortex damage perform well. A version of the self-ordered task has recently been used with monkeys, where lesions confined only to the principal sulcus produced severe deficits in performance, even though spatial memory is irrelevant to the task (Petrides, 1988).

Memory of Temporal Order

Another prominent theory of frontal cortex function is that it is specialized for the memory of temporal order information (e.g., Milner et al., 1985). For example, there is a potential for *proactive interference* from previous trials during A$\overline{\text{B}}$ and delayed response testing as the same two hiding places are used throughout. Once the reward has been hidden at well A on at least one trial and at well B on at least one trial, one might consider the task to be one of temporal order memory: "Where was the reward hidden most recently?"

Evidence for this viewpoint includes: When adult patients are shown a series of pictures, patients with frontal cortex damage can tell you which of two pictures they saw before, but not which of the two pictures they saw most recently (Corsi, cited in Milner, 1971). When asked about well-known events from the last several decades, patients with frontal cortex damage are impaired in recalling the order in which the events occurred, yet are unimpaired in their recognition and recall of the events (Shimamura et al., 1990). Indeed, all tasks sensitive to frontal cortex damage in the monkey require temporal discrimination (e.g., "I have seen the reward hidden at A and at B. Where was it hidden most recently?"), although the spatial component has been emphasized in theoretical discussion of these tasks. Monkeys with frontal cortex damage, human infants, and infant monkeys generally perform well at the first location (even though spatial memory is required here as elsewhere); errors appear when the location of the reward changes, i.e., when memory of temporal order is first required.

Most tasks diagnostic of frontal cortex damage in humans appear to require resistance to proactive interference (e.g., the Wisconsin Card Sort: "Which sorting criterion is the correct one now?", and the self-ordered pointing task: "Which stimuli have I already pointed to?").

If dorsolateral prefrontal cortex is specialized solely for the memory of temporal relationships, however, why then are there cells in dorsolateral prefrontal cortex that code the left-right location of stimuli or responses? Why, too, does damage to dorsolateral prefrontal cortex produce more profound deficits on spatial tasks (e.g., delayed spatial alternation) than on nonspatial tasks (e.g., delayed object alternation)?

Tulving and Schacter (e.g., Schacter, 1987; Tulving, 1989) have suggested that frontal cortex is critical for the memory of both space and time, specifically memory of the spatial or temporal context in which information is acquired.

Relational Memory

Spatial and temporal information (e.g., left, right; earlier, later) are inherently relational. Perhaps memory for relational information in general is dependent on dorsolateral prefrontal cortex and develops between 7½ and 12 months of age in human infants. Evidence consistent with this includes: Patients with frontal cortex damage often do well on typical delayed recall tests but fail delayed comparison tests where they must judge whether a color they saw earlier is the same shade as the color they see now, or whether a tone they just heard is the same pitch as the tone they hear now (Prisko, cited in Milner, 1964). Patients with frontal cortex damage are notoriously poor at relating two pieces of information together (e.g., Barbizet, 1970; Heilman and Valenstein, 1972). Grossman (1982) administered eight visual and auditory reversal tasks (i.e., tasks that required that subjects appreciate the relation between original and transformed states) mediated by linguistic and nonlinguistic symbol systems to adults with localized brain damage. He found no domain-specific deficits; rather, patients with frontal cortex damage were impaired across the board on the reversal tasks regardless of modality or content. Similarly, memory for space and/or time might not be a unique ability but might be a subset of relational memory in general.

It would make sense if relational memory were more difficult than single item memory, as it requires remembering a relation between two things. Perhaps memory of information that is inherently relative, i.e., that requires relating one thing to another (e.g., left, right; smaller, bigger; softer, louder) matures later and more slowly than memory of individual items (e.g., red, girl, circle). Perhaps, too, memory of any relative information, spatial or not, requires involvement of dorsolateral prefrontal cortex.

The idea that memory of space, time, or relational information in general might have a unique developmental trajectory, appear later (i.e., between 7½ and 12 months), and be sensitive to different experimental parameters[7] than memory for other, nonrelational information (e.g., color or shape) has never been considered by developmental psychologists, although it deserves investigation.[8]

Memory Plus Inhibition

I have argued that dorsolateral prefrontal cortex is required whenever *any information at all* must be remembered within each trial as long as the task *also* demands inhibition of a prepotent response (Diamond, 1985; 1988). That is, it may not matter whether one must remember temporal, spatial, relational, color, or object information. The critical factor may be whether the task demands *both memory and inhibition of a dominant response.*

Evidence for the role of inhibition is extremely strong: All memory tasks linked to dorsolateral prefrontal cortex in the monkey also impose an inhibitory demand. The *pattern* of error on the A$\overline{\text{B}}$ and delayed response tasks (i.e., errors confined to reversal trials and the trials immediately thereafter) shown by infants or by prefrontally operated monkeys cannot be accounted for by forgetting alone, for the delay is equal on all trials but errors are not equally distributed over trials (Diamond, 1985; Diamond and Goldman-Rakic, 1989). Indeed, monkeys with lesions of the hippocampal formation, who have impaired memory, never show this pattern of error on A$\overline{\text{B}}$ (Diamond et al., 1989b). Moreover, when a task requires memory, but not inhibitory control, human infants perform well months before they first succeed on A$\overline{\text{B}}$ or other tasks dependent on dorsolateral prefrontal cortex (e.g., Baillargeon et al., 1985; Fagan, 1970), and monkeys with lesions of dorsolateral prefrontal cortex also perform well (as on the delayed nonmatching to sample task [e.g., Mishkin et al., 1962; Bachevalier and Mishkin, 1986]).

Note, if dorsolateral prefrontal cortex is necessary whenever a task requires both memory *and* inhibition, then success on delayed *matching* to sample should depend on dorsolateral prefrontal cortex involvement, and this appears to be the case. Monkeys with lesions of lateral frontal cortex fail delayed matching to sample, although they succeed at delayed nonmatching to sample (Mishkin et al., 1962). In delayed matching to sample, a sample object is presented, a brief delay is imposed, and then the subject is given the choice of reaching to the object that matches the sample or to a novel object. A reach to the matching object is rewarded. Infants (e.g., Fantz, 1964; Fagan, 1970; Diamond, 1990a) and monkeys (e.g., Brush et al., 1961; Harlow, 1950) have a natural preference for novel stimuli. Therefore, to succeed at delayed matching to sample an infant or monkey must not only remember what he or she has seen but must inhibit the tendency to reach to the new object. (Hence, the importance of using different objects on each trial—for if the objects have been seen on previous trials then neither object will be novel and there will be no response bias to inhibit— and the importance of giving subjects sufficient time with the sample so they begin to get bored with it.)

Delayed nonmatching to sample is formally similar to delayed matching to sample (only the rule is different: "Reach to the familiar object" for delayed matching to sample, "reach to the new object" for delayed nonmatching to sample). However, inhibitory control is not required for delayed nonmatching to sample, as the natural preference is to reach to the new object. Hence, delayed nonmatching to sample requires only memory, not inhibitory control. It is dependent on the hippocampal neural circuit, not dorsolateral prefrontal cortex (Mishkin et al., 1962; Zola-Morgan and Squire, 1986; Zola-Morgan et al., 1989). On the other hand, delayed matching to sample requires both memory and inhibitory control; performance here appears to be impaired by lesions to either the hippocampal system or to dorsolateral prefrontal cortex (Mishkin et al., 1962).

Inhibition
Perhaps memory is not one of the abilities dependent on dorsolateral prefrontal cortex at all, and not one of the abilities developing between 7½ and 12 months. Since the delays at which dorsolateral prefrontal cortex is typically required are so brief (e.g., 2–5 seconds on $A\overline{B}$ and delayed response), perhaps this might better be described as "maintaining attention" than "memory." If one conceives of the ability to span a few seconds' delay as an ability to resist distraction and maintain focused attention, then one might conceive of $A\overline{B}$ and delayed response as requiring, not memory plus inhibition, but two types of inhibition (the ability to resist distraction and to resist repeating a rewarded response). Memory may not be required for the object retrieval task, as the goal object is always visible (although memory of which sides of the box have been tried and found closed is probably still important). It is clear, though, that the object retrieval task imposes a strong demand on inhibitory control: The pull to reach straight to the visible goal must be inhibited if the subject is to detour around the transparent box to the opening. For example, subjects perform significantly better on object retrieval when an opaque box is used; i.e., when they cannot see the goal object through a closed side of the box and so do not have to fight the tendency to reach straight to the object (Diamond, submitted; Taylor et al., 1990b). Inhibition is certainly an ability required by all three tasks on which infants improve between 7½ and 12 months: $A\overline{B}$, delayed response, and object retrieval.

However, just as a memory demand alone does not appear to be sufficient to require dorsolateral prefrontal cortex involvement, neither is a simple inhibitory demand sufficient. For example, even before 7½–12 months, infants are able to inhibit their tendency to reach impulsively for any new object (Fox and Bell, 1990). Infants and prefrontally operated monkeys succeed on AB̄ and delayed response if there is no delay (no requirement to hold something in mind), even on reversal trials where the pull to reach back to where they were previously reinforced must be inhibited (e.g., **infants:** Gratch and Landers, 1971; Harris, 1973; Gratch et al., 1974; Fox et al., 1979; **monkeys:** Harlow et al., 1952; Battig et al., 1960; Fuster and Alexander, 1971). Still, it is possible that "memory plus inhibition" is not the best way to characterize the abilities maturing between 7½ and 12 months or the abilities dependent on dorsolateral prefrontal cortex. Fox and Bell (1990), for example, characterize the ability as "inhibition of a response in the presence of distraction." Further work is needed to help us better understand the underlying abilities and choose among these competing hypotheses.

To better understand the abilities subserved by any neural circuit, or developing during any particular period of life, control tasks must be used. Ideally, they should differ in one way only from the tasks of interest. Examples of such pairs of tasks are delayed nonmatching to sample and delayed matching to sample, or delayed response for spatial location and delayed response for color or objects. In this way, hypotheses can be rigorously tested and eliminated.

What Roles Do Different Regions and Pathways Within the Same Neural Circuit Play in Subserving the Functions of the Circuit?

For example, how do the different regions of frontal cortex, the caudate nucleus, and the cingulate contribute to performance of various tasks? How distinct are the abilities they subserve? How does maturation of these and other related areas affect performance of tasks linked to dorsolateral prefrontal cortex?

The caudate nucleus is a major output structure of dorsolateral prefrontal cortex. Damage to the caudate, as in parkinsonism, appears to result in many frontal cortexlike deficits (Taylor and Saint-Cyr, 1986; see also Lees and Smith, 1983; Stern et al., 1983; Benecke et al., 1987). There has been much suggestion that many of the changes early in life in functions attributed to frontal cortex are due to maturation of the caudate, rather than to maturation of frontal cortex itself (Goldman and Rosvold, 1972; Villablanca et al., 1979; Vicedomini et al., 1982; 1984). It is critical to determine, especially during infancy and early childhood, the extent to which the caudate is important for performance of tasks linked to frontal cortex.

A pathway that may be undergoing important changes even as early as 7½–12 months is the callosal connection between the frontal cortices in each hemisphere. Over this age period infants become able, for the first time, to do one action with one hand while simultaneously doing something else with the other hand, such as raising the object retrieval box and, at the same time, reaching for the toy inside (Diamond, 1990b). This complementary use of the two hands may well be dependent on maturation of the interhemispheric connections via the corpus callosum between the right and left frontal cortex, especially between the supplementary motor areas.

Human adults (Luria, 1973; Laplane et al., 1977) and monkeys (Brinkman, 1984) with lesions of the supplementary motor area have difficulty with the complementary use of the two hands. Their hands tend to do the same thing, making bimanual coordination difficult. For example, patients with damage to the supplementary motor area have great difficulty making a fist with one hand while simultaneously turning their other hand palm up. They either do the same thing with both hands or execute the movements sequentially. This is very similar to the behavior seen in 7½–9-month-old infants. When they raise the object retrieval box with both hands, for instance, these infants have great difficulty not lowering the second hand when one hand goes down to reach in the box. By 8½–9 months, infants can solve this sequentially by first raising the box and then reaching in, but not until 9½–10 months can they simultaneously raise the box and reach inside. Simultaneous integration of the movements of the two hands probably requires inhibitory projections via the corpus callosum so that the tendency of one hand to do the same thing as the other hand can be suppressed. Adults who were born without a corpus callosum (congenital acallosals) have difficulty suppressing "associated movements"; i.e., they have difficulty inhibiting one hand from doing what the other is doing (Dennis, 1976), and the inhibitory control of callosal fibers on movement has been well documented (e.g., Asanuma and Okamoto, 1959).

I hope the guidelines presented here may be of some help to those doing research on brain-behavior relations in development. The importance of converging evidence from diverse experimental approaches, of divergent validity, and of looking at the qualitative, as well as quantitative, aspects of performance cannot be overemphasized. It is important not to stop simply with linking a task to a neural system, but to understand what abilities are required by that task and how that neural system functions to subserve one or more of those abilities. Work on humans should be supplemented by work with nonhuman primates, work on one neural region should be supplemented by work on other related and unrelated neural regions, work on one age range by work on older and younger ages, and work with one behavioral task by work with other tasks. Many questions remain to be answered, and there is room for much fruitful collaboration. I am convinced that work in neuroscience will continue to help us better understand how the mind changes as a child grows up, and that work in developmental psychology will continue to help us better understand how the brain makes complex cognitive operations possible.

NOTES

1. Infants make a characteristic error on the A$\overline{\text{B}}$ task, from which the task derives its name. They typically reach correctly at the first place the reward is hidden, well A, but when the reward is then hidden at well B, infants still search at well A, although they just saw the reward hidden at B moments earlier. That is, they are correct when the reward is

hidden at A but not when it is hidden at B; they reach to A but not to B. Hence, the name of the task "A-not-B."

2. It will be important in future work to determine the contributions of the supplementary motor area and premotor cortex to performance of the object retrieval task, as well as to determine the relative contributions of the subregions of dorsolateral prefrontal cortex (the sulcus principalis and the periarcuate region). Delayed response appears to depend most crucially on sulcus principalis; it will be important to determine whether the same is true for object retrieval.

3. More precisely stated, the functioning of other neural circuits should not be related *in the same ways* to the tasks. See guideline #5. Almost any task is going to require multiple abilities, such as visual processing, memory, and motor programming. More than one neural circuit will then be required for successful performance of the task, but the functioning of each neural circuit will affect task performance in different ways and be sensitive to different task parameters.

4. More precise information about changes in dopamine levels specifically in prefrontal cortex during development, or in human infants as opposed to infant monkeys, is not yet known.

5. The delayed nonmatching to sample task assesses recognition memory for objects: First a sample object is presented at the center of the testing area. In order to insure that the subject has seen the sample, the subject must displace it to retrieve a reward underneath. Then an opaque screen is lowered and a delay typically is imposed. The screen is then raised revealing the familiar sample object and a new object the subject has never seen before (one to the left of midline and the other to the right). If the subject displaces the new object (i.e., the one that does *not* match the object presented before the delay) a hidden reward is revealed for the subject to retrieve. The left-right position of the new and familiar objects is varied randomly over trials.

The testing procedure currently used, with different junk objects on every trial ("trial-unique stimuli"), was independently devised by Gaffan (1974) and by Mishkin and Delacour (1975). Delayed nonmatching to sample is used because monkeys find it difficult to learn delayed *matching* to sample, given their natural preference to reach to the new object (Harlow, 1950; Brush et al., 1961; Mishkin et al., 1962; Gaffan et al., 1984). Young children show this same preference (Diamond, in press, b).

6. Children cannot be tested on delayed nonmatching to sample, using the same procedure as used with monkeys or adult patients, until about 12 months of age.

7. For example, might memory for space and/or time be disrupted by delays of only 2–5 seconds when it first appears, while memory for other information is only disrupted by longer delays of $\geq$ 15–30 seconds from the very outset? When monkeys with lesions of dorsolateral prefrontal cortex fail memory tasks they do so at delays of only 2–5 seconds; if the task is not sensitive to dorsolateral prefrontal cortex damage at those delays, it is unlikely to be sensitive to it at longer delays (e.g., Diamond and Goldman-Rakic, 1989). Monkeys with hippocampal lesions, on the other hand, usually succeed at delays under 15–30 seconds, even on tasks specifically sensitive to hippocampal damage (e.g., Mishkin, 1978; Zola-Morgan et al., 1989).

8. Somewhat distant, though related questions have been investigated using the A$\overline{\text{B}}$ task, where psychologists have shown that 9-month-old infants tend to encode relative position, rather than absolute location or particular body movement (Bremner and Bryant, 1977; Butterworth, 1975); and infants can learn to associate the color of the cover over a hiding place with the toy and so they will reach to that color regardless of where the toy is hidden. (Bremner, 1978; Butterworth et al., 1982, expt. 2).

Piaget (1952 [1936]) characterized much of the change occurring in the latter part of the first year as the development of the ability to "put into relation." Certainly, infants begin to be able to relate two objects in play (Fenson et al., 1976) and to relate reaching one place and looking another during this period (Millar and Schaffer, 1972; Diamond, submitted). Holding relational information in memory might be part of this general development.

ACKNOWLEDGMENTS

Work discussed here was supported by NIMH R01 (MH-41842), NIMH F32 (MH-09007), BRSG (RR07054 & RR07083), NSF (BNS-8013-447), and by grants from the Sloan Foundation, and the McDonnell Center for Studies of Higher Brain Function at Washington University School of Medicine to the author, by NICHD (HD-10094) to Jerome Kagan, and by NIMH (MH-00298 & MH-38456) to Patricia Goldman-Rakic. Grateful thanks are offered to David Sparks for comments on an earlier version of the paper.

REFERENCES

Akert K. Comparative anatomy of the frontal cortex and the thalamocortical connection. *In* Warren JM, Akert K (eds), The Frontal Granular Cortex and Behavior, New York: McGraw-Hill, 1964, pp. 372–396.

Anden NE, Carlsson A, Dahlstrom A, Fuxe K, Hillarp NA, Larsson K. Demonstration and mapping out of nigro-neostriatal dopamine neurons. Life Sciences 3:523–530, 1964.

Andersen RA. Visual and visual-motor functions of the posterior parietal cortex. *In* Rakic P, Singer W (eds), Neurobiology of Neocortex, New York: John Wiley & Sons, 1988, pp. 285–295.

Asanuma H, Okamoto K. Unitary study on evoked activity of callosal neurons and its effect on pyramidal tract cell activity on cat. Japanese Journal of Neurophysiology 9:437–483, 1959.

Bachevalier J. Ontogenetic development of habit and memory formation in primates. *In* Diamond A (ed), The Development and Neural Bases of Higher Cognitive Functions. New York: Annals of the New York Academy of Sciences 608:457–484, 1990.

Bachevalier J, Mishkin M. An early and a late developing system for learning and retention in infant monkeys. Behavioral Neuroscience 98:770–778, 1984.

Bachevalier J, Mishkin M. Visual recognition impairment follows ventromedial but not dorsolateral prefrontal lesions in monkeys. Behavioural Brain Research 20:249–261, 1986.

Bachevalier J, Ungerleider LG, O'Neill B, Friedman DP. Regional distribution of [3H] naloxone binding in the brain of a newborn rhesus monkey. Developmental Brain Research 25:302–308, 1986.

Baillargeon R, Spelke ES, Wasserman S. Object permanence in five month old infants. Cognition 20:191–208, 1985.

Barbizet J. Prolonged organic amnesias. *In* Barbizet J (ed), Human Memory and its Pathology. San Francisco: W. H. Freeman & Co, 1970, pp. 25–93.

Battig K, Rosvold HE, Mishkin M. Comparison of the effects of frontal and caudate lesions on delayed response and alternation in monkeys. Journal of Comparative and Physiological Psychology 53:400–404, 1960.

Benecke JC, Rothwell JC, Dick JPR, Day BL, Marsden CD. Disturbance of sequential movements in patients with Parkinson's disease. Brain 110:361–379, 1987.

Benton AL. Differential behavioral effects of frontal lobe disease. Neuropsychologia 6:53–60, 1968.

Bremner JG, Bryant PE. Place versus response as the basis of spatial errors made by young infants. Journal of Experimental Child Psychology 23:162–171, 1977.

Brickson M, Bachevalier J. Visual recognition in infant rhesus monkeys: Evidence for a primitive memory system. Society for Neuroscience Abstracts 10:137. 1984.

Brinkman C. Supplementary motor area of the monkey's cerebral cortex: Short- and long-term deficits after unilateral ablation and the effects of subsequent collosal section. Journal of Neuroscience 4:918–929, 1984.

Brown RM, Crane AM, Goldman PS. Regional distribution of monoamines in the cerebral cortex and subcortical structures of the rhesus monkey: Concentrations and in vivo synthesis rates. Brain Research 168:133–150, 1979.

Brozoski T, Brown RM, Rosvold HE, Goldman PS. Cognitive deficit caused by depletion of dopamine in prefrontal cortex of rhesus monkey. Science 205:929–931, 1979.

Bruner JS, Kaye, Lyons K. The Growth of Human Manual Intelligence: III. The Development of Detour Reaching. Center for Cognitive Studies, Harvard University, Unpublished manuscript, 1969.

Brush ES, Mishkin M, Rosvold HE. Effects of object preferences and aversions on discrimination learning in monkeys with frontal lesions. Journal of Comparative and Physiological Psychology 54:319–325, 1961.

Burns RS, Chiueh CC, Markey SP, Ebert MH, Jacobowitz DM, Kopin IJ. A primate model of parkinsonism: Selective destruction of dopaminergic neurons in the pars compacta of the substantia nigra by N-methyl-4-phenyl-1,2,3,6-tetrahydropyridine. (Proceedings of the National Academy of Science), Neurobiology 80:4546–4550, 1983.

Butterworth G. Spatial location codes in determining search errors. Child Development 46:866–870, 1975.

Chelune GJ, Baer RA. Developmental norms for the Wisconsin Card Sorting Test. Journal of Clinical and Experimental Neuropsychology 8:219–228, 1986.

Chugani HT, Phelps ME, Mazziotta JC. Positron emission tomography study of human brain functional development. Annals of Neurology 22:487–497, 1987.

Cowie VA. Neurological and psychiatric aspects of phenylketonuria. In Bickel H, Hudson F, Woolf L (eds), Phenylketonuria and Some Other Inborn Errors of Amino Acid Metabolism. Stuttgart: Verlag, 1971.

Dennis M. Impaired sensory and motor differentiation with corpus callosum agenesis: A lack of callosal inhibition during ontogeny? Neuropsychologia 14:455–469, 1976.

Diamond A. Rate of maturation of the hippocampus and the developmental progression of children's performance on the delayed non-matching to sample and visual paired comparison tasks. In Diamond A (ed.), The Development and Neural Bases of Higher Cognitive Functions. New York: Annals of the New York Academy of Sciences 608:394–426, 1990.

Diamond A. Developmental time course in human infants and infant monkeys, and the neural bases of inhibitory control in reaching. In Diamond A (ed), The Development and Neural Bases of Higher Cognitive Functions. New York: Annals of the New York Academy of Sciences 608:637–676, 1990b.

Diamond A. Frontal lobe involvement in cognitive changes during the first year of life. In Gibson KR, Petersen AC (eds), Brain Maturation and Cognitive Development: Comparative and Cross-Cultural Perspectives. New York: Aldine de Gruyter, 1991a, pp. 127–180.

Diamond A. Neuropsychological insights into the meaning of object concept development. In Carey S, Gelman R (eds), The Epigenesis of Mind: Essays on Biology and Knowledge. Hillsdale, NJ: Lawrence Erlbaum Associates, 1991b, pp. 67–110.

Diamond A. Retrieval of an object from an open box: The development of visual-tactile control of reaching in the first year of life. Monographs of the Society for Research in Child Development. (submitted).

Diamond A. Development of the ability to use recall to guide action, as indicated by infants' performance on A$\overline{B}$. Child Development 56:868–883, 1985.

Diamond A. Differences between adult and infant cognition: Is the crucial variable presence or absence of language? *In* Weiskrantz L (ed), Thought Without Language. Oxford: Oxford University Press, 1988, pp. 337–370.

Diamond A, Boyer K. A version of the Wisconsin Card Sort Test for use with preschool children, and an exploration of their sources of error. Journal of Clinical and Experimental Neuropsychology 11:83, 1989.

Diamond A, Cruttenden L, Neiderman D. Why have studies found better performance with multiple wells than with only two wells on A$\overline{B}$? Society for Research in Child Development Abstracts 6:227, 1989a.

Diamond A, Doar B. The performance of human infants on a measure of frontal cortex function, the delayed response task. Developmental Psychobiology 22:272–294, 1989.

Diamond A, Goldman-Rakic, PS. Evidence for involvement of prefrontal cortex in cognitive changes during the first year of life: Comparison of performance of human infants and rhesus monkeys on a detour task with transparent barrier. Neuroscience Abstracts (Part II) 11:832, 1985.

Diamond A, Goldman-Rakic PS. Comparative development in human infants and infant rhesus monkeys of cognitive functions that depend on prefrontal cortex. Neuroscience Abstracts 12:742, 1986.

Diamond A, Goldman-Rakic PS. Comparison of human infants and rhesus monkeys on Piaget's A$\overline{B}$ task: Evidence for dependence on dorsolateral prefrontal cortex. Experimental Brain Research 74:24–40, 1989.

Diamond A, Towle C, Boyer K. Developmental progression on a test of hippocampal memory function in adult monkeys and human amnesic patients (the delayed nonmatching to sample task) in children aged 1–5 years. (in prep).

Diamond A, Zola-Morgan S, Squire L. Successful performance by monkeys with lesions of the hippocampal formation on A$\overline{B}$ and object retrieval, two tasks that mark developmental changes in human infants. Behavioral Neuroscience 103:526–537, 1989b.

Divac I, Bjorklund A, Lindvall O, Passingham R. Converging projections from the mediodorsal thalamic nucleus and mesencephalic dopaminergic neurons in three species. Journal of Comparative Neurology 180:59–71, 1978.

Divac I, Rosvold HE, Szwarcbart MK. Behavioral effects of selective ablation of the caudate nucleus. Journal of Comparative and Physiological Psychology 63:184–190, 1967.

Dobson JC, Williamson ML, Azen C, Koch R. Intellectual assessment of 111 four-year-old children with phenylketonuria. Pediatrics 60:822–827, 1977.

Donaldson M. Children's Minds. New York: Norton, 1978.

Douglas RJ. The hippocampus and behavior. Psychological Bulletin 67:416–442, 1967.

Eckenhoff MF, Rakic P. Nature and fate of proliferative cells in the hippocampal dentate gyrus during the life span of the rhesus monkey. Journal of Neuroscience 8:2729–2747, 1988.

Elsworth JD, Deutsch AY, Redmond DE Jr, Sladek JR, Roth RH. Differential responsiveness to 1-methyl-4-phenyl-1,2,3,6-tetrahydropyridine toxicity in sub-regions of the primate substantia nigra and striatum. Life Sciences 40:193–202, 1987.

Fagan JF III. Memory in the infant. Journal of Experimental Child Psychology 9:217–226, 1970.

Fagan JF III. The paired-comparison paradigm and infant intelligence. *In* Diamond A (ed), The Development and Neural Bases of Higher Cognitive Functions. New York: Annals of the New York Academy of Sciences, 608:337–364, 1990.

Fantz RL. Visual experience in infants: Decreased attention to familiar patterns relative to novel ones. Science 146:668–670, 1964.

Fox NA, Bell MA. Electrophysiological indices of frontal lobe development: Relations to cognitive and affective behavior in human infants over the first year of life. *In* Diamond A (ed), The Development and Neural Bases of Higher Cognitive Functions. New York: Annals of the New York Academy of Sciences, 608:677–704, 1990.

Fox N, Kagan J, & Weiskopf S. The growth of memory during infancy. Genetic Psychology Monographs 99:91–130, 1979.

Funahashi S, Bruce CJ, Goldman-Rakic PS. Mnemonic coding of visual space in the monkey's dorsolateral prefrontal cortex. Journal of Neurophysiology 61:1–19, 1989.

Fuster JM, Alexander GE. Neuron activity related to short-term memory. Science 173:652–654, 1971.

Gaffan D. Recognition impaired and association intact in the memory of monkeys after transection of the fornix. Journal of Comparative and Physiological Psychology 86:1100–1109, 1974.

Gaffan D, Gaffan EA, Harrison S. Effects of fornix transection on spontaneous and trained non-matching by monkeys. Quarterly Journal of Experimental Psychology 36b:285–303, 1984.

Gaiter JL. The Development of Detour Reaching in Infants. Ph.D. dissertation, Brown University, Providence, RI, 1973.

Goldman PS. Functional development of the prefrontal cortex in early life and the problem of neuronal plasticity. Experimental Neurology 32: 366–387, 1971.

Goldman PS. Recovery of function after CNS lesions in infant monkeys. Neuroscience Research Progress Bulletin 12:217–222, 1974.

Goldman-Rakic PS. Circuitry of primate prefrontal cortex and regulation of behavior by representational knowledge. *In* Plum F, Mountcastle V (eds), Handbook of Physiology 5:373–417, 1987.

Goldman-Rakic PS, Brown RM. Postnatal development of monoamine content and synthesis in the cerebral cortex of rhesus monkeys. Developmental Brain Research 4:339–349, 1982.

Goldman PS, Nauta WJH. Autoradiographic demonstration of a projection from prefrontal association cortex to the superior colliculus in the rhesus monkey. Brain Research 116:145–149, 1976.

Goldman PS, Nauta WJH. An intricately patterned prefronto-caudate projection in the rhesus monkey. Journal of Comparative Neurology 171:369–386, 1977.

Goldman PS, Rosvold HE. Localization of function within the dorsolateral prefrontal cortex of the rhesus monkey. Experimental Neurology 27:291–304, 1970.

Goldman PS, Rosvold HE. The effects of selective caudate lesions in infant and juvenile rhesus monkeys. Brain Research 43:53–66, 1972.

Goldman-Rakic PS, Schwartz ML. Interdigitation of contralateral and ipsilateral columnar projections to frontal association cortex in primates. Science 216:755–757, 1982.

Gratch G. Recent studies based on Piaget's view of object concept development. *In* Cohen LB, Salapatek P (eds), Infant Perception: From Sensation to Cognition Vol. 2. New York: Academic Press, 1975.

Gratch G, Appel KJ, Evans WF, LeCompte GK, Wright NA. Piaget's stage IV object concept error: Evidence of forgetting or object conception? Child Development 45:71–77, 1974.

Gratch G, Landers WF. Stage IV of Piaget's theory of infant's object concepts: A longitudinal study. Child Development 42:359–372, 1971.

Grossman M. Reversal operations after brain damage. Brain and Cognition 1:331–359, 1982.

Haaxma R & Kuypers HGJM. Intrahemispheric cortical connexions and visual guidance of hand and finger movements in the rhesus monkey. Brain 98:239–260, 1975.

Harlow HF. Analysis of discrimination learning by monkeys. Journal of Experimental Psychology 40:26–39, 1950.

Harlow HF, Davis RT, Settlage PH, Meyer DR. Analysis of frontal and posterior association syndromes in brain damaged monkeys. Journal of Comparative and Physiological Psychology 54:419–429, 1952.

Harris PL. Perseverative errors in search by young infants. Child Development 44:28–33, 1973.

Heilman KM, Valenstein E. Frontal lobe neglect in man. Neurology 22:660–664, 1972.

Holtzman NA, Kronmal RA, van Doornink W, Azen C, Koch R. Effect of age at loss of dietary control on intellectual performance and behavior of children with phenylketonuria. New England Journal of Medicine 34:593–598, 1986.

Hudson FP, Mordaunt VL, Leahy I. Evaluation of treatment begun in first three months of life in 184 cases of phenylketonuria. Archives of Disease in Childhood 45:5–12, 1970.

Jacobsen CF. Functions of the frontal association areas in primates. Archives of Neurology and Psychiatry 33:558–560, 1935.

Jacobsen CF. Studies of cerebral function in primates: I. The functions of the frontal association areas in monkeys. Comparative Psychology Monographs 13:3–60, 1936.

Johnson PB, Angelucci A, Ziparo RM, Minciacchi D, Bentivoglio M, Caminiti R. Segregation and overlap of callosal and association neurons in frontal and parietal cortices of primates: A spectral and coherency analysis. Journal of Neuroscience 9:2313–2326, 1989.

Johnson TN, Rosvold HE, Mishkin M. Projections of behaviorally defined sectors of the prefrontal cortex to the basal ganglia, septum and diencephalon of the monkey. Experimental Neurology 21:20–34, 1968.

Kemp JM, Powell TPS. The connexions of the striatum and globus pallidus: Synthesis and speculation. Philosophical Transactions of the Royal Society, London 262:411–457, 1970.

Koch R, Azen C, Friedman EG, Williamson ML. Paired comparisons between early treated PKU children and their matched sibling controls on intelligence and school achievement test results at eight years of age. Journal of Inherited Metabolic Disease 7:86–90, 1984.

Krause WL, Helminski M, McDonald L, Dembure P, Salvo R, Freides D, Elsas LJ. Biochemical and neuropsychological effects of elevated plasma phenylalanine in patients with treated phenylketonuria, a model for the study of phenylalanine in brain function in man. Journal of Clinical Investigation 75:40–48, 1985.

Kretschmann HJ, Kammradt G, Krauthausen I, Sauer B, Wingert F. Growth of the hippocampal formation in man. Bibliotheca Anatomica 28:27–52, 1986.

Kunzle H. An autoradiographic analysis of the efferent connections from premotor and adjacent prefrontal regions (Areas 6 and 9) in *Macaca fascicularis*. Brain, Behavior, and Evolution 15:185–234, 1978.

LaMotte RH, Acuna C. Defects in accuracy of reaching after removal of posterior parietal cortex in monkeys. Brain Research 139:309–326, 1978.

Laplane D, Talairach J, Meininger V, Bancaud J, Orgogozo JM. Clinical consequences of corticectomies involving the supplementary motor area in man. Journal of Neurological Science 34:310–314, 1977.

Lees AJ, Smith E. Cognitive deficits in the early stages of Parkinson's disease. Brain 106:257–270, 1983.

Leonard CM. The prefrontal cortex of the rat. I. Cortical projection of the mediodorsal nucleus. Efferent connections. Brain Research 12:321–343, 1963.

Luria AR. Higher Cortical Functions in Man. New York: Basic Books, 1977.

Markowitsch HJ, Pritzel M. Comparative analysis of prefrontal learning functions in rats, cats, and monkeys. Psychological Bulletin 84:817–837, 1977.

Millar WS & Schaffer HR. The influence of spatially displaced feedback on infant operant conditioning. Journal of Experimental Child Psychology 14:442–453, 1972.

Milner B. Effects of brain lesions on card sorting. Archives of Neurology 9:90–100, 1963.

Milner B. Some effects of frontal lobectomy in man. In Warren JM, Akert K (eds), The Frontal Granular Cortex and Behavior. New York: McGraw-Hill, 1964, pp. 313–334.

Milner B. Interhemispheric differences in the localization of psychological processes in man. British Medical Bulletin 27:272–277, 1971.

Milner B, Petrides M, Smith ML. Frontal lobes and the temporal organization of memory. Human Neurobiology 4:137–142, 1985.

Mishkin M & Delacour J. An analysis of short-term visual memory in the monkey. Journal of Experimental Psychology: Animal Behavior 1:326–334, 1975.

Mishkin M. Memory in monkeys severely impaired by combined but not by separate removal of amygdala and hippocampus. Nature 273:297–298, 1978.

Mishkin M, Prockop ES, Rosvold HE. One-trial object-discrimination learning in monkeys with frontal lesions. Journal of Comparative and Physiological Psychology 55:172–181, 1962.

Mishkin M, Vest B, Waxler M, Rosvold HE. A reexamination of the effects of frontal lesions on object alternation. Neuropsychologia 7:357–364, 1969

Mitchel IJ, Cross AJ, Sambrook MA, Crossman AR. Neural mechanisms mediating 1-methyl-4-phenyl-1,2,3,6-tetrahydropyridine-induced parkinsonism in the monkey: Relative contributions of the striatopallidal and striatonigral pathways as suggested by 2-deoxyglucose uptake. Neuroscience Letters 63:61–65, 1986.

Moll L, Kuypers HGJM. Premotor cortical ablations in monkeys: Contralateral changes in visually guided reaching behavior. Science 198:317–319, 1977.

Nauta WJH. Some efferent connections of the prefrontal cortex in the monkey. In Warren JM, Akert K (eds), The Frontal Granular Cortex and Behavior New York: McGraw-Hill, 1964, pp. 159–193.

Nauta WJH. The problem of the frontal lobe: A reinterpretation. Journal of Psychiatric Research 8:167–187, 1971.

Niki H. Differential activity of prefrontal units during right and left delayed response trials. Brain Research 70:346–349, 1974.

Overman WH. Performance on traditional match to sample, non-matching to sample, and object discrimination tasks by 12 to 32 month-old children: A developmental progression. In Diamond A (ed), The Development and Neural Bases of Higher Cognitive Functions. New York: New York Academy of Sciences, 608:365–393, 1990.

Pandya DN, Kuypers HGJM. Cortico-cortical connections in the rhesus monkey. Brain Research 13:13–36, 1969.

Pandya DN, Vignolo LA. Interhemispheric projections of the parietal lobe in the rhesus monkey. Brain Research 15:49–58, 1969.

Pandya DN & Vignolo LA. Intra- and interhemispheric projections of the precentral, premotor and arcuate areas in the rhesus monkey. Brain Research 26:217–233, 1971.

Passingham RE. Premotor cortex: Sensory cues and movement. Behavioural Brain Research 18:175–185, 1985.

Passler MA, Isaac W, Hynd GW. Neuropsychological development of behavior attributed to frontal lobe functioning in children. Developmental Neuropsychology 1:349–370. 1985.

Pennington BF, VanDoornick WJ, McCabe LL, McCabe ERB. Neuropsychological deficits in early treated phenylketonuric children. American Journal of Mental Deficiency 89:467–474, 1985.

Perret E. The left frontal lobe of man and the suppression of habitual responses in verbal categorical behaviour. Neuropsychologia 16:527–537, 1974.

Petrides M. Deficits on self-ordered temporal memory task after dorsolateral prefrontal lesions in the monkey. Society for Neuroscience Abstracts 14, 1988.

Petrides M, Milner B. Deficits in subject-ordered tasks after frontal- and temporal-lobe lesions in man. Neuropsychologia 20:249–262, 1982.

Piaget J. The Origins of Intelligence in Children. (Cook M, Trans.) New York: Basic Books, 1952. (Original work published, 1936.)

Porrino L, Goldman-Rakic PS. Brain stem innervation of prefrontal and anterior cingulate cortex in the rhesus monkey revealed by retrograde transport of HRP. Journal of Comparative Neurology 205:63–76, 1982.

Primrose DA. Phenylketonuria with normal intelligence. Journal of Mental Deficiency Research 27:239–246, 1983.

Quintana J, Yajeya J, Fuster JM. Prefrontal representation of stimulus attributes during delay tasks. I. Unit activity in cross-temporal integration of sensory and sensory-motor integration. Brain Research 474:211–221, 1988.

Rakic P, Nowakowski RS. The time of origin of neurons in the hippocampal region of the rhesus monkey. Journal of Comparative Neurology 196:99–128, 1981.

Rose JE, Woolsey CN. The orbitofrontal cortex and its connections with the mediodorsal nucleus in rabbit, sheep and cat. Research Publication of the Association for Research on Nervous and Mental Disease 27:210–232, 1948.

Rosvold HE. The frontal lobe system: Cortical-subcortical interrelationships. In Konorski J, Teuber HL, Zernicki B (eds), Functions of the Septo-Hippocampal System. Warsaw: Polish Sci. Pub, 1984, pp. 439–460.

Rovee-Collier C. The ontogeny of learning and memory in human infancy. In Kail R, Spear NE (eds), Comparative Perspectives on the Development of Memory. Hillsdale, NJ: Lawrence Erlbaum, 1984, pp. 103–134.

Saint-Cyr JA, Wan RO, Doudet D, Aigner TG. Impaired detour reaching in rhesus monkeys after MPTP lesions. Neuroscience Abstracts (Part I) 14:389, 1988.

Saunders RC. Monkeys demonstrate high level of recognition memory in delayed nonmatching to sample with retention intervals of 6 weeks. Society for Neuroscience Abstracts 15:342, 1989.

Schacter DL. Implicit memory: History and current status. Journal of Experimental Psychology: Learning, Memory & Cognition 13:501–518, 1987.

Schonen S de, Bresson F. Developpement de l'atteinte manuelle d'un objet chez l'enfant. Omportements 1:99–114, 1984.

Schwartz ML, Goldman-Rakic PS. Callosal and intrahemispheric connectivity of the prefrontal association cortex in rhesus monkey: Relation between intraparietal and principal sulcal cortex. Journal of Comparative Neurology 226:403–420, 1984.

Selemon LD, Goldman-Rakic PS. Longitudinal topography and interdigitation of corticostriatal projections in the rhesus monkey. Journal of Neuroscience 5:776–794, 1985.

Selemon LD, Goldman-Rakic PS. Common cortical and subcortical targets of the dorsolateral prefrontal and posterior parietal cortices in the rhesus monkey: Evidence for a distributed neural network subserving spatially guided behavior. Journal of Neuroscience 8:4049–4068, 1988.

Shimamura AP, Janowsky JS, Squire LR. Memory for the temporal order of events in patients with frontal lobe lesions and amnesic patients. Neuropsychologia 28:803–814, 1990.

Squire LR, Zola-Morgan S. The neurobiology of memory: The case for correspondence between the findings for human and non-human primates. *In* Deutsch JA (ed), The Physiological Basis of Memory. New York: Academic Press, 1983.

Squire LR, Zola-Morgan S, Chen KS. Human amnesia and animal models of amnesia: Performance of amnesic patients on tests designed for the monkey. Behavioral Neuroscience 102:210–221, 1988.

Stern Y, Langston JW. Intellectual changes in patients with MPTP-induced parkinsonism. Neurology 35:1506–1509, 1985.

Stern Y, Mayeux R, Rosen J, Ilson J. Perceptual motor dysfunction in Parkinson's disease: A deficit in sequential and predictive voluntary movement. Journal of Neurology, Neurosurgery, and Psychiatry 46:145–151, 1983.

Stroop JR. Studies of interference in serial verbal reactions. Journal of Experimental Psychology 18:643–662, 1935.

Taylor AE, Saint-Cyr JA. Frontal lobe dysfunction in Parkinson's disease. Brain 109:845–883, 1986.

Taylor AE, Saint-Cyr JA, Lang AE. Memory and learning in early Parkinson's disease: Evidence for a "frontal lobe syndrome." Brain and Cognition 13:211–232, 1990a.

Taylor JR, Roth RH, Sladek JR, Jr, Redmond DE, Jr. Cognitive and motor deficits in the performance of the object retrieval detour task in monkeys (cercopithecus aethiops sabaeus) treated with MPTP: Long-term performance and effect of transparency of the barrier. Behavioral Neuroscience 104:564–576, 1990b.

Tourian AY, Sidbury JB. Phenylketonuria. *In* Stanbury JD, Wyngaarden JB, Fredrickson D (eds), The Metabolic Basis of Inherited Disease. New York: McGraw-Hill, 1978, pp. 240–255.

Towle C, Diamond A. Developmental progression in children aged 1–5 years on the delayed non-matching to sample task, a test of hippocampal memory function in adult monkeys and human amnesic patients. Paper presented at the Society for Research in Child Development, Biennial Meeting, April 18–21, Seattle, WA, 1991.

Tulving E. Remembering and knowing the past. The crucial difference between remembering personal experiences and knowing impersonal facts. American Scientist 77:361–368, 1989.

Van Essen DC. Visual areas of the mammalian cerebral cortex. Annual Review of Neuroscience 2:227–263, 1979.

Vicedomini JP, Corwin JV, Nonneman AJ. Behavioral effects of lesions to the caudate nucleus or mediodorsal thalamus in neonatal, juvenile, and adult rats. Physiological Psychology 10:246–250, 1982.

Vicedomini JP, Isaac WL, Nonneman AJ. Role of the caudate nucleus in recovery from neonatal mediofrontal cortex lesions in the rat. Developmental Psychobiology 17: 51–65, 1984.

Villablanca JR, Olmstead CE, Levine MS, Morcus RJ. Effects of caudate nuclei or frontal cortical ablations in kittens. Experimental Neuropsychology 61:615–634, 1979.

von Bonin G, Bailey P. Neocortex of Macaca mulatta. Urbana: University of Illinois Press, 1947.

Warren JM, Akert K. The Frontal Granular Cortex and Behavior. New York: McGraw-Hill, 1964.

Wellman HM, Cross D, Bartsch K. A meta-analysis of research on stage 4 object permanence: The A-not-B error. Monographs of the Society for Research in Child Development 5(3), 1987.

Welsh MC, Pennington BF, Ozonoff S, Rouse B, McCabe ERB. Neuropsychology of early-treated phenylketonuria: Specific executive function deficits. Child Development 61:1697–1713, 1990.

Werner JS, Perlmutter M. Development of visual memory in infants. Advances in Child Development and Behavior 14:2–56, 1979.

Williamson M, Dobson JC, Koch R. Collaborative study of children treated for phenyl-ketonuria: Study design. Pediatrics 60:815–821, 1977.

Wilson FAW, Goldman-Rakic PS. Effect of spatial and color cues on delayed-related neuronal responses in prefrontal cortex. Abstracts of the Society for Neuroscience 15:71, 1989.

Wozniak RH & Balamore U. Speech-action coordination in young children. Developmental Psychology 20:850–858, 1984.

Zola-Morgan S, Squire LR. Memory impairment in monkeys following lesions limited to the hippocampus. Behavioral Neuroscience 100:155–160, 1986.

Zola-Morgan S, Squire LR, Amaral DG. Lesions of the hippocampal formation but not lesions of the fornix or mammillary nuclei produce long-lasting memory impairment in monkeys. Journal of Neuroscience 9:897–912, 1989.

VIII
Rehabilitation of the Frontal Lobe Damaged Patient

19

The Relationship of Frontal Lobe Damage to Diminished Awareness: Studies in Rehabilitation

GEORGE P. PRIGATANO

Research on mechanisms underlying the association of frontal lobe physiology and anatomy with complex behavioral activities in humans and nonhuman primates has been active for a number of years as witnessed by the previous chapters and numerous papers and volumes on the "frontal lobes" (e.g., Fuster, 1980; Perecman, 1987; Pribram and Luria, 1973; Stuss and Benson, 1986; Warren and Akert, 1964). Yet, despite this impressive effort to understand the contribution of the frontal lobes to human behavior and mental processes, there has been a paucity of studies specifically aimed at the utilization of this knowledge for rehabilitation purposes. For example, Newcombe's (1985) review on rehabilitation of neuropsychologic impairments does not include any discussion of what can be done for patients who have disorders of "executive function" secondary to frontal lobe pathology. This is because such a literature does not exist and there seems to be a latent, if not manifest, pessimism regarding substantially helping such individuals.

The frontal lobes have been considered so important for guiding attention, sustaining motivation, and for social adaptation (see Fuster, 1980; Goldstein, 1942; Luria, 1948/1963; Stuss and Benson, 1986) that significant damage to these regions of the brain may automatically spell a poor rehabilitation and psychosocial outcome (see Luria, 1948/1963 for a discussion of this point). Although this point of view can be questioned (Prigatano, 1988a), the purpose of this paper will not be to document what can be done for various neuropsychologic problems associated with frontal lobe pathology. (There have been a few efforts that address components of this problem, e.g., Stuss et al., 1987; von Cramon and von Cramon, 1989.) Rather, the discussion will focus on one problem that has been neglected and yet may hold promise for improving the psychosocial outcome for this group of patients. That problem is altered self-awareness after brain injury. It will be considered in the light of rehabilitation work with patients who have focal frontal lesions as well as those who have frontal damage in the presence of diffuse cerebral injury. The problem will be placed in a brief historical perspective as well and its theoretical implications considered. Methodologic issues and future areas of investigation will be outlined.

NEUROPSYCHOLOGIC REHABILITATION AND THE PROBLEM OF DIMINISHED AWARENESS

Neuropsychological rehabilitation after brain injury attempts to facilitate recovery by actively working on the restoration of higher cerebral functions (Luria, 1948/1963), teaching compensatory skills to cope with permanent alterations of brain function (Goldstein, 1942), and helping the individual understand residual impairments and resultant disabilities. In addition, an attempt is made to help the individual develop a sense of renewed commitment to life in the face of their personal tragedy (Prigatano and Others, 1986; Prigatano, 1989). These activities may help the person avoid significant pyschosocial and psychiatric complications that often occur when rehabilitation is not instituted or when previous rehabilitation efforts have failed (Prigatano and Others, 1986; Prigatano, 1991).

The efficacy of such work has been evaluated by Prigatano and colleagues (1984), Ben Yishay and associates (1987), and Ben Yishay and Prigatano (1990). These studies suggest that approximately 50% of neuropsychologically treated patients are able to be gainfully employed 2 years posttrauma. The stability of that employment figure over several years is, however, unknown. Yet, if it remains at the 30–40% level, this would be a substantial contribution to these patients' care. Less than 10% of severe traumatic brain-injured (TBI) patients may be working 10 to 15 years postinjury (Thomsen, 1984). Improved emotional control, ability to interact successfully with others, and enhanced acceptance/awareness of residual abilities may be especially important for successful long-term psychosocial adjustment (e.g., maintaining work) after significant brain injury (see Ben Yishay's data reported in Ben Yishay and Prigatano, 1990).

DISORDERS OF AWARENESS: A BRIEF REHABILITATION AND THEORETICAL PERSPECTIVE

Disturbances in awareness of neurologic and neuropsychologic changes after brain injury have been recognized in neurology, psychiatry, and neuropsychology for some time. While the clinical observations of Von Monakow, Anton, Pick, Babinski, and Marie are often cited as the first neurologic reports of impaired awareness following brain injury (Prigatano, 1988b), Bisiach and Geminiani (1991) cite a letter from antiquity documenting unawareness of apparent cortical blindness some 2,000 years before Von Monakow's 1885 report. More recently, McGlynn and Schacter (1989) have reviewed disturbances in awareness in various neuropsychologic syndromes. An edited text will soon appear on disorders of awareness as seen from neurologic, neuropsychologic, and contemporary cognitive and clinical psychology perspectives (Prigatano and Schacter, 1991).

What has been the contribution of rehabilitation-oriented observations in understanding the problem of altered awareness after brain injury? Moreover, what specific role does frontal lobe pathology play in this class of disturbances? Goldstein (1952; pp. 246–247) believed that "Personality structure is disturbed particularly by lesions of the frontal lobes, the parietal lobes and the insula Reili; but it also is disturbed by diffuse damage to the cortex." Based on his diagnostic and rehabilitation experience with brain-injured soldiers, Goldstein felt that "extensive lesions of the frontal lobes" do not produce deficits in behavior that typically occur in over-routinized or customary daily activities. Patients may appear "a little slow" and rigidly direct their attention to one thing at a time, but they can carry out many daily activities in a stereotypic fashion. Such patients are described, however, as being "concrete" in their approach to problems and exhibiting an impairment in their abstract attitude. When this impairment results in a failure to cope with environmental demands, the patient may experience a catastrophic reaction. Goldstein (1952) described in some detail the "protective mechanisms" that brain-injured patients *automatically* rely on to avoid the catastrophic reaction. He emphasized that these protective mechanisms were not the same thing as the defensive mechanisms discussed by psychiatrists to explain how "ego" processes cope with anxiety. Under these protective mechanisms, he listed social withdrawal, excessive and fanatic orderliness, and unawareness of neurologic deficit. He had this to say about the awareness problem:

> We very often observe that a patient is totally unaware of his defect—such as hemiplegia or hemianopsia—and of the difference between his state prior to the development of the symptom and his present state. This is strikingly illustrated by the fact that the disturbance of these patients plays a very small role in their complaints. We are not dealing simply with a subjective lack of awareness, for the defects are effectively excluded from awareness, one might say. This is shown by the fact that they produce very little disturbance—apparently as the result of compensation. . . . As a matter of fact, a patient may get to a catastrophic condition when we make him aware of his defect or when the particular situation does not make possible an adequate compensation. (p. 258)

Luria (1943/1963) was also impressed with disorders of awareness that he encountered in diagnostic and rehabilitation settings. He approached the problem, however, from a somewhat different perspective. He saw the frontal lobes as playing a major role in human motivation and the awareness problem was related to this basic disturbance. Luria (1948/1963) pointed out that patients with diffuse and bilateral frontal lobe lesions seem unable to initiate and sustain effort in working on a variety of rehabilitation activities compared to nonfrontal brain-injured patients. Disturbances in "goal-directed behavior" were at the heart of frontal lobe impairments and robbed the patient of the necessary neural templates to actively engage rehabilitation efforts.

Unlike patients with superior temporal lobe injuries or parietal injuries, extended practice at systematic retraining activities often seemed fruitless with

Table 19-1   Pattern of Mental Tension During Experiments with Changes in the "Level of Demands"

Type of curves	Normal subjects (%)	Patients with frontal lobe lesions (%)
Relationship found between mental tension and success or failure	96	6
No relationship found between mental tension and success or failure	0	87

From Luria, A. J. (1963). Restoration of Function After Brain Injury (p. 238). The Macmillan Company, New York. Reprinted with permission.

frontal lobe patients because of their lack of "drive" accompanying purposeful acts. Luria (1948/1963) cites the early work of Zeigarnik to show how patients with massive frontal lobe lesions demonstrate a lack of "mental tension" when performing various tasks. Table 19–1 is taken from Zeigarnik's work but was published in Luria's (1948/1963) book.

Luria (1948/1963) notes that in normals there is a certain "mental tension" that accompanies goal-directed behavior, but no such tension seems to be felt in the majority of patients with extensive frontal lobe lesions. Some years later, Luria (1970) expanded his concept of the function of the frontal lobes to state that they are "involved in the formation of intentions and programs of behavior" (p. 68). The introduction of the concept of "intentions" set the state for modern day conceptualizations about disturbances in awareness associated with frontal lobe pathology.

Pribram (1980) connects the phenomenon of intentions to self-consciousness or self-awareness. He suggests that consciousness refers primarily to a state of attention. Being "conscious" of something means attending to a stimulus. Self-consciousness refers to attending to the "self." "Pribram (1980) suggests that intentions and intentionalities make up self-consciousness. That is, the capacity or the state to intend some action or to prefer to perceive some stimulus (i.e., intentionality) constitutes the 'stuff' out of which self-consciousness or self-awareness emerges." (Prigatano, 1988a, p. 341).

Disturbances of frontal lobe activity may have a negative impact on the ability to integrate feelings ("loss of mental tension") with a plan of action even though the patient *may want* to achieve a certain goal. In this sense, frontal lobe patients are not necessarily unmotivated (i.e., they still have wants or desires); yet, many have lost their ability to integrate and act on the vital connection between being in a state of tension and engaging a plan of action to reduce that tension.

CLINICAL EXAMPLES FROM REHABILITATION

A clinical example will help clarify this point. A young man suffered diffuse cerebral injury with clear bilateral frontal contusions secondary from a fall. His computerized tomography (CT) scan revealed bilateral frontal atrophy several weeks postinjury (see Fig. 4.1 in Prigatano and Others, 1986). This patient had a vocational goal. He *wanted* to be a helicopter pilot or a short-order cook! Yet, he could not develop a plan to achieve either goal, nor did he experience any feeling (humor or tension) in making such a seemingly disconnected vocational choice. However, when given a specific step-by-step plan for action, he could demonstrate that he was motivated to do certain things even though the integration of "feelings" and a plan of action was impaired. For example, he also stated that he wanted to do yard work at his parents' home and agreed to mow their lawn several times, but with no corresponding behavioral follow-through. Despite repeated requests on the part of his parents, he did not initiate the action. When given a specific plan of action and literally helped to initiate that plan, he carried out the activity of going out to the garage, starting the lawn mower, placing it next to the lawn, and he proceeded to cut the grass with precise detail. Yet, he seemed to lack a subjective sense of pleasure over completing the job in a manner similar to what he had previously demonstrated.

Patients vary in the extent of their neuropathological lesions and their premorbid cognitive and personality characteristics (a greatly neglected problem for research in this field). Yet, the phenomenon of frontal lobe patients showing disturbances in intentions and consequent awareness has become progressively recognized in many rehabilitation settings.

When I first encountered this problem, I felt that it was secondary to an impairment of the abstract attitude, as Goldstein (1942) had earlier suggested. Another patient demonstrated, however, that his lack of insight into himself could exist in the presence of essentially normal performance on a well-accepted abstract reasoning task. While the patient committed less than 30 errors on the Halstead Category Test, he had incredible lack of insight into his socially inappropriate behavior and the impact that it had on others (for a discussion of this see Prigatano, 1991).

Based on these clinical experiences, a few patients who sustained severeTBI with known or suspected frontal injuries were asked to rate themselves on a simple question that dealt with their ability to perceive how the effects of their brain injury affected their day-to-day functioning. What made it even more interesting was that these ratings were done *after* these patients had undergone intensive rehabilitation (see Prigatano, 1991). To our initial surprise, each of the patients who was deemed a "treatment success" reported that he or she did *not* completely appreciate the impact of the brain injury on everyday functioning (on a scale from 1 to 10, they rated themselves a 9). In contrast, all treatment failures said that they were totally aware of the consequences of their brain injury on day-to-day life (rating themselves as a 10). Staff members agreed with the "treatment successes," but were in strong disagreement with the "failures" (Table 19–2; also for a discussion of this see Prigatano, 1991).

Fordyce and Roueche (1986) reported that TBI patients with known or suspected frontal and anterior temporal injuries typically rate themselves as more competent than their relatives. The patients' ratings of their behavioral competencies were unrelated to whether or not they were "vocationally active" or "inactive." Family and rehabilitation staff ratings of the patients' behavioral competencies were, however, associated with the patients' vocational status.

Table 19–2 Comparison of Staff and
Patient Ratings on Awareness of
Implications After Brain Injury

	Patient ratings	Staff ratings
"Success"		
DB (6 mos)	9	9
BW (6 mos)	9	9
ML (12 mos)	9	9
AM (6 mos)	8	6
"Failure"		
SD (6 mos)	10	2
(12 mos)	10	6
TW (6 mos)	10	4
(12 mos)	10	8
CP (6 mos)	10	6
(12 mos)	9	4

From Prigatano, G. P. (1991). Disturbances of self-awareness of deficit after traumatic brain injury. *In* G. P. Prigatano, D. L. Schacter (eds). Awareness of Deficit After Brain Injury: Clinical and Theoretical Issues. Oxford University Press, New York. Reprinted with permission.

These observations suggested that altered self-awareness in TBI patients with frontal lesions was an important rehabilitation and theoretical problem (Prigatano and Others, 1986). In the context of that work, clinical research projects were initiated to study this phenomenon.

AWARENESS DEFICIT IN TBI PATIENTS: FRONTAL LOBE INJURIES IN THE PRESENCE OF DIFFUSE DAMAGE

A growing literature on the neuropathology of severe and moderate TBI secondary to acceleration/deceleration injuries emphasizes two facts: Prefrontal (including orbital-frontal) and anterior temporal lobe injuries frequently occur (see Prigatano and Others, 1986; Ruff et al., 1989) and diffuse axonal damage is common (Povlishock, 1989). As a group, these patients can be notoriously unaware of certain residual higher cerebral impairments and their psychosocial impact. Oddy and colleagues (1985), for example, reported that 7 years post severe craniocerebral trauma 40% of patients' relatives described these patients as childish and "refusing to admit to difficulties." This refusal to admit to difficulties may well be more than defensive denial as McGlynn and Schacter (1989) have used that term. As a group, there seems to be a strong element of what might broadly be called organic unawareness (Prigatano, 1991).

A common finding in TBI patients with neuroradiographic evidence of "frontal lobe pathology" is they frequently fail to recognize behavioral limitations postinjury. Utilizing the Patient Competency Rating Scale (PCRS) (see Prigatano and Others, 1986) TBI patients were asked to rate on a five-point scale their behavioral competencies. A rating of four or five meant they perceived themselves as being able to do the task fairly easily or with complete ease. A rating of three meant that they perceived themselves as being able to do the task, but with some difficulty. A rating of one or two meant that they perceived themselves as unable to do the task or could do it only with extreme difficulty.

Given our clinical experience plus animal research (Franzen and Myers, 1973) and studies on human frontal lobe disturbance (Brown, 1985), it was assumed that a high incidence of socially inappropriate behaviors would frequently be seen following extensive prefrontal and anterior temporal lobe injury—injuries that are common in TBI as mentioned previously. Consequently, it was predicted that a randomized group of TBI patients seen for neuropsychologic assessment would overestimate their social competency skills but not overestimate skills involved in basic activities of daily living (ADL). Ten items on the PCRS were selected as being items in which TBI patients would overestimate their behavioral competencies versus relatives' ratings. These items included such things as adjusting to unexpected changes; handling arguments with people they know well; and recognizing when something they have said upsets others.

In addition, another eight items were selected from the scale that were predicted to reveal essentially no difference between patients' and relatives' perception of competency. These items included such things as dressing one's self, care of personal hygiene, and the ability to remember names of people they often see. Sixty-four TBI patients and relatives were studied. Mean chronicity (time from injury) was 16.0 months. The average Glasgow Coma Score was 9.68, but there was great variability (see Prigatano et al., in press, for details). The hypotheses were strongly supported when looking at the mean differences of patients' ratings versus relatives' ratings on these groups of items. Table 19–3 illustrates these findings.

These 64 patients were then subdivided into three groups (Prigatano and Altman, in press). Group 1 overestimated their behavioral competencies on the PCRS as compared to their relatives' ratings. Group 2 showed behavioral ratings similar to relatives' reports on this scale. Group 3 underestimated their behavioral competencies.

Group 1 had a greater incidence of bilateral and multiple site lesions than groups 2 and 3. However, they did not show greater impairment on tests of abstract reasoning (such as the Wisconsin Card Sorting Test) or measures of memory impairment (both verbal and nonverbal measures). However, group 1 was bilaterally slow in speed of finger tapping, with significant differences occurring in the speed of the left hand, suggesting possible greater involvement of the right posterior frontal lobe. There was a trend for a greater incidence of frontal and parietal lesions in Group 1 patients. But the sample size was too small to obtain reliable statistical differences.

Table 19–3 Patient Competency Rating Scale (PCRS)

Expect Difference				(Freq. analysis across subject)		
			Mean Diff	P>R	P=R	R>P
Item #Content						
6		Personal finances	+.578	32	17	15
9		Work when bored	+.219	26	21	17
16		Adjust to unexpected changes	+.188	25	23	16
17		Handling arguments	+.547	34	13	17
20		Acting appropriately	+.109	19	33	12
23		Recognizing when upset by something	+.516	34	17	13
24		Scheduling daily activities	+.250	24	26	14
27		Control temper	+.375	28	21	15
28		Keep from being depressed	+.250	29	18	17
29		Keep emotions from affecting daily activities	+.203	21	29	14

$$\overline{X} \text{ Diff} = \frac{3.235}{10} = .324$$

Expect no Differences

Item #						
1		Prepare meals	+.234	22	28	14
2		Dressing self	+.031	9	49	6
3		Personal hygiene	−.047	11	39	14
4		Washing dishes	+.250	17	39	8
5		Doing laundry	+.156	15	36	13
11		Remembering names of people seen often	−.125	25	14	25
19		Controlling crying	−.297	25	26	13
30		Controlling laughing	−.250	11	31	22

$$\overline{X} \text{ Diff} = \frac{.048}{8} = .006$$

$$T = 3.86, \text{ D.F.} = 63, p = .000$$

From Prigatano, G. P., Altman, I. M., and O'Brien, K. P. Behavioral limitations traumatic brain injured patients tend to underestimate. The Clinical Neuropsychologist, 4:163–176, 1990. Reprinted with permission.

Other studies have also reported TBI patients' tendencies to underestimate the severity of their higher order deficits (for review: Prigatano, 1991). As noted previously, this does not seem to be a pure function of abstract reasoning capacity. It is also interesting to note that in patients with Alzheimer's disease, early in the course of this illness the patient is often acutely aware of subtle higher cerebral dysfunctions. As the disease progresses and it is assumed that there is greater frontal lobe involvement and greater diffuse injury, the patient clearly shows a lack of awareness of the severity of the disability (see Prigatano, 1987a). This point has been made by McGlynn and Schacter (1989) with other patient groups in which frontal lobe impairment is known or suspected. Isolating the specific contribution of frontal lobe disorders to awareness has been, however, difficult.

AWARENESS AFTER SURGICAL REMOVAL OF A FRONTAL VERSUS PARIETAL-OCCIPITAL OLIGODENDROGLIOMA

A rehabilitation project for a 36-year-old male who underwent surgical resection of a right frontal oligodendroglioma is the subject of a report (O'Brien et al., 1989). The patient and his wife underwent a program to educate both of them about the predictable behavioral problems following frontal lobe damage and to help them develop a daily routine to aid the husband with problems in initiation and planning. Interestingly, the patient's awareness of his behavioral limitations, as measured by the PCRS, improved following the rehabilitation program.

A comparison was then made of this patient's ratings of his competencies to that of another man who suffered an identical neoplasm in the right posterior-occipital region. This man was a little older (48 years) with a similar, bright normal, premorbid intelligence. Both had stable psychosocial adjustment pre- and postsurgery. Both had dedicated and reliable spouses who could make useful judgments about their husbands' behavior.

Eight months postsurgery the "frontal patient" had a measured Verbal IQ of 126 and a Performance IQ of 92. Yet, that patient could only achieve four out of six categories on the Wisconsin Card Sorting Test. The parietal-occipital lobe patient, 6 months postsurgery had a Verbal IQ of 112 and a Performance IQ of 93. Unfortunately, the Wisconsin Card Sorting Test was not administered to him at that time. The frontal and parietal lobe patients had Wechsler Memory Scale Memory Quotients of 101 and 109, respectively. Speed of finger tappings was 56 taps for the right hand and 50 taps for the left hand for the frontal patient. The parietal lobe patient had 61 taps for the right hand and 48 taps for the left hand.

Their awareness of disabilities was measured in two ways. First, areas of good agreement between spouse and patient on behavioral problems were identified. Good awareness was considered to exist when the patient and spouse identified a problem area and had identical ratings as to the severity of the problem. Poor awareness was defined as existing when a patient identified a behavioral skill as posing *no* problem or only a mild problem for him, whereas the patient's spouse saw him as having more difficulty with that particular dimension. In this way, the specific behavioral competencies in which patients had good versus poor awareness were assessed.

Tables 19–4 and 19–5 present the findings obtained. It can be seen that, 8 months postsurgery for a right frontal oligodendroglioma, both the patient and spouse recognized that the patient had trouble with initiation, planning, and adjusting to unexpected changes. This is quite compatible with what is known about the higher "executive" functions mediated by the frontal lobe. The patient with the parietal-occipital lesion did not report problems in these areas and his wife agreed. In contrast, the parietal patient reported difficulties with higher order visuomotor tasks such as driving a car, and higher order visuospatial difficulties such as dealing with the math associated with personal finances.

Perhaps even more interesting, the frontal lobe patient showed areas of poor awareness precisely in higher order social interactions and in the control of emotions. For example, the patient felt that he had no trouble controlling his crying,

Table 19–4   Awareness of Behavioral Problems in a "Frontal Patient" 8 Months
Postsurgery

PCRS item		Patient's rating	Wife's rating
Good awareness			
# 6	Managing personal finances	3	3
# 7	Keeping appointments on time	2	2
# 8	Starting conversations in a group	3	3
#13	Remembering important things I must do	2	2
#16	Adjusting to unexpected changes	3	3
#24	Scheduling daily activities	2	2
Poor awareness			
# 9	Staying involved in work activities when tired or bored	2	1
#12	Remembering my daily schedule	3	2
#17	Handling arguments with people I know well	4	3
#19	Controlling crying	5	2
#23	Recognizing when something I say or do has upset someone else	4	3
#26	Consistently meeting my daily responsibilities	2	1
#28	Keeping from being depressed	4	2
#29	Keeping my emotions from affecting my ability to go about the day's activities	4	3

while the wife reported that crying was a major problem. The patient reported only minimal difficulty in recognizing when he has said something to upset others, while the wife reported this behavior to be a frequent occurrence. Also, the patient described himself as being nondepressed, whereas the wife said he was very depressed. This is interesting in light of the fact that pseudodepression is often noted in frontal lobe patients (Blumer and Benson, 1975).

In contrast, the patient with the parietal-occipital lesion had absolutely no difficulties perceiving changes in social interaction except perhaps in participating in groups and accepting criticism from others. His difficulties were in perceiving higher order visuospatial problems involved in self-care activities.

These observations are, of course, tentative. Yet, they suggest that different types of awareness problems exist in the presence of frontal versus parietal lesions (as Pribram, 1987 had previously suggested). Assuming that the frontal lobes are especially important for the modulation of emotions and the control of behavioral responses appropriate for social adaptation, it may be precisely in these areas that frontal lobe injury affects awareness the most. Furthermore, since the definition of "one's self" is at least in part obtained by comparing and contrasting one's characteristics with others', frontal lobe lesions may particularly affect the highest perceptions of one's own self-functioning. That is, it may be precisely in the area of making judgments about one's personality as well as one's interactions with others that the effects of frontal lobe damage on awareness are most severe. Further research, of course, will need to explore this possibility.

Table 19–5 Awareness of Behavioral Problems in a "Parietal-Occipital Patient" 6 Months Postsurgery

PCRS item		Patient's rating	Wife's rating
Good awareness			
# 6	Handling personal finances	—	2
#14	Driving a car if I had to	1	1
Poor awareness			
# 1	Preparing meals	4	3
# 2	Dressing	5	3
# 3	Care of personal hygiene	4	3
# 4	Washing dishes	4	3
# 5	Doing laundry	4	3
#15	Getting help when confused	4	3
#18	Accepting criticism from others	4	2
#22	Participating in group activities	4	3

METHODOLOGIC AND RESEARCH ISSUES

There are notable methodological problems in studying altered awareness after brain injury. One problem is in the establishment of a definition of the phenomenon that can be empirically investigated. In clinical research, impaired awareness was defined as existing when the patient's verbal report of a behavioral competency was deviant from a reliable observer's report of the patient's competency (as witnessed in a variety of everyday settings). Obviously, the need to demonstrate reliable ratings by the patient and the observer is the first methodologic step to systematic research in this area. Next, obtaining ratings on behavioral items that are sensitive to frontal lobe pathology is the second major goal. As the reliability of self-reports and the selection of appropriate items emerge, the third step is then to determine whether or not these items validly represent what patients do in the "real world." That is, do the subjective or verbal reports of patients and relatives match-up with behaviors in various environmental settings? Questions of reliability, content validity, and concurrent validity are therefore of key importance in this initial phase of research investigation. A few studies have appeared in the literature that document that TBI patients can reliably self-report their perceptions on questionnaires (e.g., Kinsella et al., 1988). It has also been our impression that by the time the patients are involved in postacute rehabilitation programs (between 6 months and several years posttrauma), they are fairly consistent in their reports unless there is significant overall intellectual and memory impairment.

To separate an "awareness" problem from a judgment or perceptual problem, it is important to have patients rate other individuals' behavioral competencies. If frontal patients can reliably and validly judge others' behavior, but not their own, this is evidence of a specific disturbance in "self" or "subjective" awareness.

It is also important to determine in what specific areas of behavioral functioning does the patient show "good" versus "poor" awareness. It is predicted that it is precisely in the area of the highest integrated functions of certain brain regions that awareness will be the poorest (Bisiach et al., 1986).

In addition to obtaining self-reports and judgments on others, it is important to obtain convergent behavioral and psychophysiologic measures that may underlie altered self-awareness after frontal lobe injury. Pribram and Luria (1973) approached this problem in their edited text *The Psychophysiology of the Frontal Lobes.* Knight (this volume) also discusses the relationship of evoked potential studies of attention and orientation in frontal lobe patients. Using such measures when the patient is intending some action or expecting to perceive some stimulus may be quite illuminating in understanding the psychophysiology of impaired awareness after frontal lobe injury.

In addition to psychophysiologic measures and self-reports, it is important to take into consideration the premorbid behavioral characteristics of the individual. Luria (1948/1963) emphasized this point. When one is interested in determining whether or not the intentions of an individual have been altered as a result of frontal lobe pathology, it is important to have some idea of what were stable "premorbid" intentions and to evaluate whether or not they have been changed. In this regard, it has long been recognized that premorbid cognitive and personality functioning are important contributors to the symptom picture, but they have not been systematically investigated. It has been difficult to identify what dimensions of premorbid status are relevant and interact with lesion location and lesion etiology in producing the symptom picture. Two general classes of behavioral phenomena should be considered when evaluating premorbid personality. The first centers around "objective" evidence regarding the premorbid capacity to behave in a socially acceptable fashion (i.e., history of arrest, failure to complete high school, etc.). The second has to do with the personal or "subjective" experiences of the individual that are long standing and well entrenched. For example, asking patients what they stood up for or fought against in their adolescent years may give insight into long-term belief systems. Second, inquiry into their favorite fairy tales may provide leads as to how the patients began to conceptualize their world early in life and what major "intentions" emerged.

Postmorbid behavioral changes are also important. Luria (1948/1963) discussed the phenomenon of loss of "mental tension" after frontal injuries. It would be useful to measure psychophysiologic indices as well as verbal reports of "tension" after such injuries, especially while carrying out various tasks. This would provide convergent information on how this dimension affects intentions and goal-directed (problem-solving) behavior. As noted elsewhere, engaging the patients and increasing their "tension" can be an important part of neuropsychologic rehabilitation (Prigatano and Others, 1986; Prigatano, 1987b).

Along these lines, two other dimensions may be important. One is the overall "energy level" of the patients and their easy fatigability. Clinically, this dimension seems to relate to poor frustration tolerance. Second, the ability to visualize options and future plans is very important for learning delayed response for future gratification. Many frontal lobe patients, for example, cannot adequately answer the question, "What are your plans for the future?"

Finally, the question of how rehabilitation efforts affect impaired awareness and long-term psychosocial outcome needs to be evaluated. Some patients may be unaware of their cognitive and personality difficulties but can be directed into a line of work that they accept and maintain (this is what the supportive employment model assumes). However, these individuals may be the exception. It is often the case that impaired awareness negatively affects the ability to maintain employment and engage rehabilitation. When patients have trouble doing a job and this is brought to their attention, they become irritated with the supervisor or coworker or become indifferent. Consequently, they are fired or quit a job because they do not fully appreciate how they have been affected and the impact it has on work competence. The importance of self-awareness in work maintenance, therefore, is a very important area of future research.

A second dimension is the relationship of awareness to maintaining interpersonal relationships. Many "frontal" patients are childlike, impulsive, irritable, and do not fully appreciate the severity of these problems nor the impact they have on others. The patient is, then, frequently seen as selfish or childish and not capable of empathizing with others' feelings. Consequently, they lose friendships while having very little insight as to why this occurs.

TOWARD A DEFINITION OF ALTERED AWARENESS AFTER BRAIN INJURY AND ITS THEORETICAL IMPLICATIONS

Stuss and Benson (1986) defined self-awareness or consciousness in the following manner: "Self consciousness or self-reflectiveness is that attribute of the human which not only allows awareness of the self, but also realizes the position of the self within the social milieu." They argued that the frontal lobe plays an exceptionally important role in this venture.

Schacter and Prigatano (1991) agree with Frederiks (1969) that it is exceedingly difficult—if not impossible—to provide a clear, concise, or universally acceptable definition of consciousness or awareness. In an effort to move toward such a definition, we submit the following ideas:

> Self-awareness is the capacity to perceive the "self" in relatively objective terms while maintaining a sense of subjectivity. This is a natural paradox of human consciousness. On the one hand it strives for objectivity—that is, perceiving a situation, object, or interaction in a manner quite similar to the others' perception while at the same time, maintaining a sense of private, subjective, or unique interpretation of an experience. This latter aspect of consciousness implies a feeling state as well as a thought process. Self-awareness, or awareness of higher cerebral functions, thus involves an integration of "thoughts" and "feelings." (Prigatano and Schacter, 1991, p. 14.)

Thoughts and feelings can only be indirectly measured. They make up the "intentions" Luria (1970) referred to when talking about the contribution of the frontal lobes to mental life and behavior. Self-report measures, actual behavioral competency measures, and psychophysiologic measures converge on the awareness problem, but they lead to a level of inference that is often difficult for scientists to accept. However, such "acceptance" may be necessary in order to study this difficult, but important problem. The methodologic issues raised in the preceding section and the research issues advanced are in concert with this conclusion. What are the theoretical implications of the model proposed?

Mesulam (1985) has suggested a reconceptualization of cortical and subcortical tissue. The question should be asked: How do various brain regions respond to different types of stimuli? Classic neurology refers to primary sensory/motor regions while other cortical areas are defined as "association cortex." Mesulam suggests that in addition to the primary sensory motor cortex, association cortex can be subdivided into unimodal and heteromodal cortex. Unimodal cortex responds primarily to one type of stimuli but at a complex level. For example, the inferior portion of the temporal lobe responds primarily to visual stimuli, but complex visual stimuli (for example, line orientation), the heteromodal cortex, responds to multiple types of stimuli and at times responds simultaneously to these stimuli.

It should be noted that the heteromodal cortex includes regions of the brain that are last to develop phylogenetically and ontogenetically (see Figure 6 in Mesulam, 1985). These regions are in close proximity to what Mesulam (1985) refers to as the paralimbic belt. This region of brain is least organized in its laminar structure but is very important for the registration of internal bodily states. The heteromodal cortex, therefore, may provide an interface between perceptual information and thought processes and those "internal" perceptions called feeling states. It may be precisely in the region of the heteromodal cortex that an integration of the thoughts and feelings that underlie intentions occurs. The frontal lobes have an important role to play in this regard. Other areas of the brain may contribute, however, to this and it is interesting to note that disturbances of awareness have been reported in lesions affecting other areas of the "heteromodal cortex." For example, the classic state of anosognosia for hemiplegia is frequently seen after an inferior parietal lobular lesion (Critchley, 1953). This is, within Mesulam's analysis, heteromodal cortex. Cases of anosognosia for jargon aphasia have been reported after superior temporal lobe (again heteromodal cortex) regions have been lesioned (Lebrun, 1987). Massive lesions to the prefrontal regions can produce childlike and socially inappropriate behaviors that the patient may not fully appreciate. These latter problems have readily come to the attention of clinicians faced with the rehabilitation of patients who suffer serious traumatic brain injury (Prigatano and Others, 1986).

These theoretic ideas have two corollaries that can be tested experimentally: (1) Depending on the region of heteromodal cortex, there may be different types of awareness problems present; (2) the amount of heteromodal cortex damage may relate to the severity of the awareness problem and its recovery course. For example, bilateral and diffuse lesions may produce greater awareness difficulties than unilateral or focal lesions. Lesions in the inferior parietal lobe may affect awareness of body parts and higher order visuospatial and motor skills. Lesions in the prefrontal cortex may specifically affect awareness of socially inappropriate behaviors. Varying degrees of abstract reasoning deficits may be present depending on the amount of brain dysfunction present and associated brain locations that have been negatively affected.

These ideas may help explain divergent observations made by investigators and potentially provide direction for understanding the multiple variables contributing to the phenomenom of disordered awareness after brain injury. The next step is to develop research methods for uncovering and studying this important dimension of human behavior in order to aid the rehabilitation process.

REFERENCES

Ben-Yishay Y, Silver SM, Piasetsky E, Rattok J. Relationship between employability and vocational outcome after intensive holistic cognitive rehabilitation. The Journal of Head Trauma Rehabilitation 2(1):35–48, 1987.

Ben-Yishay Y, Prigatano GP. Cognitive remediation. In Rosenthal M, Griffith ER, Bond MR, Miller JD (eds), Rehabilitation of the Adult and Child with Traumatic Brain Injury: Edition 2. Philadelphia: F.A. Davis Company, 1990, pp. 383–409.

Bisiach E, Vallar G, Perani D, et al. Unawareness of disease following lesions of the right hemisphere: Anosognosia for hemiplegia and anosognosia for hemianopia. Neuropsychologia 24(4):471–482, 1986.

Bisiach E, Geminiani G. Anosognosia related to hemiplegia and hemianopia. In Prigatano GP and Schacter DL (eds), Awareness of Deficit After Brain Injury: Clinical and Theoretical Issues. New York: Oxford University Press, 1991.

Blumer D, Benson DF. Personality changes with frontal and temporal lobe lesions. In Benson DF and Blumer D (eds), Psychiatric Aspects of Neurologic Disease. New York: Grune & Stratton, 1:151–170, 1975.

Brown JW. Frontal lobe syndromes. In JAM Frederiks (ed), Handbook of Clinical Neurology. Clinical Neuropsychology. New York: Elsevier Science Publishers, 1(45):23–41, 1985.

Critchley M. The Parietal Lobes. New York: Hafner Publishing Company, 1953.

Fordyce DJ, Roueche JR. Changes in perspectives of disability among patients, staff, and relatives during rehabilitation of brain injury. Rehabilitation Psychology 31(4):217–229, 1986.

Franzen EA, Myers RE. Neural control of social behavior: Prefrontal and anterior temporal cortex. Neuropsychologia 11:141–157, 1973.

Frederiks JAM. Consciousness. In Vinken PJ, Bruyn GW (eds), Handbook of Clinical Neurology: Disorders of Higher Nervous Activity. Amsterdam: Elsevier/North-Holland, 3:48–61, 1969.

Fuster JM. The Prefrontal Cortex: Anatomy, Physiology, and Neuropsychology of the Frontal Lobe. New York: Raven Press, 1980.

Goldstein K. Aftereffects of Brain Injury in War. New York: Grune & Stratton, 1942.

Goldstein K. The effect of brain damage on the personality. Psychiatry 15:245–260, 1952.

Kinsella G, Moran C, Ford B, Ponsford J. Emotional disorder and its assessment within the severe head injured population. Psychological Medicine 18:57–63, 1988.

Lebrun Y. Anosognosia in aphasics. Cortex 23:251–263, 1987.

Luria AR. Restoration of Function After Brain Injury, OL Zangwill (ed. and trans). New York: Pergamon Press, 1963. (Original work published in 1948 by Medgiz, Moscow).

Luria AR. The functional organization of the brain. Scientific American 222:66–78, 1970.

McGlynn SM, Schacter DL. Unawareness of deficits in neuropsychological syndromes. Journal of Clinical and Experimental Neuropsychology 12(2):143–205, 1989.

Mesulam M-M. Principles of Behavioral Neurology. Philadelphia: F.A. Davis Company, 1985.

Newcombe F. Rehabilitation in clinical neurology: neuropsychological aspects. In JAM Frederiks (ed), Handbook of Clinical Neurology. Neurobehavioral Disorders. New York: Elsevier Science Publishers, 2(46):609–642, 1985.

O'Brien KP, Prigatano GP, Pittman HW. Neurobehavioral education of a patient and spouse following right frontal oligodendroglioma excision. Neuropsychology 2:145–159, 1989.

Oddy M, Coughlan T, Typerman A, Jenkins D. Social adjustment after closed head injury: A further follow-up seven years after injury. Journal of Neurology, Neurosurgery, and Psychiatry 48:564–568, 1985.

Perecman E (ed). The Frontal Lobes Revisited. New York: IRBN Press, 1987.

Povlishock JT. Structural aspects of brain injury. In Bach-y-Rita P (ed), Traumatic Brain Injury. New York: Demos Publications, 1989, pp. 87–96.

Pribram KH. Mind, brain, and consciousness: The organization of competence and control. In Davidson J and Davidson R (eds), The Psychobiology of. New York: Plenum Press, 1980, pp. 47–61.

Pribram KH. The subdivision of the frontal cortex revisited. In Perecman E (ed), The Frontal Lobes Revisited. New York: IRBN Press, 1987, pp. 11–40.

Pribram KH, Luria AR (eds). Psychophysiology of the Frontal Lobes. New York: Academic Press, 1973.

Prigatano GP, Fordyce DJ, Zeiner HK, Roueche JR, Pepping M, Wood B. Neuropsychological rehabilitation after closed head injury in young adults. Journal of Neurology, Neurosurgery, and Psychiatry 47:505–513, 1984.

Prigatano GP and Others. Neuropsychological Rehabilitation After Brain Injury. Baltimore: The Johns Hopkins University Press, 1986.

Prigatano GP. The neuropsychology of aging. BNI Quarterly 3(3):38–44, 1987a.

Prigatano GP. Recovery and cognitive retraining after craniocerebral trauma. Journal of Learning Disabilities 30:603–663, 1987b.

Prigatano GP. Emotion and motivation in recovery and adaptation after brain damage. In Finger S, LeVere TE, Almli CR, Stein DG (eds), Brain Injury and Recovery: Theoretical and Controversial Issues. New York: Plenum Press, 1988a, pp. 335–350.

Prigatano GP. Anosognosia, delusions, and altered self awareness after brain injury. BNI Quarterly 4(3):40–48, 1988b.

Prigatano GP. Work, love, and play after brain injury. Bulletin of the Menninger Clinic 53(5):414–431, 1989.

Prigatano GP. Disturbances of self-awareness of deficit after traumatic brain injury. In Prigatano GP, Schacter DL (eds), Awareness of Deficit After Brain Injury: Clinical and Theoretical Issues. New York: Oxford University Press, 1991.

Prigatano GP. Deficits in social and vocational functioning after TBI. In N Brooks (ed), Closed Head Injury: Psychological, Social, and Family Consequences. 2nd edition. New York: Oxford University Press, (in press a).

Prigatano GP, Altman IM. Impaired awareness of behavioral limitations after traumatic brain injury. (submitted for publication).

Prigatano GP, Altman IM, O'Brien KP. Behavioral limitations traumatic brain injured patients tend to underestimate. Clinical Neuropsychologist 4:163–176, 1990.

Prigatano GP, Schacter DL. Awareness of Deficit After Brain Injury: Clinical and Theoretical Issues. New York: Oxford University Press, 1991.

Ruff RM, Buchsbaum MS, Troster AI, Marshall LF, Lottenberg S, Somers LM, Tobias

MD. Computerized tomography, neuropsychology, and positron emission tomography in the evaluation of head injury. Neuropsychiatry, Neuropsychology, and Behavioral Neurology 2(2):103–123, 1989.

Stuss DT, Benson DF. The Frontal Lobes. New York: Raven Press, 1986.

Stuss DT, Delgado M, Guzman DA. Verbal regulation in the control of motor impersistence: A proposed rehabilitation procedure. Journal of Neuro Rehab 1(1):19–24, 1987.

Thomsen IV. Late outcome of very severe blunt head trauma: A 10–15 year second follow-up. Journal of Neurology, Neurosurgery, and Psychiatry 47:260–268, 1984.

von Cramon D, von Cramon G. Frontal lobe lesions in patients: Therapeutical approaches. *In* Steinbuchel Nv, Poppel E, Cramon Dv, Palitzsch M (eds), International Symposium Brain Damage and Rehabilitation—A Neuropsychological Approach. Germany: Munich, 1989, p. 25.

Warren JM, Akert K. The Frontal Granular Cortex and Behavior. New York: McGraw-Hill, 1964.

IX
Epilogue

20
Concluding Comments

ANTONIO R. DAMASIO

THE RIDDLE

The frontal lobe has been more reluctant to yield its physiologic secrets than any other sector of the human brain. Hans-Lukas Teuber once wrote about the "recurrent perplexity" caused by studying the frontal lobe and about how the problems it posed "seemed to exceed" those encountered in the study of other brain regions. He entitled his 1964 paper "The Riddle of Frontal Lobe Function in Man," and although his text closed on an optimistic note and with a proposal for solving the riddle, most investigators have continued to think of the frontal lobes as an enigma and preferred to spend their scientific lives behind the central sulcus.

The reason usually invoked to explain all this despair is the immense complexity of frontal lobe structure and the failure to isolate its general purpose. This is easy enough to accept considering that the totality of the frontal lobe, including its prefrontal, premotor, motor, and limbic sectors, constitutes almost half of the entire cortical mantle and that extensive damage to its components, especially the prefrontal, seems to leave intact so many fundamental psychologic functions. And yet, vision, memory, language, or attention are not exactly simple, and legions of investigators have been consistently committed to their elucidation. Perhaps a more satisfactory explanation is that complexity of frontal lobe function has not been met by heuristic models powerful enough to cope with it. Be that as it may, I now sense that the tide is changing. As I reflect on the early history of frontal lobe investigations summarized by Arthur Benton, and on the record of new results from Teuber's era to the present, I believe that the suspense is over and that the solution to the enigma is in sight.

AN ENIGMA NO MORE

Following Benton's illuminating history of frontal lobe research up to the 1950s, the contributions in this volume fall in three large areas. The first area is the anatomy of the frontal cortices in human and nonhuman primates; the second is the physiology of frontal cortices as disclosed by electrophysiologic studies in both humans and animals, and through the lesion method in neuropsychologic studies, again in both humans and animals; the third area is clinical.

One might have thought that everything there is to be known about frontal lobe structure at the macroscopic level is known already. Hanna Damasio's chapter indicates that this is not quite so. For example, as fastidious a neuro-anatomist as Brodmann was, he never completed the mapping of cytoarchitec-tonic areas in the frontal region, and it was left for Elizabeth Beck to chart the orbital region many years later. The main problem discussed in Hanna Dama-sio's chapter, however, is the need for detailed landmarks to recognize prefrontal structures when it comes to using the modern neuroimaging techniques avail-able for human studies in vivo.

The chapters by Helen Barbas and Deepak Pandya and by Patricia Gold-man-Rakic and Harriet Friedman discuss important developments in micro-scopic neuroanatomy of frontal cortices as studied in nonhuman primates. The issue here is the description of intricate patterns of corticocortical and cortico-subcortical connectivity, in relation to different frontal cytoarchitectonic fields. These contribute important new information on the topic, but it is clear that much needs to be learned about these connectional patterns. In fact, one might say that progress in the understanding of frontal lobe function depends largely on the availability of additional detailed knowledge of connectional anatomy. One might also add that vital progress will be hindered if the studies remain confined to nonhuman primates. We must tackle the problem of neural connec-tions in the *human* brain, because it is altogether unlikely that all or even most human patterns are comparable to those of the monkey.

There are several approaches to the understanding of brain physiology and most are represented in this volume. In the chapters by Joaquin Fuster and Gol-man-Rakic/Friedman, the authors review their extensive findings in single cell recording experiments. Despite differences in nomenclature and interpretation, the essence of this important body of work establishes that dorsolateral prefron-tal cortices in nonhuman primates are involved in temporal processing. In short, they have a role to play in neural activity that occurs long after the stimuli that have prompted it have been removed from the scene. Whether the account emphasizes general temporal integration or focuses on the notion of working memory, both chapters offer unequivocal support for the role of dorsolateral frontal cortices in many varieties of delayed processing. Naturally, one wishes that the next wave of studies using these powerful tools and experimental para-digms will include sampling of other prefrontal fields, most especially the ven-tromedial. Admittedly, that will not be easy but there is little doubt that it is necessary. But let me make clear that progress in this area has been remarkable. In fact, it is difficult to think of a better example of integration of pertinent lines of evidence—physiology, anatomy, chemistry, psychology—than what can be found in Goldman-Rakic's work.

The chapter by Robert Knight also draws on electrophysiologic methods, but this time evoked potentials are the technique and the subjects are humans. The material serves the important purpose of linking attentional processes and frontal cortices and uses paradigms that are readily replicable in humans with and without neurologic lesions. Yet another bridge to the human frontal lobe is offered in the chapter by Marlene Oscar-Berman, Patrick McNamara, and Morris Freedman. Focusing on classic delayed-response tasks they establish some parallels between neuropsychologic experiments in nonhuman primates and a host of clinical measurements in patients with frontal damage.

Although rarely considered under the heading of physiology, the lesion method is one of the main avenues to the understanding of neural function in both humans and animals. Three chapters in this volume offer important new information based on this approach. Michael Petrides reviews the results of some fascinating learning experiments in monkeys with circumscribed ablations of dorsolateral prefrontal cortices. Tim Shallice and Paul Burgess turn to humans with frontal lobe damage and discuss their impairments in tasks that call for multistep organization of behavior. They discuss the results in the perspective of a theory of decision making that is eminently testable. The Shallice and Burgess account shares one concept with the theory I have proposed in collaboration with Daniel Tranel and Hanna Damasio. The concept is that of a *marker* on the basis of which a particular thought process or action can be interrupted or started. In our chapter we advance the notion that the nature of the marker is somatic, more specifically a somatic state that is generated in connection with certain representations and, by its very presence, manages to alter behavior. It can do so consciously, by influencing a deliberate decision, or nonconsciously, by interfering with subcortical mechanisms in charge of appetitive or aversive behaviors.

The volume is also rich in contributions in the neuropsychology, neurology, and psychiatry related to the human frontal cortices. Shimamura, Janowsky, and Squire approach the highly pertinent problem of the contribution of frontal lobe damage to memory disorders. There is a direct application of this knowledge in the diagnosis of neuropsychologic disorders caused by frontal damage, but the issue is just as important for the basic understanding of memory in general. In other words, even conventional forms of memory cannot be understood fully in terms of the hippocampal or cerebellar systems. The chapter by Donald Stuss contributes to this same topic by focusing on interference effects on memory. The study he reports relies on a particular group of patients with frontal lobe damage, those who were treated with frontal leukotomies for their psychiatric conditions.

Harvey Levin and his colleagues Felicia Goldstein, David Williams, and Howard Eisenberg concentrate on the largest group of patients with frontal lobe dysfunction, those with head injury, and discuss the diagnostic problems they raise. In a chapter that is thematically related, George Prigatano contributes his perspective on neuropsychologic rehabilitation after frontal lobe damage. As it turns out, this is perhaps most relevant in patients with head injury, a large and young cohort of patients for whom appropriate management procedures are sorely needed. To the efforts in these chapters should be added the contribution by Neary and Snowden on the characterization of a demential syndrome related to frontal lobe damage. In fact, numerous neurologic conditions as varied as head injury, tumors, and degenerative disease can cause preponderant damage and dysfunction in prefrontal cortices and lead to a demential syndrome of the frontal type.

The attempt to link structure and function of the prefrontal cortices to a variety of psychiatric syndromes began in earnest with Egas Moniz and with his development of prefrontal leukotomy. That the connection was real was certainly proven by the successes of this surgical intervention as implemented according to Moniz's original design, in its early years. In general, it has been difficult to approach this relationship in a rigorous and methodologically powerful manner. In this volume two distinct contributions prove that the link can be established in an effective way. Sergio Starkstein and Robert Robinson use the lesion method to relate affective disorder and human frontal lobe structures damaged by stroke, while Daniel Weinberger, with his colleagues Karen Berman and David Daniel, uses dynamic imaging methods to study the activity of prefrontal cortices in patients with schizophrenia.

In short, this collection brings together, under the same cover, virtually all the issues and authors that first come to mind in relation to current frontal lobe research. Even a cursory consideration of the range of topics justifies the optimism I professed in my opening paragraph.

The material in this volume does not produce the final view on the human frontal lobes. Yet it reveals enough of neuroanatomy, neurophysiology, and pathophysiology to leave readers with some sound ideas about what the frontal cortices do and do not do. In other words, there is no longer any enigma. What remains, nonetheless, is the call for a general perspective on the varied prefrontal lobe functions, an assignation of value and hierarchy to those functions, and perhaps a strategic plan for how to distribute research efforts in this area. I would like to close by outlining my general views on these issues.

THE HUMAN PREFRONTAL CORTICES

Primary Functions

I propose that, from an evolutionary perspective, the prefrontal cortices have developed to perform a primary goal: *To select the responses most advantageous for the organism in a complex social environment.* The *primary value* used for the selection is the *state of the soma,* understood as a combination of the state of viscera, internal milieu, and skeletal musculature. The *primary signal* used for the process of response selection is a somatic response, which we call a *somatic marker.*

The human prefrontal cortices are also dedicated to this primary goal. But the neural devices that support it have been expanded and co-opted to perform several associated goals relative not only to the social domain but to other domains of knowledge. The associated goals include (1) the *guidance of multistep behaviors,* (2) *decision making,* (3) *planning,* and (4) *creativity.*

The Theory of Somatic Markers

The development of the theory behind this view draws on our study of patients with damage to ventromedial frontal cortices. In spite of previously normal personalities, those patients develop defects in decision making that result in an abnormal social conduct, and repeatedly lead to punishing consequences (see the chapter by A. Damasio, Tranel, and H. Damasio). I have proposed that the disorder is due to an inability to activate somatic states linked to punishment and reward, which ought to have been reactivated in connection with anticipated *outcomes* of response options. Failure to reactivate pertinent *somatic markers* deprives the individual of a warning signal for deleterious consequences relative to responses that might nevertheless bring immediate reward. Alternatively, a somatic marker may signal an advantageous outcome relative to a response that might bring immediate pain. In the negative example, I believe that activation of somatic markers forces attention to future negative consequences, leads to conscious suppression of the responses leading to them, and thus promotes selection of biologically advantageous responses. Somatic markers also trigger nonconscious inhibition of response states. This is carried out by engaging subcortical neurotransmitter systems linked to appetitive behaviors. In this volume, my colleagues and I offer preliminary support for this theory in an investigation of patients with frontal damage.

Origin and Nature of the Somatic Marker Mechanism

The neural device that supports response selection is a complex neural network constituted by varied prefrontal fields and interacts with nonfrontal cortices and subcortical units. The ventromedial sector is of special importance. It is too early to say whether both left and right ventromedial sectors are required for the device, or if the operation, as I suspect, is more connected to the right ventromedial sector. Outside of the ventromedial sector I also suspect that right prefrontal cortices have an edge. The device is tuned by critical learning interactions throughout development. Most important among those is the learning of conjunctions between social events and the somatic state of the organism at the time of the event, and at the time in which the consequences of the event took place.

It should be noted that the learning of such conjunctions has been critical for many nonhuman species throughout evolution, and that this permitted the development of an automatic signaling system alerting the animal for a possible danger or for a possible opportunity for food, shelter, or sex. The importance of such a signaling system in subhuman species in which representational and reasoning powers are limited goes without saying. The signaling system provided an automated decision-making device in which somatic states played a privileged role as a guide to behavior that resulted in survival of the individual and the species. But it is clear from our studies in patients such as EVR (see Chapter 11, this volume, for reference) that such a signaling system must also exist in humans and that it is still playing an important role in decision making. Our contention is that the complex, deliberate systems that humans use for decision making and planning are rooted in terms of neural architecture and cognitive processing, on a primitive, automated device. When the device fails, the superimposed levels of the system do not operate efficiently. In fact, we have argued that such a basic device becomes all the more critical to behavioral guidance in an environment as rich in contingencies as are the human social environments.

To confer the best possible advantages in humans, this device is tuned to conjunctions between *future outcomes* of response options and *somatic states.*

I believe that the primary signaling device has been co-opted for realms of cognitive operation that are no longer immediately related to basic biologic needs and serves them too with behavioral guidance, decision making, planning, and creativity. This would be ideal to help individuals to navigate through elaborate behavioral sequences with numerous steps in time. The signal marker would still be a somatic response albeit not necessarily conscious.

Using the Somatic Marker

In humans, the system that generates somatic markers has many avenues of action. For instance, it is likely that it acts on a conscious level, marking outcomes of responses as positive or negative and thus leading to deliberate avoidance or seeking of a certain response option. But it is also likely that the device operates covertly by inhibiting or exciting subcortical neurotransmitter systems that mediate appetitive or aversive behaviors. It is through this latter mode that the device would operate to provide subtle markers on the basis of which we can interrupt an ongoing action or thought, start another action or thought, in short, force our attention on a given set of representations as opposed to another. This may be, incidentally, the kind of marker system that Shallice has in mind when he discusses his model of decision making. Although he has not yet proposed any link between his markers and mine, I suspect that the underlying physiology must be the same, i.e., conscious or nonconscious somatic signaling on the basis of which an attention shift is triggered.

Support Functions in Prefrontal Cortices

In order to operate normally, the response selection device that I outline here requires some of the operations that other investigators have proposed as the central functions of prefrontal cortices. For example, in order to make a response selection relative to multiple environmental contingencies, the prefrontal cortices must perform *integrations over time,* as Fuster has suggested. This is because the selection process must be based on a multifarious display of recalled information from (1) past experience, (2) projected future scenarios, and (3) somatic states that are triggered by the latter and take place concurrently. Evidently, such a process requires the holding on-line of numerous representations by means of a powerful working memory. In turn, this allows a large set of representational components to coincide in time. It is critical for the system to hold sizable sets of activity, occurring in discrete anatomic regions, across *long delays,* i.e., across many thousands of milliseconds after the triggering stimulus is no longer present. Without this capacity, whose neurophysiologic underpinnings have been the focus of Goldman-Rakic's contributions, it would not be possible to become conscious of different alternatives for action and of different outcomes of those actions, nor would there be a way for the pertinent representations to generate somatic markers.

There are several other types of prefrontal operation that would support the central function outlined here. For instance, Brenda Milner has shown how right prefrontal cortices in the human are associated with *memory for the frequency of events* or for the *temporary placement* of events. Shallice and Evans have shown how prefrontal cortices are related to the process of *estimation,* e.g., estimating sizes, amounts, frequencies, and so on. Milner, Benton and others have shown that the prefrontal cortices are related to *categorization of knowledge* on the basis of arbitrary criteria. Presumably prefrontal cortices can categorize most entities and events according to any distinctive feature of those entities or events. An example is the categorization of words by their initials, or by their lengths, or the categorization of social events by their emotional valence, e.g., wedding and birthday parties versus funerals and executions. I believe all of these operations exist to support the general decision-making role of prefrontal cortices, but in and of themselves they permit the imagination on which scenario development, planning, and creativity are rooted.

Another prefrontal operation that I see linked to its primary goal is the *monitoring of ongoing actions,* e.g., movements or speech production. This is the sort of ability that permits us to monitor our actions and anticipate potential error, e.g., monitor the upcoming trajectory of our hand holding a crystal glass so that it can anticipate and avoid collision with a hard object that would lead to breakage; or the anticipation that an upcoming comment on a given social or political problem will be offensive to someone in the audience you are addressing. It is not difficult to see that self-consciousness requires this operation.

In sum, in my proposal, the prefrontal cortices evolved to give the organism its best protection. This goal was first implemented in a relatively simple social environment dominated by opportunities for food, sex, and shelter, and by the avoidance of predators. Later, a host of contingencies in ever more complex environments were connected by learning with the original set, and the original neural mechanism for response selection was co-opted for decision making at newer and more elaborate levels. In the later process, the abilities to plan and create emerged, and so did self-consciousness. I believe the prefrontal cortices arose to perform these biologic roles, and that most operations that both clinical neurology and neuropsychology have attributed to these structures have surfaced so that the primary prefrontal assignments might be discharged.

ACKNOWLEDGMENTS

This study was supported by The Mathers Foundation.

Index

A$\overline{\text{B}}$ task, 368
  developmental changes during infancy, and,
    340, 341, 344, 346, 348, 349*t*
  rewards and, 368–69
Ablation, prefrontal
  behavioral effects, 19–21
  bilateral, personality effects, 13–14
Abscess, brain, 174
Abstract attitude, 22
Abstract designs
  drawing of, in closed head injury, 331
  response to, after frontal cortex excision, 263–
    69
Abstract reasoning
  in dementia of frontal lobe type, 310
  in Parkinson's disease, 240
  in schizophrenia, 279
Acceleration/deceleration injuries, traumatic
    brain injury and, 386
Acetylcholinesterase, reduced activity of, 242
Acquired sociopathy, 218, 226–27
Action
  appraisal of, interference and, 158
  cognitive control of, 125
  ongoing, 407
Action space, assessment of, 202
Affective disorder, following stroke. *See* Stroke
Afferent projections to frontal cortex, laminar
    origin of, 50
Akathesia, 206
Akinesias, 200, 210, 312
  directional. *See* Directional akinesia
  endo-evoked, 201, 202, 210
  exo-evoked, 202, 210
  limb, 207, 208, 209
  mixed, 201, 202
  spatial, 201
  types of, 201–3
Akinetic mutism, 209
Alcoholism. *See also* Korsakoff's syndrome,
    alcoholic
  in dementia of frontal lobe type, 315–16

Allesthesia, 205
Allochiria, motor, 205–6
Alzheimer's disease, 11, 174
  comparison with dementia of frontal lobe
    type, 311–12
  delayed-response and delayed alternation
    performance deficits in, 241, 246, 247
  cholinergic dysfunction and, 245
  catecholamine dysfunction and, 244
  neuropsychologic syndrome differentiated
    from, 306. *See also* Dementia, of frontal
    lobe type
Amnesia, 174, 209
  anterograde, 180, 247
    in anterior communicating artery disease,
      240
    declarative memory in, 192
    frontal, 322–23. *See also* Dysexecutive
      syndrome
    memory for temporal order of events in,
      187–188
    metamemory in, 185, 186
    neurological profile in, 176, 177f, 180–81
    release from proactive interference in, 183–84
    retrograde, 174
    source memory in disorders in, 189–90
    for words, 9
Amnesic deficit, 159
Amphetamine, in schizophrenia, regional
    cerebral blood flow effects of, 282–83
Amplitude disinhibition, 141, 141f
Amygdala, 225
  main afferents, 299
  mania after stroke and, 298–99
  metabolic activity, working memory and, 85–
    86
Amyotrophic lateral sclerosis (ALS), 304
Amytal, 300
Angular gyrus, cortical visual center in, 13
Animal behavior, studies on, historical
    perspective, 19–21
Anomia, 248

Italic letter *t* denotes a table.